Victorian Incurables:
A History of the Royal Hospital
for Neuro-Disability, Putney

Lois

With all good wishes

Gordon Coose

Victorian Incurables:
A History of the Royal Hospital
for Neuro-Disability, Putney

by

G.C. COOK,

MD, DSc, FRCP, FRCPE, FRACP, FLS
Visiting Professor, University College, London

The Memoir Club

First published in 2004 by
The Memoir Club
Whitworth Hall
Spennymoor
County Durham

British Library Cataloguing in
Publication Data.
A catalogue record for this book
is available from the
British Library.

ISBN: 1 84104 090 8

Typeset by George Wishart & Associates, Whitley Bay.
Printed by CPI Bath.

To the patients at the Royal Hospital
– past, present, and future.

Contents

Illustrations and Tables

Preface

IN THE MID-NINETEENTH CENTURY, individuals with diseases which were at that time considered incurable, e.g. rheumatism, 'paralysis', deformity, and spinal disease or injury, were by no means welcomed into or retained in *general* hospitals; the major problem was the lengthy period of time required between admission and death.[1] Such cases were, therefore, classified as *incurable*. The *Royal Hospital for Incurables* (RHI) was the first hospital specifically designed for this category of patient (in 1854), but by the 1880s and 90s (the latter days of Victoria's reign) there were many similar institutions throughout Britain. Large houses were often utilised – for example Mauldeth Hall, near Manchester, was used by the 'Northern Counties Hospital and Home for Incurables', whilst the 'Arboretum' at Leamington Spa was occupied by the 'Royal Midland Counties Home for Incurables'. *The British Home and Hospital for Incurables* was in effect a sister-institution of the RHI. It was originally founded in a house at Clapham Rise, London, but moved to a new building in Streatham (a semi-rural district) which was erected in 1892-4; this had been designed by Arthur Cawston (1857-94) and after he accidentally shot himself it was completed by Edwin T. Hall FRIBA (1851-1923). The exterior has a neo-Tudor façade. The *new* building was officially opened by the Princess of Wales (later Queen Alexandra: 1844-1925) on 3 July 1894 (i.e. 40 years after foundation of the RHI); there were two three-storey ward blocks with rooms for 50 patients and resident staff. Here, as at the RHI, there were spacious raised terraces from which the patients could appreciate the surrounding gardens. This institution still bears the name *British Home and Hospital for Incurables* and is situated in Crown Lane, Streatham, London SW16 3JB; it remains a Charity (like the RHN) and possesses a mere 125 beds.[2]

Throughout this book therefore, the term *incurable* should be accepted in a mid-Victorian connotation, i.e. a *long-stay* patient who could not be accommodated in one of the *general* (acute) hospitals of England.[3]

It is important to emphasise the pioneering rôle of the RHI in this *new* arena, without which the specialty (which now incorporates rehabilitation medicine) might never have 'got off the ground'. Although the RHI was originally founded as 'an asylum for the reception of patients who were dismissed from ... various hospitals as past cure',[4] it was available only 'for the relief of persons above the pauper class [who were] suffering from incurable maladies'.[5]

Domestic comfort was from the outset of paramount importance in hospitals (homes) for incurables, although in design the traditional elements of *general* hospitals were usually incorporated e.g. pavilion planned wards (recommended by Florence Nightingale) and a wide linking corridor running the entire length of the building – for easy movement of beds and wheelchairs.

Although the Royal Hospital seems today to be a haven of peace and tranquillity, this has certainly not always been the case. Like most pioneering institutions it has seen its fair share of squabbles, disagreements and downright criticism; some of these are highlighted in this book.

In the late nineteenth century management of the RHI frequently came under criticism – not least for its staunch adherence to a controversial voting system; whereas this brought in much needed funds from subscribers, it undoubtedly failed to ensure acceptance of many of the most needy! Attempts by the all-male hierarchy to keep women out of the board room is in itself an interesting story. The major potential obstacle however in its 150-year history was undoubtedly the threat, in the light of the 1946 *National Health Service Act*, of a loss of identity, individuality, and its voluntary status; a takeover by the then Minister of Health (Aneurin Bevan) was narrowly avoided.

I have also addressed the part played by Charles Dickens in the genesis of the RHI, and that of Florence Nightingale who gave a great deal of advice (I have transcribed seven of her letters for the first time) on a proposed hospital at Coulsdon, Surrey, and on the appointment of the longest-serving Matron in the history of the Charity.

This text is primarily a history of the *Royal Hospital for Incurables* written to mark its 150th year; in 1918 *Home* was incorporated in its title, and not until much later (in 1995) was its name changed for the last time (not without a great deal of controversy), to the Royal Hospital for Neuro-disability.

Although there is no formal link between the RHN and the modern hospice movement, demarcation is a blurred one, for care of the incurable and dying has taken place since time immemorial, and was perhaps at its zenith in the medieval monasteries of Europe.[6]

At its foundation, Queen Victoria had already reigned for nearly two decades. The Prime Minister was the fourth Earl of Aberdeen (1784-1860) (whose grandson was to become a President of the RHI); he is best known for his declaration of the Crimean War – which the British public simply did not want! Widespread use of anaesthesia had yet to come, while smallpox and other infectious diseases remained major causes of mortality.

Other matters of interest have involved the rejection, for reasons unknown, of the 'elephant man' in 1886, and the ghost (not awfully well documented) of Melrose Hall – the definitive venue of the Hospital.

The hospital has always attracted support (financial and otherwise) from people of influence, including numerous members of the Royal Family – this has contributed enormously to its success over 150 years.

The early history of the RHI has been summarized by an anonymous correspondent in the *City Press* for 1922.[7] Until now, no in-depth history of this pioneering institution (the RHI) has been written. In attempting to do this, I have drawn from several short texts[8] as well as perusing a great deal of archival material, much in possession of the relatively newly named Royal Hospital for Neuro-disability. I have read from the minutes of the Board of Management (Appendix 2), which assembled fortnightly, and less so on those of the House Committee which met weekly. I am especially indebted to Robert Sproats for much help with access to the archival material.

G.C. COOK
Royal Hospital for Neuro-disability
West Hill, Putney, London, SW15 3SW
August 2003

References and Notes

1. H. Richardson (ed.) *English Hospitals 1660-1948; a survey of their architecture and design.* Swindon: Royal Commission of the Historical Monuments of England 1998. 130-1.
2. E.T. Hall, 'The British Home and Hospital for Incurables, Streatham, SW', *Academy Architecture and Architectural Review*, 1912; 42: 118.
3. One of the greatest literary achievements of Henry Charles Burdett (1847-1920) was a massive four-volume work entitled *Hospitals and asylums of the World* (1891-93); this included architectural details of the various establishments for incurables in Britain. *See also:* G.C. Cook, 'Henry Charles Burdett [1847-1920]: outstanding hospital administrator, successful secretary of the Seamen's Hospital Society and notable philanthropist.' *J med Biog.* 2001; 9: 195-207; G.C. Cook, 'Henry Currey FRIBA (1820-1900): leading Victorian hospital architect, and early exponent of the "pavilion principle".' *Postgrad Med J.* 2002; 78: 352-359.
4. Anonymous, 'The Royal Hospital for Incurables', *Times, Lond.* 1871; 16 March: 10; Anonymous, 'A Place Apart: The Royal Home for Incurables', *City Press* 17 June 1932.
5. Anonymous, 'Royal Hospital for Incurables', *Times, Lond.* 1886; 10 May: 9.
6. G. Goldin, 'A protohospice at the turn of the Century, St Luke's Hospital, London, from 1893 to 1921', *J Hist Med Allied Sci* 1981; 36: 383-415; C.M.S. Saunders, *Personal Communication.*
7. Anonymous, 'Royal Hospital for Incurables: no help from public funds', *City Press* 17 June 1922.
8. Anonymous, '*The Royal Hospital for Incurables designed for the permanent care and comfort of those who by Disease, Accident, or Deformity are hopelessly disqualified for*

the duties of life (London: RHI, 1868): 229; E.D. Maclagan, *The Royal Hospital and Home for Incurables: three lectures delivered to the patients of the Hospital, on 6th, 13th and 27th November 1946* (London: RHI 1946): 5, 9, 10; A.E. Stokes-Roberts, *A short history of the Royal Hospital and Home for the Incurables, Putney* (London: RHHI, 1972) 56; Anonymous, *Notes and sketches past and present: a century in the life of the Royal Hospital and Home for Incurables* (London, RHHI, 1954): 32; N. Alvey, 'The Royal Hospital and Home, Putney', *Local Historian* 1994; 24: 15-26.

Prologue

When in 1863 (soon after Andrew Reed's death), the Management Committee of the Royal Hospital for Incurables (RHI) decided to purchase Melrose Hall, they had committed the Institution to a location south-west of London which had a rich and interesting history – past, present and future. West Hill, Putney, was until the mid-eighteenth century little more than a track. At about this time, several substantial houses were erected and it became temporarily a highly aristocratic neighbourhood. On the north of West Hill, for example, were the Clock House (1760), which was demolished in the late 1880s, and Colebrook Lodge (1764); the latter, which was built on land near Tibbet's Corner, was the home of Sir William Fordyce (1724-92), an eminent and wealthy physician. But the grandest house, West Hill (later Melrose Hall), built on the site of a former edifice – which now forms a diminutive portion of the Royal Hospital for Neuro-disability (RHN) – was situated on the south side and its estate adjoined Wimbledon Common (probably dating from Saxon times), Putney Heath, and Wimbledon Park (owned by the Earls Spencer). In 1827 the Marquess of Stafford, who later became the first Duke of Sutherland, bought 117 acres of Lord Spencer's estate at Wimbledon Park – which included woods and game cover. His son, the second Duke, made further purchases and ultimately owned most of South Field. In 1842 he sold the entire area to John Augustus Beaumont (1806-86), a property developer, who intended converting it into a building estate.[1] The RHI bought Melrose Hall from him in 1863.

On 6 June 1863 (i.e. during the same year that the RHI moved to Melrose Hall), Holy Trinity Church was consecrated by the Lord Bishop of Winchester (Samuel Wilberforce (1805-73) – who is perhaps better known while Bishop of Oxford for his opposition to Darwin's theory of evolution. Windows in the church were donated by the Rücker family (east) and the Goldschmidts (north) who lived locally. (Mme Goldschmidt was better known as Jenny Lind – the Swedish nightingale (1821-87)). This, with its imposing steeple (which was added in 1888) – visible for miles around – has therefore been a close neighbour of the RHN since its removal there; in a way they have grown up together!

In March 1925, Bath House (now demolished), situated at the upper end of West Hill and adjoining Tibbet's Corner, which had been built sometime between 1876 and 1885, was purchased to accommodate the *Ross Institute &*

Hospital for Tropical Diseases to commemorate the discoveries of Sir Ronald Ross (1857-1932), who had demonstrated the rôle of the mosquito in transmitting the malaria parasite to *Homo sapiens* in 1897-8 and for which he received the Nobel Prize for Medicine and Physiology in 1902, the first British recipient of this award. Ross died in this hospital and his funeral service took place in Holy Trinity Church.[2]

References and Notes

1. D. Gerhold, *Wandsworth Past* (London: Historical Publications Ltd); R. Milward, *Wimbledon: a pictorial history* (Chichester, Sussex: Phillimore, 1994). *See also*: Anonymous, 'Shelter where feeble feet –' (London: RH, 1917): 38.
2. G.C. Cook, 'Aldo Castellani FRCP (1877-1971) and the founding of the Ross Institute & Hospital for Tropical Diseases at Putney', *J med Biog.* 2000; 8: 198-205; G.C. Cook. 'A difficult metamorphosis: the incorporation of the Ross Institute & Hospital for Tropical Diseases into the London School of Hygiene and Tropical Medicine' *Med Hist* 2001; 45: 483-506.

CHAPTER 1

Early days of the Royal Hospital
for Incurables (RHI)

QUEEN VICTORIA had been on the British throne for a mere seventeen
years of her 64-year reign; the Crimean (Russian) War had just begun;
there were still fifteen years to elapse before the publication of the most
controversial book of the nineteenth century, Charles Darwin (1809-82)'s
Origin of species by natural selection. Whose idea was it at that time to found a
hospital for 'incurables', and what were the diseases from which the patients
suffered? Miss Lucy Begg, matron of the RHI from 1909 to 1930, when
speaking to an *international nurses' meeting* in 1927, 'told how the founder, taken
as a boy to see the statue of John Howard [1726(?)-90 – the great eighteenth
century philanthropist], was inspired to do something for the poor and
suffering'. She had probably obtained this information from the biography
written by two of his sons. Although there were widespread mutterings in the
mid-nineteenth century for appropriate care and facilities for this 'special'
group, the major catalyst seems to have been the celebrated novelist Charles
Dickens (1812-70; fig 1.1) who was the editor of the weekly journal *Household
Words*. Dickens was probably reflecting popular opinion of the time.
Nevertheless, he (or one of his literary contemporaries) wrote a short article in
the first volume of *Household Words* entitled: 'No hospital for Incurables':

> It is an extraordinary fact that among the innumerable medical charities with
> which this country abounds, there is not one for the help of those who of all
> others most require succour, and who must die, and do die in thousands,
> neglected, unaided. There are hospitals for the cure of every possible ailment or
> disease known to suffering humanity, but not one for the reception of persons past
> cure. There are, indeed, small charities for incurables scattered over the country –
> like the asylum for a few females afflicted with incurable diseases, at Leith, which
> was built and solely supported by Miss Gladstone; and a few hospital wards, like
> the Cancer ward of Middlesex, and the ward for seven incurable patients in the
> Westminster; but a large hospital for incurables, does not exist.

Dickens (or a contemporary writer) then proceeded to outline a case report:

> The case of a poor servant girl which lately came to our knowledge, is the case of
> thousands. She was afflicted with a disease to which the domestics of the middle
> classes, especially, are very liable - white swelling [probably tuberculosis] of the
> knee. On presenting herself at the hospitals, it was found that an operation would
> be certain death; and that, in short, being incurable, she could not be admitted.

1

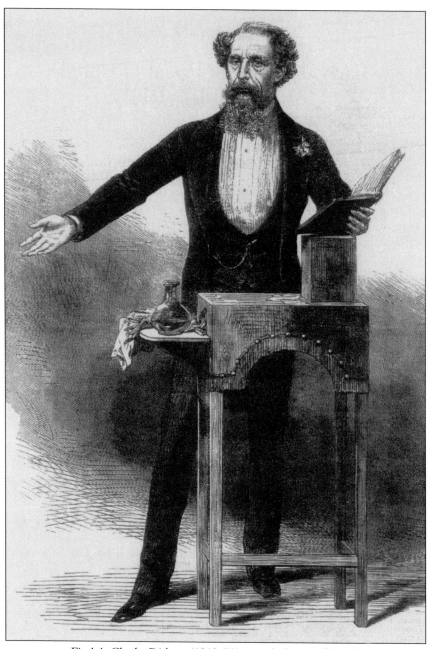

Fig 1.1: Charles Dickens (1812-70) towards the end of his life.
(Engraving in the Illustrated London News 1870; 56 (19 March): 301.

She had no relations; and crawling back to a miserable lodging, she lay helpless till her small savings were exhausted. Privations of the severest kind followed; and despite the assistance of some benevolent persons who learnt of her condition when it was too late, she died a painful and wretched death.

The writer then reverted to the *urgent* need for such an institution:

It is indeed a marvellous oversight of benevolence that sympathy should have been so long withheld from precisely the sufferers who most need it. Hopeless pain, allied to hopeless poverty, is a condition of existence not to be thought of without a shudder. It is a slow journey through the Valley of the Shadow of Death, from which we save even the greatest criminals.

When the law deems it necessary to deprive a human being of life, the anguish, though sharp, is short. We do not doom him to the lingering agony with which innocent misfortune is allowed to make its slow descent into the grave'.[1]

The Royal Hospital for the Care of Incurables was founded four years after Dickens' article was written (in 1854). Three preliminary meetings were held at the London Tavern, Bishopsgate Street – on 13, 20 and 27 July of that year. In addition to the founder, Dr Andrew Reed (Chapter 2), Messrs Munk, Peek, Millard, and the 4th Marquis of Townshend were present at those meetings, and they were joined at the last by Mr Davies; the Chairman at all of the meetings was Peek.[2] Then came a public meeting, on 31 of that month (when the Charity was officially inaugurated), held in the Egyptian Hall of the Mansion House; this was chaired by the Lord Mayor of London. At this meeting various resolutions were passed. The Hon. Edmund Phipps moved (this was 'unanimously adopted') that 'it was most desirable to found such an institution as the one proposed. If any evidence … was required of the necessity of such an institution, it would be found in the number of persons who apply for relief at existing hospitals, and were refused because their illness was so long standing, or who were discharged because they were incurable, or their case would take up so long a time, and who therefore had to become out-patients, and return to a home where … the comforts were such as would lend to a cure.'

The names of the officers of the new institution (Appendix 1) were read out and adopted:

Treasurer: Samuel Gurney Jun. Esq.,
Provisional Secretary: Rev. Andrew Reed, DD,

Board of Directors:

Mr Geo. Alexander	Mr Thomas Dakin
Mr Percy Anderson	Mr David Davies
Mr John Bedmead	Mr Wm. Dobinson
Thos. Calloway RCS	Hon. E. Scott Gifford
John Conolly MD, DCL	Dr J.H. Gladstone

Mr R.A. Gray	Hon. Edmund Phipps
Mr R. Habberfield	Mr Chas. Reed
Mr Thomas B. King	Mr George Stagg
W.J. Little, MD	Mr W.W.F. Synge
Mr H.W. Masters	Mr James Taylor
Mr Wm. Millard	Mr W.J.Thompson
Mr George Moore	Mr J.A.S. Townsend [sic]
Mr William Munk	Mr Alderman Wise
Mr Wm. Peek	Mr R. Woodhouse

It was also announced at that meeting that 'upwards of £2000' had already been contributed to the Charity, and this contained several donations of £100 or more. At a Board Meeting on 11 January 1855, Mr Frederic Andrew was 'appointed as [full-time] Sub-Secretary and Collector, subject to three months notice on either side'.[3]

Subsequent meetings that year were held either at the City of London Tavern or 11 Poultry; it was agreed that the Board should meet on the second and fourth Thursdays of each month at 3.00 p.m. There were two initial appeals for voluntary donations, and the constitution was, at that time, clearly set out (Chapter 3).[4]

Accommodation at Carshalton 1854-57

Clearly, a suitable venue for the newly-established institution was a major priority; at a Board Meeting held on 26 October 1854 Reed was able to announce that: 'Mr [Samuel] Gurney [a wealthy Quaker] had proposed a house in his possession at Carshalton [north of Epsom] as suitable for occupation as a temporary Hospital' [figs. 1.2 and 1.3] and it was agreed that 'the Secretary and Mr Woodhouse [chairman of this particular meeting] should accompany Mr Gurney on a visit to the premises.' The minutes of the following meeting (31 October) contain a description of this: 'the ground floor was already occupied and would probably not be included in any engagement; the part at disposal would accommodate about 40 patients [who would pay £30-£75 per annum for maintenance] – the rent would not exceed £60 per annum.' At a meeting on 9 November, unanimous consent was given to a proposal from Gurney (later the subject of legal quibbling): 'That the house be taken from year to year, subject to three months notice, ending at times on either side. The rent to be £40 per annum. The first and second floors to be wholly given up to the Board, with the use of the kitchen, the passage room, and the garden.' At the same meeting the following was also agreed: 'That Mr Gurney, and such ladies as he might approve, form a Ladies' Committee for the oversight of domestic affairs. The matter of furniture to be left to the discretion of the ladies and officers.'[5]

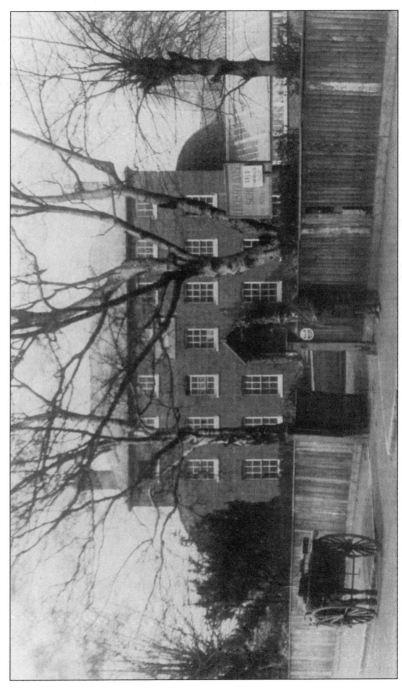

Fig 1.2: The original 'home' of the RHI – in Carshalton – from 1854-57 (date unknown, but probably early twentieth century).
(Courtesy Sutton Central Library)

5

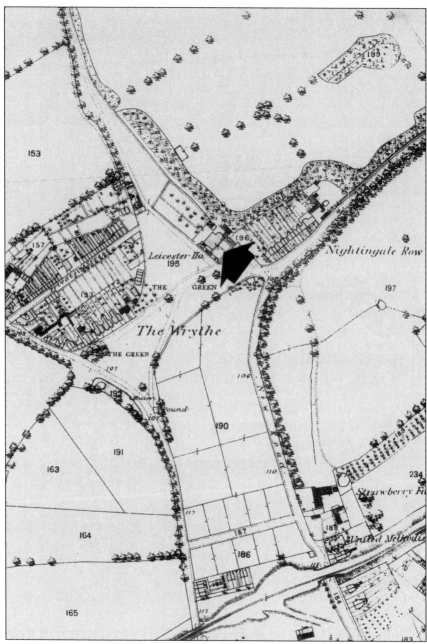

Fig 1.3: The location of the original 'home' of the RHI – Leicester House in Carshalton. (Ordnance Survey 1868 (1st ed.) 25" map, sheet XIII)

Carshalton, therefore, became the first site for the Royal Hospital for Incurables – in a building subsequently to become Leicester House (figs 1.2 and 1.3), which was demolished in 1928.[6] Much later, the 1878-79 *Annual Report* reminded the Subscribers that 25 years had by then elapsed since the Hospital at Carshalton was opened – at a cost of £63=00 a year in rent. A later *Report* (1898-99) referred to this building [the old workhouse] rather romantically as a '... small house [hired in] the lavender fields of Carshalton'.[7]

The workhouse movement dates back to 1723 (the first poor-law institutions having been established soon after the dissolution of the monasteries), when by Act of Parliament (the Workhouse Test Act), a system to care for the pauper was introduced throughout the country; churchwardens and overseers, with the consent of local residents, were empowered to build a workhouse, and refusal to enter was deemed a disqualification for 'relief'. The Carshalton building had been erected in 1792 and was subsequently used as the *new* workhouse. Some ten years earlier, the parish of Mitcham had established a similar institution. Both buildings were 'red-brick structures in whose unornamented façades were three tiers of plain rectangular windows, of progressively diminishing size as they rose to the roof. The two upper storeys each had seven windows, but, on the ground floor, there was a door instead of a central window.'

In 1834, the *Poor Law Amendment Act* was passed by Parliament; it received Royal Assent on 14 August of that year. This had resulted from a Report of a *Royal Commission* on the Poor Laws. These buildings provided for the poor (the pauper) throughout the country, by the administration of parochial funds, and were under the superintendence of a central board, the Poor-Law Commissioners; they were enabled to build unions and unite two or more parishes. Another section of the Act stated that overseers were no longer to have full command, but a Board of Guardians (usually local businessmen, shopkeepers or farmers) was elected by ratepayers of the grouped parishes. Underlying the Act was the principle of 'deterrance'. In consequence of this legislation the 'inmates' of this workhouse were removed to the Union Workhouse at Epsom.

Between 1841 and 1854 (when the newly-formed RHI took it over) this building belonged to the Metropolitan Convalescent Asylum; their objective was 'to provide an asylum, in the country, for the temporary residence of the convalescent and debilitated poor'. The *raison d'être* was that restoration of health for London residents was impracticable either in a *general* hospital or in their 'unhealthy and ill-provided homes', but that this was rapidly effected by pure (country) air – which was relatively free from miasmas – rest, and a nutritious diet. In 1854, this institution had moved to new premises at Walton on the Hill.

Brightling, writing in 1872, has outlined the RHI's occupancy between 1854 and 1857: 'each case was arranged for as it seemed to need; for one the ground floor, for another a sun-lit chamber; for all, cheerful society, good books and nourishing diet; nurses to the sick and weak, readers for the bedridden; and each [patient] would retain little articles of furniture of their own – worthless it might be in the eyes of the stranger, but of priceless value …'.

An anonymous local poet wrote:

> It's built of red brick and covered with slate;
> if you want to get in you must ring at the gate.
> It's established for people who long have been ill
> Past curing by physic or surgical skill.

After the removal of the RHI, in 1857, to Putney House (see below), it was used until 1866 as a British School (a non-conformist counterpart of the Church of England's 'National Schools') – the Leicester House School; the principle patron of this venture was also Samuel Gurney.[8]

A Matron for the Carshalton-based Hospital

The 'situation' of matron was offered at a meeting held on 14 December 1854 to Mrs Anne Crossthwaite who accepted for a period of 6 months beginning on 1 January 1855. At a Board Meeting almost a year later it was resolved: 'That the salary of the Matron be fifty pounds a year, to date from Midsummer last.' However, she was not to occupy this position for long for in August 1856, a letter from her indicated that owing to 'delicate health' she wished to resign at Michaelmas. It was immediately suggested that Mrs Eliza Bellringer, 'lately Matron of the Asylum for Idiots' might be a suitable person to succeed her and she was duly appointed 'at a salary of £60 a year'. The change of matrons took place on 29 September.[9] Names of subsequent matrons are recorded in Chapter 11 and Appendix 1.

Patients and the first office-holders

Chapter 4 gives details of the first 100 applicants for admission (including their diagnoses). On 22 March 1855: 'Dr Reed stated that one patient had already entered the Hospital, and that the remaining three would do so in a few days.'[10]

The first *Annual Meeting* (and 3rd election) of the newly formed Charity was held rather more than one year after foundation of the hospital (on 26 November 1855), again at the City of London Tavern. At a meeting of the Board on 22 November, the following names had been submitted by Reed 'for adoption at this Annual Meeting'.

President: The Right Hon., the Earl of Harrowby

Vice-Presidents:
His Grace, the Duke of Devonshire, KG
His Grace, the Duke of Bedford, KG

His Grace, the Duke of Leeds
The Most Noble, the Marquis of Landowne, KG
The Most Noble, the Marquis of Bristol
The Right Hon., the Earl of Albermarle
The Right Hon., the Earl of Ferrers
The Right Hon., the Earl Spencer, KG
The Right Hon., the Earl of Leicester
The Right Hon., the Viscount Palmerston, MP, GCB
The Right Hon., the Viscount Sydney
The Right Hon., the Viscount Canning
The Right Hon., the Lord Robert Grosvenor, MP, GCB
The Right Hon., the Lord Southampton
The Right Hon., the Lord Panmire, KT, GCB
The Right Hon., William Francis Cowper, MP
Colonel, the Hon. Peregrine F. Cust
Baron Lionel De Rothschild, MP
Sir John Villiers Shelley, Bart., MP
Sir Robert Peel, Bart., MP
Admiral Sir Augustus W.J. Clifford, Bart., CB
Sir James Clark, Bart., MD, FRS
Sir William Clay, Bart., MD
Sir James Hudson, KCB
Captain Townshend, RN, MP
John Conolly Esq., MD, DCL
R. Bernal Osborne, Esq., MP
Martin Tucker Smith, Esq., MP
James Luke, Esq., FRCS
Apsley Pellatt, Esq., MP
David Wise, Esq., Alderman

Board of Directors:
Geo. W. Alexander, Esq.
Percy Anderson, Esq.
Wm. E. Arundell, Esq.
Wm. Chas Caldwell, Esq.
Thos. Dakin, Esq.
David Davies, Esq.
William Dobinson, Esq.
The Hon. J.T.T.W. Fiennes
The Hon. E. Scott Gifford
J.H. Gladstone, Esq.
R.A. Gray, Esq.

R. Habberfield, Esq.
Thos. B. King, Esq.
The Right Hon., the Lord Kingsdale
Wm. Millord, Esq.
Geo. Moore, Esq.
Wm. Munk, Esq.
The Hon. Edmund Phipps
Charles Reed, Esq.
W.W.F. Synge, Esq.
Geo. Stagg, Esq.
Joseph Tanner, Esq.
Joseph Taylor, Esq.
J.V.S. Townshend, Esq.
Sir Henry Vane, Bart
Rev. Wm. Woodhouse

It was recommended at the same meeting that the current *Treasurer* and
'*Gratuitous*' *Secretary* (Reed) be re-elected.[11]

Escalating accommodation problems
In August 1855 there was considerable discussion on the possible purchase of
an estate at Slough (known as the Royal Hotel) which belonged to the
Railway; it was considered 'that £5000 was a fair sum for the premises *as they
stood*, excepting … the plot of ground reserved upon the auction plan for the
Directors of the Railway Company'. This offer was however declined and,
since greater accommodation was felt imperative, attention immediately turned
to an estate 'a few miles from Croydon, adjoining and using the trunk line of
the London and Brighton Railway'. This estate amounted to 40 acres, and had
initially been 'purchased by the Committee of the Asylum for Fatherless
Children' (Chapters 2 and 7). Reed felt that one-half of this estate could be
acquired for £2,500. An alternative plan was suggested by Woodhouse; he was
aware that 'an estate at Wimbledon, lately the property of Lord Cottenham,
and comprising a Mansion, and about 15 acres of park land was [also] for sale'.
This estate was however later rejected owing to the fact that it was 'in a state of
great dilapidation'.[12]

There were rapid developments regarding the 'Croydon plan' at a meeting
in December 1855; Reed reported that the 'Orphan Board' were 'prepared to
look at £2750'. However, a Special Meeting of the Board of the New Asylum
for Fatherless Children (20 December 1855) resolved their readiness 'to accept
the offer previously made by the Royal Hospital of £2,500 for the Land in
question, viz. the 20 acres lying nearest the Railway, and that the terms of
payment [i.e. £500 paid as a deposit] be as stated in this Board's minute of the

22 November 1955'. This offer seems to have been readily acceptable to the initial RHI Board (see below).[13]

As accommodation in the house at Carshalton was rapidly becoming too limited, an urgent need for a new and larger venue was continually raised at Board Meetings. At a meeting in June 1856 it was decided to go ahead and purchase the 'portion of land ... situated at Coulsdon in the County of Surrey', but the Charity lacked sufficient funds for erecting a building. A later minute states that £200 was paid as a deposit on the Coulsdon Estate, and it was resolved to pay a second instalment of £300.[14]

On 28 August 1856, the minutes contain a report of an inspection of an 'estate at Putney'. Later that year it was stated that 'several places had been seen', and that 'lately an estate near Croydon' with 28 rooms and 43 acres of land, 'near the site of the proposed building' (at a rent of £261) should be considered. Some premises at Southall constituted a further possibility. In late 1856, Dr Reed reported on the Ordnance School at Carshalton (accompanied by 30 acres of land which was administered by the War Department) – which would probably be let in the near future at £350.[15]

Early Progress of the Charity

Fig. 1.4 summarises numbers of in- and out-patients during the first years of the RHI's existence.

The second *Annual Meeting* (and fifth election) was held in late 1856 – again

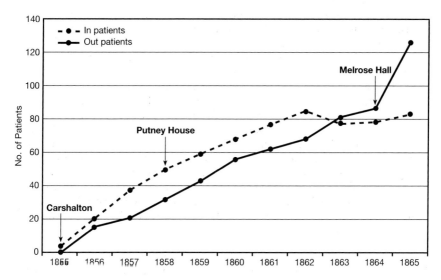

Fig 1.4: Numbers of 'home' (inpatients) and 'extra' (outpatients) patients during the first decade of the RHI.

at the City of London Tavern, when the Rt. Hon. The Viscount Raynham MP took over the treasureship from Samuel Gurney, Esq. In addition to Munk, Luke and Little (Chapter 5), Seymour (later Sir Francis) Haden FRCS (Chapter 5) was added to the list of Medical Staff as a Visiting Surgeon. The Board of Directors was re-elected with few alterations; additional names were: John H. Allen, Esq. and H. Percy Andaum [sic] Esq., with the deletion of R. Habberfield, Esq.[16]

A fund-raising dinner was reported in the newspapers of the day; *The Times* of 7 June 1856 informed its readership:

> On Thursday evening the anniversary dinner of this Charity [essentially a fund-raising occasion], established two years ago for the permanent care of persons who by disease, deformity, or accident are hopelessly disqualified for the duties of life, was held at the London Tavern, under the presidency of Mr. Charles Dickens.

There were almost a hundred individuals on this occasion and they included, in addition to Reed (Chapter 2), the 4th Marquis of Townshend (1798-1877), Baron Tenterden (1834-82), Viscount Raynham (later the 5th Marquis of Townshend) (1831-99), Lord Alfred Paget (1816-88), Sir John Boileau FRS (1794-1869), Francis Ramsbottom FRCP (1801-68), William Little FRCP (1810-94), and John Conolly MD (1794-1866).

At this dinner, Dickens outlined the *history* of this fledgling institution:

> ... he had the high privilege to give a toast which recognized the immense social importance and great Christian humanities of [the hospital]. ... It was the distinguishing feature of this institution that it entered into competition with none of the existing hospitals, but came in aid of every one of them. There was not an establishment for the treatment of the sick in this city [London] from the doors of which some unfortunate persons, altogether disqualified for the duties of life, were not driven away. The Royal Hospital had scarcely achieved the second year of its existence; but, nevertheless, it had obtained 'a local habitation and a name', and in one of the prettiest places in the environs of London. There was nothing about the institution which partook of sectarianism; its principle was to know no distinction in religion; and there were now 44 patients under its protecting care. It divided itself into two branches, affording, first, to those objects of charity a home for life who had no other home [the 'home' or inmates], and, secondly, assisting with regular donations and kind counsels such patients as had friends to relieve them in part and give them shelter, feeling that they could not bear that sharpest pain – the separation from those they loved [the 'extra', or outpatients].

The necessity for such an institution (the 'subscriptions and donations [then] amounted' to almost 900*l* (£)) was, he continued, highlighted by the fact that out of 87 applications received during the previous month, the managers were able to accommodate a mere 10 of them.[17]

The *second* anniversary dinner (subscriptions then amounted to 1,270*l* [£]) was held – also at the City of London Tavern – again with Dickens presiding. In addition to many of the distinguished men who had been guests a year before, were: The Hon. Edmund Phipps (1808-57), Sir Charles Smith (1786-1858), and John Mechi (1803-80). Dickens spoke enthusiastically of a visit he had made to the 'temporary hospital [in an old workhouse] at Carshalton', although it 'required enlargement, and needed many appliances'.[18]

Yet another *Special* Board Meeting was held in May 1857 at which a letter from Charles Dickens was read (by the chairman, Viscount Raynham) in relation to the Carshalton building which was in need 'of full ventilation and to other inconveniences which rendered the place, in his view, very undesirable for its present purpose'.

Putney House – 1857-64
The Carshalton venue had thus become too small to accommodate the rapidly-expanding number of 'inmates'.

In February 1857 (i.e. a mere 2½ years after inauguration of the Charity), a *Special* Meeting had been convened 'to consider what steps should be taken to provide a dwelling adapted to the probable requirements of the Hospital for the next five or seven years'. Reed clearly had 'accommodation for 150 persons' in mind, and this could be completed by Michaelmas (i.e. in the autumn); the envisaged cost of a building (on the 'estate belonging to the Charity') would be £5000-£7000. The meeting failed to take a definite decision, and the matter was postponed until another *Special* Meeting met in early March. At this meeting it was resolved that '... the estate as marked on the plan be rented for five years at £250 per annum, and that information should be desired respecting the recupation (sic) of the adjoining ground.

On 11 June, Dr Reed (together with Mr Moore) 'had pursued the business of the premises at Putney, and he was happy to say that the terms of the lease were all but finally arranged'. Later that month, Reed was able to report that 'possession had been taken of Putney House [fig 1.5] [and that with one exception] *the whole family* [my italics] had been safely removed [from Carshalton], while, on 25 February 1858, Woodhouse was able to report 'that the House Committee had met at Putney House [present were: Moore, Allen, Davies, Hall, and himself].[19]

Putney House (now demolished) was a spacious mansion in Richmond Road (now Upper Richmond Road); the RHI were tenants there from 1857 until 1865.

The *third* annual meeting (and 7th election) was held on 25 November 1857, with Lord Raynham presiding. It was indicated that there were then 61 (about to rise to 71) patients of the institution, whereas at the previous annual meeting, the number had been a mere 43. Receipts for the previous year amounted in total to 3,953*l*. 16*s*. 10*d*., and the 'disbursements' were outlined in detail. In an anonymous report, *The Times* referred to the fact that 'a more commodious premises' had been obtained at Putney and in order to acquire funding for a permanent venue they had 'secured an estate of 20 acres at Stoat's Nest … on the trunk line of the Brighton and Dover Railway.'[20] 1889-90 and 1898-9 *Annual Reports* of the RHI mention rather romantically something of the early history of the RHI. The second 'Home' of the institution was: 'the historic "Putney House" in Upper Richmond Road (now demolished) where Byron went to school [and] which has lately gone the way of many a mansion in that once secluded village, now a thickly peopled suburb of the ever widening metropolis', and the 1898-9 *Annual Report* records: '… a removal was made [from Carshalton] to Old Putney House, the school-day scene of troops of boys under the care of the well-known Dr Trimmer [in 1857].

A short time after this building was 'acquired', a smaller building known as the Branch Hospital was also taken over.

An annexe to Putney House
At a Board Meeting on 24 March 1859, 'Dr Reed introduced the question of *additional* premises, stating that he had seen a house at Putney 'in every way suitable [as an annexe to Putney House] including the offices; the rent for a term of three years would be £80 a year'. The matter was pursued at the next Meeting, when it was resolved: '(I) 'That the present house [Putney House] being full, it is desirable to provide additional room for the requirements of the family, and (II) That the house in Putney [situated in Clarendon Road] spoken of at the last meeting be taken [on the conditions stated], subject to the approval of a sub-committee consisting of Messrs. Hall, Osborne, and Taylor, who should be requested to visit the house and communicate their opinion to Dr Reed, who would take action accordingly'! This committee duly recommended that the house be taken, with the provisos that as little expense as possible be incurred in furnishing, …and that the present sub-matron (at Putney House) be removed to the new house, to take charge, under the superintendence of the Head Matron, and that no additional staff of nurses be engaged, the Sub-Committee being of the opinion that by removing the more helpless and bed-ridden of the patients to the new premises, a better classification of the inmates could be made. There seems to have been however a lengthy battle to persuade the previous occupant to remove his furniture from the building!

At a meeting on 28 April it was recorded that Mr Vale ' was willing to sign a memorandum prepared by Mr Taylor in accordance with the request of the Board. It was arranged to exchange the agreements early in the following week.' A month later, 'The Sub-Committee, after inquiring as to the furniture necessary for the Branch House, presented a list of articles, which was approved, and the Sub-Committee were authorised to procure the things specified in the list.' At the July meeting, it was resolved 'That the accts. for furniture etc. for the Branch House should be at once paid on being certified by Mr Osborne or Mr Wright.'[21]

At a meeting in January 1862, it was resolved: 'That the House Committee be requested to make inquiries for a larger house than the one at present used as the Branch.'[22]

Larger and more steps to acquire a permanent venue

A more permanent and larger venue was urgently required, and it was resolved at a meeting held in February, 'That enquiry be made whether an Estate at Putney, known as the "Limes" be to let, and on what terms.' A later meeting however was told that the 'Limes' had already been sold.[23] About this time, the Board was told that 'a view of Putney House [was to be] published in the *Illustrated London News*' (fig 1.5).[24]

In April: 'It was reported by the Secretary that the house next to the Branch was to be let' but it was considered by the Board that 'no action should be taken'. At the same meeting 'The Secretary stated that no answer had been received from the purchasers of the 'Limes', or of Addiscombe College'; the Board was later notified that the new owners of the 'Limes' 'would *not* [let the premises] for the purposes of the Hospital'; however, interest was shown in the latter property. These buildings 'comprised a mansion [which 'lay between two roads leading from Croydon, St James' and the Addiscombe roads'], a residence for [the] principal officer, six large blocks of buildings adjoining, various outbuildings, and two lodges. The whole included about 120 rooms of various size.' It was decided: 'That the Board be summoned to view this estate on Saturday 3 May, to proceed to West Croydon by the train leaving London at 1.15.' The Board duly met at Addiscombe on the appointed day, and resolved: 'That the Secretary be requested to write to the British Land Company [BLC, the owners] inquiring: 1st the acreage of that portion of the estate lying between a line bounding the space allotted for building plots, and the fence forming the boundary of the lawn. 2nd the price put upon the said portion. Also, that a special meeting of the Board be called upon receipt of the Company's reply.' When the BLC replied indicating that the property in question was priced at £30,000 this option was immediately declined![25]

In October of the same year it was minuted: 'That [other] premises in Putney Hill were seen and considered unsuitable.' Therefore, the RHI had to continue at Putney House for the time being, but on 10 March 1864, the Board agreed 'to give Notice to Quit Putney House at Michaelmas next'. This notice was duly conveyed to the RHI solicitors, Messrs Freshfields and

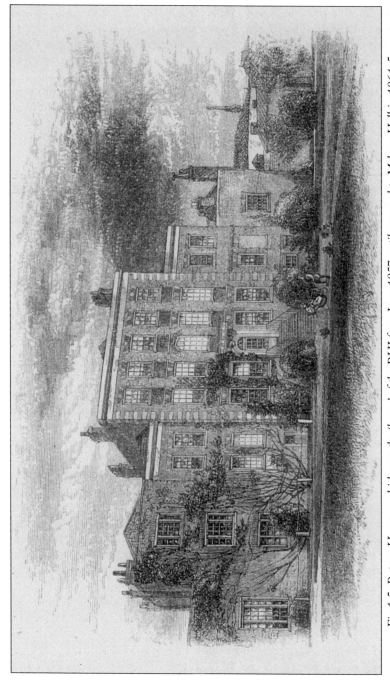

Fig 1.5: Putney House – which was the 'home' of the RHI from June 1857 until removed to Melrose Hall in 1864-5.
(From A. Reed, C. Reed (eds), Memoirs of the Life and Philanthropic Labours of Andrew Reed, D.D., with Selections from his Journals (2nd Edn. London: Strahan & Co. 1863): 425

Newman. By this time Melrose Hall (Chapter 8) had become the likely permanent venue, but owing to a delay in completion of alterations, a later minute deemed it 'advisable, to secure, if possible, a further holding of Putney House for three months, viz. to Chmas next'. This 'holding of Putney House' was indeed extended in August until 'Lady Day 1865', and later still, to 'Midsummer'.[26]

A minute in November 1857 states that: 'In the matter of the Coulsdon agreement, Dr Reed was requested to see the solicitor before the remainder of the purchase money be paid.' It was also recorded in the Board minutes that a roadway was being constructed on the Coulsdon estate.[27]

In July 1858, a letter from the Rev. J.W. Aveling revealed that the 'Board of the New Asylum had given the name of "*Reedham*" to their Estate' in order to honour Reed – the founder of the Asylum for Fatherless Children (Chapter 2).[28]

More Annual Meetings and Dinners

At a Board Meeting on 25 February 1858, it was resolved 'That Mr Charles Dickens be solicited to act as Chairman at the [*fourth*] Dinner'. He presumably declined, for by 8 April, a reply, in this context, from Lord Westminster was awaited. Both he and Mr Gladstone, MP also declined, and later in April it was decided to approach Lord Carlisle.

The *fourth* anniversary dinner (under the presidency of the seventh Earl of Carlisle [1802-64] was held in June 1858. By that time patients had been clearly divided into two 'classes' – 'home' (numbering 53) and 'extra' (32). The former consisted of persons 'received into the asylum, fed, clothed, and [were] carefully attended by ... medical and surgical staff'. The latter were 'patients ... unable, from excess of numbers, to be admitted as residents'; they were however, given an allowance of 'one guinea each per month'. The 'home' patients 'when pronounced incurable by other hospitals, [received] every attention, ..., if not to cure, at least to alleviate the maladies by which they [were] afflicted.' It was announced at that dinner that the receipts for the year 1856-57 amounted to 4,610*l*. 3*s*. 11*d*.; the expenditure had been 2,556*l*. 18*s*. 5*d*.

A more suitable (and permanent) building for the institution was (the Chairman emphasised) still sought, and 2,800*l* 'had already been devoted to the purchase of an estate at Coulsdon, beyond Croydon' (Chapter 7). (This site, although favoured by Reed and Florence Nightingale (1820-1910), was however considered by some 'inconvenient for visitors and too steep for disabled people' by many of the board members.) Later that year, in December, *The Times* referred to gratifying news that the late Mr Richard Habberfield had bequeathed the sum of 1,500*l* to the Charity in his will. And in 1863 the same newspaper recorded that 'Mr. and Madame Goldschmidt' [Jenny Lind (1821-87)]' had donated the proceeds (amounting to 500 guineas) of a grand concert held at St James's Hall. And the following month, funds were again boosted significantly by a 'grand fête and fancy fair' under the patronage of their Royal Highnesses the Duchess of Cambridge and the Princess Mary; the venue for this ambitious performance was the International Exhibition.[29]

The Charity gets into 'full swing'

Competition for 'relief' was intense; by May 1858, for example, two cases were 'declined' on the grounds of 'having received parish relief', and 'of a class bordering upon the pauper'. An introduction from a professional man was clearly of value in gaining admission to the Royal Hospital. The Vicar of Islington, for example, wrote to *The Times* describing a woman (both of whose parents had died when she was young) who suffered from a chronic incurable disease of the chest (presumably tuberculosis, or 'phthisis'), an 'internal complaint, as well as epilepsy. When once admitted, there was no guarantee of continued care; in July 1858, the Board decided, for example, that one of the inmates was 'of unsound mind, and therefore unfit to continue as an inmate of the Royal Hospital, her friends being requested to remove her without delay'.[30]

Fig 1.4 summarizes numbers of patients admitted during the first ten years of the RHI's existence. By August 1856 (i.e. after the Charity had been in operation for two years), there were 28 (14 men and 14 women) 'home' patients, and 14 (8 men and 6 women) 'extra' patients. This number had increased marginally (29 and 19, making a total of 48) by January 1857. By November (shortly before removal to Putney House) the respective numbers were 43 and 22, making a total of 65, and by January 1858 the numbers had further increased to 48 and 27, producing a total of 75. In December 1863, the terms 'inmates' and 'pensioners' were replaced with 'home' and 'out patients'.[31]

In February 1859, the Board viewed sympathetically a suggestion that a 'Free Ward' should be incorporated into the new building. This would be funded from a '… bazaar or fête [and] a free bed [would be] placed [in a wing of the permanent hospital] whenever a sufficient sum had been prescribed to maintain a patient in perpetuity.'[32]

In 1865, *The Times* gave details of the *ninth* anniversary dinner of the Charity – held at the London Tavern with G.J. Göschen MP presiding. It was emphasised that the 'proper subjects' for admission were 'incurables from other hospitals, or from their own homes, who [were] not rich enough to be properly cared for in their own houses, or in the houses of their friends, and who [were] not poor enough to be ranked with paupers in the union houses'. Göschen assured the assembled company, numbering 'upwards of 150' that he had personally inspected Melrose Hall, Putney (chapter 8) (the new home of the institution) and that it 'merited all the praise that had been passed upon it by those who had preceded him in the chair ... Although a new wing had [already] been added to the building, the competition for accommodation was exceedingly great.'[33] Subscriptions that year had amounted to 'upwards of 4,600*l*'.

Medical Care
Details of early medical 'cover' are outlined in Chapter 5. But the ratio of doctors to patients was low; Table 1.1 gives details of numbers of beds and medical officers in most of the *general* hospitals of London in 1868. Although the numbers of beds at the RHI were rather lower, numbers of medical officers (who to this day have never been resident) fell far short – making this from earliest times, primarily a 'home' rather than a hospital, in the widely-accepted meaning of the term.[34]

Patronage
By mid 1857, it was considered that the Charity was 'sufficiently advanced' to write to the Queen (Victoria) requesting her patronage (Chapter 9).
  At a meeting held on 8 April 1858, Dr Reed reported that Lord Shaftesbury (1801-85) had consented to be a Vice-President.

Fund-raising Sermons
Charity Sermons were major fund-raising events in the mid-nineteenth century (Chapter 16). It proved difficult however to find a suitable venue for the Bishop of London to preach; St Marylebone proved unsuccessful and efforts were made for St George's Hanover Square. However, sermons during the first five years of the Charity were eventually preached by the Lord Bishop (at St Andrew's Westminster) and also by the Revd. M.H. Vine, and the Revd. H.M. Bellen (sic) (at Bow Church). All three were immediately made life governors of the Charity, and the Bishop later 'consented to become a Vice-President'.
  How best to advertise the Charity was an on-going problem; in December 1863 it was agreed (by the Board) to ask permission of the South-Western Railway Company to have (advertising) boards put up at Putney Station. However, this request was declined.[35]

Early problems and domestic matters
Following foundation of the Charity in 1854, there were inevitably numerous ongoing 'teething' problems to be faced by the Board (which met fortnightly), and House Committee (weekly). Several of these will now be highlighted.
  The first sign of instability within management (Chapter 14) came on 11 February 1867; the Secretary received a letter from the Revd. William Woodhouse (a member of the Board):

Table 1.1: Numbers of beds compared with numbers of medical officers in the General Hospitals of London in 1868: derived from a memorandum in The Seamen's Hospital Society archive, dated 24 March 1868

	No. of Beds	No. of Medical Officers*
St Bartholomew's	650	24
King's College	130	13
London	570	23
University College	136	23
St Thomas's	211†	17
St Mary's	180	16
Charing Cross	135	13
Middlesex	320	20
St George's	360	21
Guy's	580	23
Westminster	200	15

*Includes those performing out-patient duties.
†This low-ish number was presumably a result of the removal from the 'old' (Borough) to the 'new' (Lambeth Bridge Road) sites.

See also: R. Farguarson. In: R. Quain (ed) *A dictionary of medicine including general pathology, general therapeutics, hygiene, and the diseases peculiar to women and children* (London: Longmans, Green and Co. 1890): 1520-21.

West Hill, Wandsworth, S.W.
February 11th 1867

Dear Sir,
A Magistrate of this district has expressed an opinion that "if the Governors of the Royal Hospital have any regards for the Charity, they will certainly have an Inquest [which was duly carried out by the Coroner] held on the body of Mrs Curtis now lying in the Institution, the remains of the third patient who has died in the same room in about twelve days. A Barrister of great experience in matters of this nature is also of the same decided opinion. I give no opinion …

Much later, the Secretary (Newton) resigned 'under a cloud'. A patient had threatened to commit suicide, and blame was attributed to Newton. His resignation was accepted in June 1906, and an advertisement for a successor issued. Seven of the sixteen applicants were interviewed and Charles Cutting of the Royal Free Hospital was appointed on a salary of £350 per annum.

Progress
The 1874 *Annual Report* began by reminding subscribers (and others) that it was a mere two decades ago (27 November 1854) since the Governors met at the City of London Tavern to hold the *first* election of the Charity. Since then, the success of the RHI could be 'traced to the fidelity with which the general scheme of its founder [had] been followed'. Success had in effect been based upon two 'sound and far-sighted' principles: (i) the Institution was placed upon a *popular* [my italics] basis, making it the property of the subscribers', and (ii) 'it allotted the benefit in accordance with the need, allowing in some cases a moderate pecuniary grant, and devoting to the most necessitous the resources of a Medical Home'.[36]

Day-to-day administration
The bulk of work undertaken by the various committees was of a trivial nature, albeit important, e.g. the recording of legacies and other financial matters, elections, organisation of the Annual Meetings and dinners, numbers of 'inmates' and outpatients – their health and deaths, ordering of provisions, including coal and wine, garden and other domestic matters. In 1861 a further 'chore' was introduced: '… a book be kept for registering the supply and consumption of wine, spirits and strong ales' (see below).[37]

Other 'domestic' matters
The nineteenth-century Minute Books contain a vast amount of detail concerning other day-to-day activities, e.g.: a minute in December 1876 states: '… it had been agreed to dispense with the signing of the Visitors' Book in certain cases, owing to the inconvenience felt by Visitors coming in carriages', and on 9 May 1877, the Earl of Shaftesbury KG (who later that month presided at the Annual Dinner) visited the RHI, staying three hours and talking to many of the 'inmates'.[38]

The free ward
This small ward (see above) was reserved for *deserving* individuals who had failed in the voting system. As there were only a limited number of beds in the *Free Ward*, places were usually only available on death of an 'inmate'. The 'Free Ward Committee' proposed, in April 1887 for example, to 'fill up Vacancies caused by the deaths of [two patients] and asking to be furnished with the names of any unsuccessful candidates who might be considered eligible.' Two candidates, whose names were forwarded by the Board, were therefore duly visited.[39]

Criteria for entry
It was proposed by the Chairman of the Hospital for Incurable Children that

cases who were 16 years and over in that hospital might be accommodated, on payment, at the RHI. This idea was however, rejected by the Board.[40]

Another request, this time to 'house' members of the Jewish faith was also declined by the Board (Chapter 15).[41]

Deaths
Death of a Board member, or of a national figure, was documented in detail; thus, on 3 December 1882, the Archbishop of Canterbury (President of the RHI) died. A resolution of condolence, which was forwarded to Mrs Tait, was acknowledged by the Revd. Randall T. Davidson (a future Archbishop of Canterbury, 1903-28). The Board duly wrote to the Revd. Montague Fowler, who was acting on behalf of the incoming archbishop 'asking His Grace [Edward White Benson – 1829-96] to accept the position of President of the Institution held by his two immediate predecessors [Archbishops Longley and Tait]'. His Grace's first reaction was that 'an Institution of this magnitude required a *resident* [my italics] Chaplain …'. After receiving details of the 'services and other religious work at the Hospital', the new archbishop merely reinforced his views. Therefore, the Board did not think it worthwhile 'to persevere in the request', and they suggested inviting either the Duke of Albany, or the Earl of Aberdeen to be president. The former rejected the invitation, but the latter (Chapter 14) fortunately accepted.[42]

The death of the Seventh Earl of Shaftesbury (see above) – who was a Vice-President of the Charity – was reported to a Board meeting on 8 October 1885. He had presided at the Annual Dinner for 1877, and 'the Incurables had a cherished place' in his wide range of activities. In March 1886 a Minute records an invitation from a sculptor to view a recently completed 'Marble Bust of the late Earl'; he was prepared to sell replicas at £5-5-0 (in plaster), or £105 (in marble).[43]

In November 1900, Andrew, the long-serving Secretary (he had served for 46 years) resigned, and in January 1901 he suddenly became seriously ill whilst working in his office at the RHI and 'lost the power of speech'. He died (presumably as a result of a cerebro-vascular accident) on 22 January. Andrew left a substantial sum (about £6,000) to the RHI; the Board resolved (on November 20 1902) that a room in the 'Old Building' should be called the 'Andrew Day Room'. There is later mention of a portrait of him. An advertisement for a new secretary was placed in *The Times* for 15, 17, 19 December 1900. He had to be between 30 and 40, and 'to reside within a mile of the Hospital'. The interviews took place on Tuesday 15 January 1901 at 2 o'clock, when David Newton was appointed.[44]

Henry Huth (the Treasurer of the RHI) died suddenly on the morning of 11 December 1878. He was of German extraction, and a 'man of means' who lived in Princes Gate. The 'Comm^ee … ordered that the flag be hoisted half-staff high.' (At the same meeting, the death of Mrs Tait, wife of the former Archbishop of Canterbury [see above], was recorded.) A note of condolence and details of the funeral (which was a strictly private one) were subsequently recorded. An obituary notice was included in the 'Supplementary edition of the Appeal' and a 'Memorial Inscription' was produced. Huth was succeeded as treasurer by John Darby Allcroft who died – after holding the position for 14 years – in August 1893; he in turn was succeeded by his son Herbert John Allcroft. Henry Ellis Esq. was appointed as temporary treasurer in the absence of a treasurer. George F. White, Esq. was then asked if his name could go to the AGM in November, as the successor. After serving on the Board for thirty years, White died in 1897. He had been a staunch supporter: '... in its day, the New Wing [Chapter 8], erected at an outlay of £30,000.'[45]

It was recorded, on 28 March 1881, that Sir Charles Reed MP (son of the Founder) had died on the 25th of that month; arrangements for representatives of the Board to attend the funeral and a 'Resolution of Condolence' were minuted. The death of the Revd. Andrew Reed (eldest son of the Founder), was later recorded – in April 1899.[46] James Best who had been Collector for forty-four years died in 1900.[47]

Distinguished friends of the RHI were also held in high regard, and their deaths were duly recorded in meticulous detail. For example, following the death of HRH the Duchess of Teck (1833-97), letters of condolence were sent to HH the Duke of Teck and HRH the Duke of York. And the death of the Duke of Clarence & Avondale (1864-92) was also recorded in the minutes.[48]

The City Offices

Like the vast majority of charities in the nineteenth century, the RHI was run very largely from a *city* office and *not* from the hospital itself. The House-Committee met at the Hospital (either Carshalton or Putney-based), but the major administrative events, including Board Meetings, Annual Dinners, and AGMs were always held in the City of London. The original city offices were situated at 10 Poultry. In the early days of the RHI, there were no cars or even telephones, so communication between the city office and the hospital was difficult. In order to get to the hospital, the city staff (including the Secretary) had to take a train from Waterloo to Putney, or alternatively go by 'underground' to East Putney.

There must however have been a good deal of dissatisfaction with the city venue for in October 1870, the Board resolved unanimously 'That [a] Sub-C[ee] be requested to negotiate and conclude an arrangement for securing [new city] offices at 1 Poultry.'[49] However, these negotiations soon broke down and at a Special Board Meeting in February 1874 (i.e. 20 years after formation of the Charity), 'the desirability of engaging new offices at No 4, Gracechurch St.'

(which consisted of 'the whole of the upper part of a house at a rent of £250 a year') was considered but again rejected.

However, as I shall show, the RHI was to prove somewhat peripatetic regarding its city offices, for a month later, 'the Committee appointed in this matter engaged offices' at 33 King St, Cheapside; [these consisted] of two rooms on the third floor, at a rent of £270 per annum, for a term of 7, 14 or 21 years, terminable at the option of either party, or for a fixed period of 21 years, as the Board might prefer ...'. A draft lease for these *new* offices was presented to the Board in May; however, this contained several 'objectionable clauses' and further negotiations were abandoned; as an alternative the Board became interested in 'rooms at 113, Queen Victoria St' at a rent of £300 annually. These rooms were also to be on lease for 7, 14 or 21 years; if the last option was accepted the rental would increase to £350 for the last 7-year period. The Board approved, a lease was prepared and it was reported at the August meeting 'that the business of the Charity had been removed to [these offices]'.[50]

In July 1887, the Board decided to 'terminate the tenancy' of these offices at Midsummer next; they could have continued for a further 7 years 'at an advanced rental of £350, the present being £300'. A suggestion was made that they 'purchase the Premises, 106 Queen Victoria St. ... for say £4000'; however, the Board declined to 'make any proposal'. A letter was read at a Board meeting in September indicating that these premises had been made over to them, and requesting the payment of rent. To find suitable *new* offices proved difficult, and in February 1888 a sub-committee suggested 'a continuation of the occupancy of the [present offices] at the present rent (£300) on an agreement for 3 years'. This offer was accepted, and several minor improvements approved. Shortly after that, these premises were sold, but the new owner had 'the interest of the Hospital at heart' and continued with the agreement. An offer to the Board to purchase the premises (they were prepared to pay up to £5000), with a lease of 61 years, was declined. They were therefore sold by auction, and the RHI had to vacate them by the following June. Negotiations subsequently took place and ultimately the Board accepted a 'New Lease' at the existent rental of £300.[51]

The lease for these premises was due to expire in Midsummer 1898. Therefore '... the secretary was directed to write to the Agent for the premises [in Queen Victoria Street], Mr [William] Jacobs of 1 Angell Court, asking whether the landlord would be disposed to renew the lease on the same terms as at present'; at their meeting in February 1898 the Board were told: ' [Jacobs] was willing to renew the lease of the offices for another period of seven years from Midsummer next, upon the same terms as at present.' Jacobs consented to a new lease for 21 years, although this was terminable at either 7 or 14 years. Meanwhile, life in the City was not without problems and a 'complaint had been made [in August 1898] of noise and obstruction created by the tenants of the ground floor, an Aluminium Company, in the common stairway.'[52]

Salaries of the clerical staff

The salaries of the clerks in the City Offices came under annual review in January of each year. In 1887, the salaries of Simmonds, Starling, Hall and Moss were £200, £200, £120 and £100, respectively; all except Starling received gratuities of £10, £5, and £5, respectively. The following year, these gratuities were increased by £20, £20, £15 and £10. In January 1889, the salaries of Hall and Moss were elevated to £130 and £110, while the gratuities to Simmonds, Starling, Hall and Moss amounted to £25, £25, £10 and £5; similar gratuities were paid in 1890 and 91, with the exception that in the latter year, Moss received £10. In 1890, the Secretary received a gratuity of 150 guineas for his work in connection with the previous Christmas Appeal (Chapter 18).

Over the following few years, salaries rose steeply, and by 1898, Simmonds and Starling were receiving £300, while Hall's salary had been raised to £200, and that of the junior clerk (Luscombe) to £100; Hall, in addition, was awarded a gratuity of £40 in respect of the Christmas appeal.[53]

In 1898 also, Starling replaced Best (see above) as Collector; Best had been partially retired since 1895, i.e. after 39 years service. In 1870, the office of Steward was abolished, and his duties were subsumed by the Governor.[54]

Water and alcohol consumption

The quality and quantity of drinking water

There was at this time increasing recognition that impure drinking water might be related to disease. John Snow (1813-58) had published his hypothesis linking the 1853-4 cholera outbreak in Soho in London with faecally-contaminated drinking water, in 1854. The three great cholera epidemics in London had occurred in 1831-2, 1848-9, and 1853-4.

In August 1859, it was decided to request the landlord of the Branch House (at Putney) 'to supply a cover to the water tank'. At a meeting in February 1858, a Board minute states: 'Upon tasting the water from the [Putney House] Well [the Committee] had thought fit to send it to an analyst for an opinion upon its quality as suitable for consumption', and in April, Lindsay Blyth of the Board of Health was duly thanked for his analysis. However, at a meeting in October 'An application from Dr Thompson for a fee of six guineas for analysing the water at Putney house [had been received, and this] was referred to Mr Wm G. Davies, as it was understood at the time that the service was to be gratuitous'! Several years later (in June 1866) 'the Secy. stated that the House C^cc ... had agreed to recommend the adoption of a system of filtration of water for drinking purposes, as well as for Surgery use according to a plan and estimate submitted by the Moulded Carbon Filter Company, Fleet St. – total cost about £27.'[55]

The quality of the water was later analysed by H.R. Gregory, Esq., a Fellow of the Institute of Great Britain and Ireland, for which a charge of four guineas was made. 'Two samples were submitted, viz: filtered and unfiltered.' Gregory wrote that 'neither of [these] samples contain any marked amount of organic impurity', and both were 'quite safe to use for drinking and domestic purposes'. The minute concluded: 'Order given to cleanse the filters through-out the building.'[56]

The day supply of water (there was no night supply) in those days left a good deal to be desired, but a minute dated May 1877 recorded 'a favourable report as to the abundance of the supply'. The following month, the well (at Melrose Hall) had been opened, and the engineer calculated 'that an unlimited supply of water could be obtained at a considerably less cost than from the Water Company'. The minutes contain numerous references to water consumption, which would obviously increase as soon as the Great Extension (Chapter 8) was opened. The Southwark and Vauxhall Water Co. had informed the RHI in April 1878 that from September, their rates were about to be increased. The overall cost of water for the RHI was escalating, and Mr Rich of Messrs Easton and Anderson met the Board to explain what was going on.[57]

In December 1882, the Board received a letter from a London solicitor, writing on behalf of a client who had purchased a portion of the Wimbledon Park Estate; this requested 'that the Hospital Authorities "stop the flow of either water or sewage" into the Pond' (which had been designed by Capability Brown). '... the C[ee] did not feel prepared [however] to accede to their request.'![58]

Alcoholism, and the consumption of 'extras' and 'stimulants'
Overindulgence in alcohol was felt to be a serious problem in the early days of the Charity; this afflicted both staff and patients. It affected staff not only at the RHI in Putney, but also at Seaside House.[59] Chapter 5 contains more information on this topic, on which there seems to have been differing opinions.

The Secretary (Andrew) informed the Board in 1898 that he 'had made preliminary inquiries about a Home for Inebriates'; the objective on this occasion was to attempt to get one of the female pensioners admitted there. He, and Starling (a clerk), had 'visited the locality where she last resided, and obtained additional information from the Police and from the parties keeping a public house, the Wargrave Arms.' They discovered that 'on the 19th Oct. last' (i.e. some 3-4 months previously) she was 'locked up and charged with drunkenness' and also that she had been refused service at the public house.

'... it was now discovered that [she] had entered the Marylebone Workhouse on the 10th inst. and was transferred to the Infirmary on the 11th. As a result of these inquiries it was agreed that her name 'must be removed from the list of Pensioners.'[60]

But in a more general sense, the excessive use of '*stimulants*' was one which repeatedly occupied the attention of the House-Committee; for example in May 1869 '... owing to the increasing consumption [two members of the House Committee] had been requested to visit the British Home for Incurables [Clapham] and other Institutions [see below] and report upon the quantities found to be used in such Institutions.' This matter again came to the fore in October, when Dr Little (who had consulted with Dr Woodhouse on this matter, concluded that: 'the amount of stimulants was not, considering the age and maladies of the patients, excessive'. At the same meeting however, it was agreed 'to forbid the purchasing or receiving of wines, spirits, or other stimulants by the inmates ...'. Later that year '... it [was] agreed to substitute by way of trial, British for French Brandy'. And a month later it was decided 'That the scale of consumption of malt liquors by the Officials had been revised, and that in some instances it had been arranged to give money in lieu of Beer.'[61]

In March of 1870 surprisingly '... it had been agreed to *increase* [my italics] the allowance of Beer to the Male Inmates to 1¹/₂ pints per day.' However, a year later '... the subject of the increased consumption of stimulants ... had [arisen again and had] engaged the attention of the [House-Committee]. In August 1871, the minutes of the Finance Committee 'desired to draw the attention of the House C[ee] to the consumption of bottled ales and spirits'. Some two months later the Board considered: '... it had been agreed to consult Dr. Munk (Chapter 5) on the subject of the consumption of *extra diet and stimulants* [my italics], the administration of which appeared to the C[ee] to be irregular and excessive.' Munk felt that '... judging from the list submitted to him, the consumption was [indeed] excessive.' At the same meeting (in November) it was recorded that 'the Governor had indeed visited the British Home for Incurables at Clapham Rise, and found that stimulants were used there in nearly the same proportion as at the [RHI]; the extras, on the other hand, shewed a much less relative consumption.' A few months later, the Board minutes state: 'That in relation to the Dietary, Dr. Munk and Dr. Woodhouse had had a long conversation on the subject of extras and stimulants, and had agreed upon considerable reductions. In the light of Munk's advice [submitted in a written report], there was 'a considerable reduction' in the use of 'stimulants' ... 'without injury to the inmates'!'[62]

The matter of 'stimulants' continued to be at the forefront of the minds of members of the Board of Management as well as the House-Committee. Figures for the 'consumption of wines, spirits, and alcoholic beverages [in July

1879] (excepting claret, and ale and porter in casks)' ordered by the medical officer are recorded in Table 1.2. This report commented that: (i) the average consumption was lower than formerly, and (ii) 'in the opinion of the House Committee the rate of consumption is justifiable on medical grounds …'. Regarding claret, the daily consumption was '150 ounces, or 6 bottles, amongst 26 patients, viz: 8 male, and 18 female, the former consuming 7 ounces, and the latter 5 ounces per day.' Claret was used (the report continued) 'in place of malt liquors by inmates who prefer it or for whom malt liquors are unsuitable'. The House-Committee further considered that 'the substitution of Claret [was] beneficial to the health of the inmates [and] in the opinion of the medical officer, [prevented] the necessity in certain cases of prescribing more expensive wine or brandy'. The report was adopted by the Board, with the important proviso that claret should *not* be included 'in the general item of house keeping' but was to remain as at the present time 'under the head of wines and spirits'.[63]

In April 1882, the Board suggested that 'Claret be discontinued as a beverage', and that an allowance in money be made to any of the staff who might wish it, in lieu of ale or porter'. It was later agreed by the House-Committee to 'offer to male members of the staff an allowance at the rate of £3, and to females of £2.10 annually in lieu of beer'. Interestingly, '[while] nearly all the female staff … accepted the offered allowance … in lieu of beer, [none] of the male staff [did]'.[64]

A few years later, in May 1889, a Board minute contains a: 'Recommendation for the reduction [in] the use of alcoholic beverages; including the limiting of beer allowed to inmates to one glass at dinner and one at supper; extension of beer money in lieu of beer to all the present staff, the same to be in future paid as an addition to wages, also that all new servants be engaged on the understanding that no beer is allowed, the matron or the steward being authorised, at their discretion, to add £2 per annum to usual wages in lieu of beer money.' This however, brought forth a letter from 15 male inmates protesting against the limitation of beer, and requesting that the allowance be raised to two glasses. This request was refused, and the quantity of claret used on the male side was 'reduced from $7^1/_2$ ozs to 5 ozs'. In February 1894 the Board agreed that 'all special diets and all beverages, i.e. beer, claret [and] milk, should be ordered by the Medical Officer …'.[65]

Although there was at this time, therefore, a great deal of discussion about the *quantity* of 'stimulants' used by the inmates (see below), there seems to have been a great deal of dissatisfaction with the *quality* of the wine also, which was in use for its restorative properties. In July 1859, for example, 'it was agreed to discontinue the use of *colonial* [my italics] wines [and it was decided to purchase] 3 doz. of port at from 25/- to 40/- and the same quantity of sherry.'

Table 1.2: An assessment of alcohol consumption in July 1879

Daily rate	No of Patients	Cases
Brandy		*Cases*
49 ozs	27	4 temporary, 6 great debility, 3 abscesses, 4 phthises, 1 hip disease and debility, 5 spinal disease, 2 bronchitis, 2 old age.
Port		
16 ozs	6	1 dying, 1 old age, 1 phthises, 2 spinal disease, 1 discretionary.
Sherry		
2 ozs	1	obstinate vomiting.
Gin		
2 ozs	1	renal disease.
Champagne		
3 pts bott	3	1 temporary, 1 abscesses, 1 dying.
Stout		
8 small bott	4	2 abscesses, 1 spinal disease, 1 lupus.
Ale		
4 small bott	2	abscesses.

NB. About 2 pints of Brandy extra per month are delivered from the stores, viz: 1 pint for occasional use and emergencies and 1 pint for household consumption.

Incidentally, the major donor of champagne in the early days of the Charity seems to have been none other than the Treasurer, Henry Huth!

References and Notes

1. **Charles Dickens** (1812-70) was one of the greatest of the Victorian novelists. He emerged as a precocious genius, and produced *Pickwick Papers* at the age of 24 years. He wrote 'for all time'. Born on 7 February 1812 at Portsea, he died on 9 June 1870 at Gadshill. He was buried in Westminster Abbey on 14 June 1870. '[Dickens] was of the people and lived among them.' He therefore occupied a unique position 'with the English and also with the American public for the third of a century'; Anonymous, *Times, Lond.* Leading article 10 June 1870. *See also.* Anonymous, *Times, Lond.* 11 June 1870; L. Stephen *Dictionary of National Biography* 1908; 5: 925-37; P. Ackroyd: *Dickens* (London: Sinclair-Stevenson, 1990): 1195; P. Ackroyd,

Dickens: public life and private passion (London: BBC 2002): 160; C. Dickens (ed). *Household Words: a weekly journal* (1850), 1: 517. Anonymous, 'International Nurses at Putney', *Nursing Times* 12 March 1927; Reed A., Reed C. (eds), *Memoirs of the Life and Philanthropic Labours of Andrew Reed D.D. with selections from his Journals.* 1863 – 2nd edn London; H.J.G. Bloom, W.W. Richardson, E.J. Harries, 'Natural history of untreated breast cancer (1805-1933): comparison of untreated and treated cases according to histological grade of malignancy. *Br Med J* 1962; ii: 213-21; I.F.W. Beckett, *Victoria's Wars* (Princes Risborough, Bucks: Shire Publications Ltd., 2nd ed. 1998): 15-22.

2. Board minutes Book 1: 1-5.
3. Ibid: 1 and 27-32.
4. Ibid: 5, 6, 7, 33, 34, 39, 41, 42, 45; Ibid: (Appeals 1 and 2): 9-15, 16-19. These two 'appeals' are extremely verbose, and the bulk of the text was incorporated in the Constitution (Chapter 3), 19-27.
5. Op cit., see note 2 above: 35-6, 39-40.
6. G.B. Brightling. *Some particulars relating to the history and antiquities of Carshalton: compiled from the best authorities.* (London: Operative Jewish Converts' Institution 1872): 25-32; A.E. Jones, *From medieval manor to London suburb: an obituary of Carshalton* (Carshalton: A.E. Jones 1970): 89-90; A.E. Jones, *An illustrated directory of Old Carshalton* (Carshalton: A.E. Jones 1973): 136-7; K.G. Harris, *History of Carshalton Work House* (Unpublished typescript (SBC 344): London Borough of Sutton Learning for Life Central Library).
7. RHI Annual Report 1978-9: (Op.cit., see note 2 above. Book 12: 406-7); RHI Annual Report 1898-9: 11; Book 21)
8. K. Morrison. 'The new Poor Law of 1834' in: *The Workhouse: a study of Poor-law buildings in England* (Swindon: Royal Commission on the Historical Monuments of England, 1999): 43-52; Board Minutes, 65: 210.
9. Op.cit., see note 2 above, Book 1: 43, 79, 208, 214.
10. Ibid: 60.
11. Ibid: 102-8.
12. Ibid: 80-1, 96.
13. Ibid: 115, 121, 126.
14. Ibid: 145, 175.
15. Ibid: 214, 223, 227.
16. Ibid: 237-9.
17. Anonymous, 'The Royal Hospital for the care of incurables', *Times, Lond.* 7 June 1856: 12.
18. Anonymous, 'The Royal Hospital', *Times, Lond.*, 22 May 1857: 12.
19. Op.cit. See note 2 above: 260, 265-6, 273-4, 306, 318, 323; Book 1: 31.
20. Anonymous, 'The Royal Hospital', *Times, Lond.*, 26 November 1857: 10.
21. Ibid. Book 2: 202, 208, 212-13, 220, 234-40, 270.

22. Ibid. Book 4: 53, 67, 81, 95, 107, 211.

23. Ibid. Book 4: 148, 174.

24. Ibid: 163-4.

25. Ibid: 187, 196-7, 201, 209.

26. Ibid. Book 4: 292; Book 5: 187, 195, 233, 234-5, 293, 368, 410.

27. Ibid. Book 1: 374, 375.

28. Ibid. Book 2: 80.

29. Anonymous, 'The Royal Hospital', *Times, Lond.*, 11 June 1858: 9; Anonymous, 'The Royal Hospital', *Times, Lond.* 11 December 1858: 10; Anonymous, 'The Royal Hospital for Incurables', *Times, Lond.*, 25 May 1863: 11; Anonymous, 'Royal Hospital for Incurables', *Times, Lond.*, 26 June 1863: 7.

30. D. Wilson. *Times, Lond.*, 23 November 1863: 11; Board minutes. Book 1: 64, 79.

31. Op.cit., see note 2 above, Book 1: 374, 396; Book 5: 152-3.

32. Ibid. Book 2: 185.

33. Anonymous, 'The Royal Hospital for Incurables', *Times, Lond.*, 8 March 1865: 12.

34. A.E. Stokes-Roberts, *A short history of the Royal Hospital and Home for Incurables Putney* (London: RHHI 1972): 3.

35. Ibid. Book 5: 130.

36. Ibid. Book 10: 240-4.

37. Ibid. Book 4: 47; Book 6: 457-8; Book 23: 233-4, 235-6, 263, 268, 269.

38. Ibid. Book 11: 313, 324. **Anthony Ashley Cooper,** seventh Earl of Shaftesbury (1801-85) was one of the great philanthropists and reformers of the nineteenth century. Educated at Harrow and Christ Church, Oxford, he became an MP (1826-51). He urged reform of the lunacy laws (1829), protection of factory operatives (1833-44), colliery workers and chimney sweeps. He also advocated ragged schools and reclamation of juvenile offenders (1848), as well as improved housing for the poor. He was also Chairman of the Sanitary Commission in the Crimea.

39. Ibid. Book 16: 8, 12, 32, 38, 42, 62, 82, 141; Op.cit. See note 2 above. Book 15: 476, 483.

40. Ibid. Book 17: 242.

41. Ibid. Book 16: 39-40.

42. **Archibald Campbell Tait** (1811-82) was Archbishop of Canterbury from 1868 until his death. He was educated at Edinburgh High School, Glasgow University and Balliol College, Oxford. In 1842, he succeeded Arnold as Headmaster of Rugby. He became Dean of Carlisle (1849) and was Bishop of London 1856-69; Op.cit. See note 2 above. Book 14: 90, 94, 170, 177, 188, 225, 233. *See also:* E. Carpenter *Cantuar. the archbishops in their office* (London, Cassell, 1974) 334-359.

43. Ibid. Book 15: 163, 182, 258.

44. Ibid. Book 22: 229, 232, 254-5, 263-4, 274, 277, 281, 308-9, 331, 341, 497; Book 23: 58.
45. Ibid. book 12: 152, 165-6, 169-70, 180, 183, 214, 224, 233; Book 18: 433-4, 439-40, 444, 464; Book 19: 14, 15, 194, 206, 250; Book 21: 176]; RHI Annual Report 1897-8.
46. Op.cit. See note 2 above. Book 13: 236, 239, 367; Book 21: 292.
47. Ibid. Book 22: 160.
48. Ibid. Book 20: 452-3; Book 18: 33.
49. Ibid. Book 8: 363.
50. Ibid. Book 10: 43, 84, 117, 138, 149, 160, 182, 191.
51. Ibid. Book 16: 41, 47, 57, 95, 168-9, 192, 202, 213, 228, 248, 278-9, 286, 331-2, 362; Book 17: 314, 334-5, 418-9, 429.
52. Ibid. Book 20: 474, 488, 534; Book 21: 29, 52, 125-6, 142, 163-4.
53. Ibid. Book 15: 429; Book 16: 143, 340; Book 17: 51, 297, 324; Book 18: 28-9, 310; Book 20: 29, 257-8, 501-2.
54. Ibid. Book 8: 149, 177, 225; Book 19: 381-2; Book 20: 38-9; *See also*: RHI Annual Report 1894-5.
55. Op.cit. See note 2 above. Book 2: 126; Book 6: 238-9.
56. Ibid. Book 20: 316.
57. Ibid. Book 11: 2-3, 321-2, 329, 384; Book 12: 468, 481; Book 13: 353, 385, 389, 397.
58. Ibid. Book 14: 93.
59. Ibid. Book 17: 44-5.
60. Ibid. Book 20: 37, 63.
61. Ibid. Book 8: 45, 147-8, 199.
62. Ibid: 242, 419; Book 9: 22, 51, 57-8, 133, 142, 152.
63. Ibid: Book 12: 340-3.
64. Ibid: Book 13: 466, 467-8, 472.
65. Ibid: Book 16: 416, 426; Book 19: 65.

CHAPTER 2

The founding father – Andrew Reed, Doctor of Divinity (1787-1862)

WHO WAS REED? Andrew Reed (1787-1862) (fig 2.1), who was to become one of the nineteenth century's major philanthropists, was born at Beaumont House, Butcher Row, St Clement Danes, London, on 27 November 1787; he was the fourth son of a watchmaker, Andrew Reed (who came from Maiden Newton, Dorset), and his wife Mary Ann (née Mullen) who before her marriage had taught at a dame school in Little Britain; later, she ran a successful china shop in Clerkenwell.

Reed was privately educated (at Mitcham and Hayes, Kent) and when 16 years old, joined the congregation of a local congregational church (where his father was a lay evangelist, who preached until the end of his life) at New Road, St George's-in-the-East. Reed was apparently present with his father at the founding of the Religious Tract Society on 10 May 1799. Although for a while (from 15 years of age) he took part in his father's business, he soon found this uncongenial, and at the age of 20 entered (as a theological student) the newly-founded ('dissenting') Hackney College.

In November 1811, Reed was ordained into the 'Independent' (i.e. Congregational) ministry and immediately became pastor of New Road chapel (which apparently had a congregation of 800 individuals, including some well-to-do City merchants and tradesmen). This church was situated near the Commercial Road, in London's 'East End'. He also became, in effect, an itinerant preacher – visiting many parts of England, and on one occasion venturing as far afield as Dublin. The possibility of his proceeding to Cambridge was considered but this course was for all practical purposes at that time barred to non-conformists. During the following seventeen years, amidst his regular duties, he built a larger place of worship, Wycliffe Chapel, which was opened on 21 June 1831; here, he held the pastorate until November 1861, resigning at the celebration of his jubilee.

In 1834, he was sent (by the Congregational Union of England and Wales – which consisted of 'Independents' and Baptists) to the congregational churches of America in order to 'promote peace and friendship between the two communities'. Before returning home, Yale University conferred on him their honorary DD degree.

Reed always played a personal role in the various charities which he founded (see below), and because this necessitated living nearby, built himself

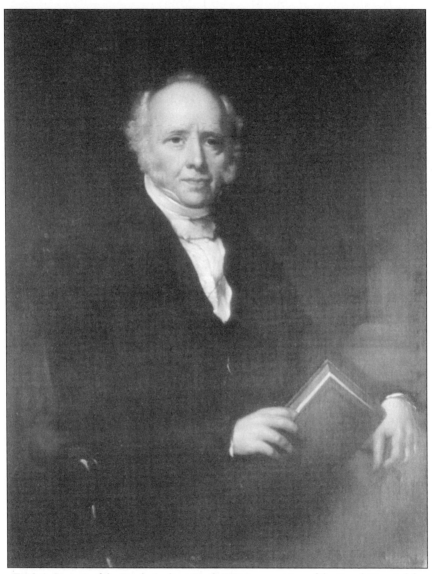

Fig 2.1: Portrait of the Revd. Andrew Reed, DD in possession of the Royal Hospital for Neuro-disability. It was painted by Beatrice Murray in about 1857.

a house at Cambridge Heath, Hackney, he and his wife having previously lived at Cheshunt. His later life was passed here, and he died there on 25 February 1862. He was interred in the Abney Park Cemetery, Stoke Newington, near the 'monument to the memory of Dr Isaac Watts'.[1]

Reed married (in April 1816) Elizabeth, eldest daughter of Jaspar Thomas Holmes of Castle Hall, Reading; there were five children of the marriage – four sons (the second of whom, Sir Charles Reed MP, FSA [1819-81],[2] was to become Chairman of the London School Board) and a daughter.

Reed's death on 25 February 1862 was announced at a Board Meeting of the RHI by the chairman (Huth) two days later; this was followed by a lengthy eulogy, a copy of which, it was resolved, should be sent to his family (this was duly acknowledged by his son, Charles). It was also resolved that Reed's death should be recorded in: *The Times, City Press, Morning Star,* and *Daily Telegraph.* The funeral service, which was to be held on 3 March, would be attended by four members of the Board: Messrs. Woolley, Hartley, Wilkinson, and Kelsey. Reed had left nothing in his Will to the RHI; this was attributed (by William Woodhouse) to the fact that this was 'made ten years since, and prior to the existence of the Charity'.

There were apparently several portraits of Reed, apart from that hanging today in the RHN. A minute of 14 November 1867 refers to 'an oil portrait of the Founder ... which was a present from the Treasurer [Huth]'. A letter from the *Asylum for Idiots* (see below) was read to the Board; this invited a deputation to be present at the unveiling (by The Earl of Shaftesbury, KG) at Earlswood of a portrait of the 'late Revd. Andrew Reed D.D.'.[3]

From 1856 to 1881, Reed's eldest son (now Sir Charles Reed) was a member of the RHI board, and for 28 years (1902-30) his grandson, Eliot Pye-Smith Reed, was also a member. Subsequent descendents (including one from the present generation) have also been active members of the Management Committee, although the non-conformist background was abandoned for the Church of England long ago.

Reed's Charities
For almost 50 years of his life, Reed was engaged in philanthropic work (table 2.1; fig 2.2).

In 1813, he published an appeal (which was supported by the Duke of Kent [1767-1820], father of Queen Victoria, and other members of the Royal Family) urging the formation of an asylum for orphans; this became (in February 1815), the *London Orphan Asylum.* The inaugural dinner of this institution was attended by the Duke of Kent. A site in Clapton (consisting of a house surrounded by eight acres) was subsequently bought for 3,500 guineas. A later building (which cost 25,000*l* (£) on this site was opened in 1825 by the Duke of Cambridge (1774-1850). In 1869, this asylum was removed to

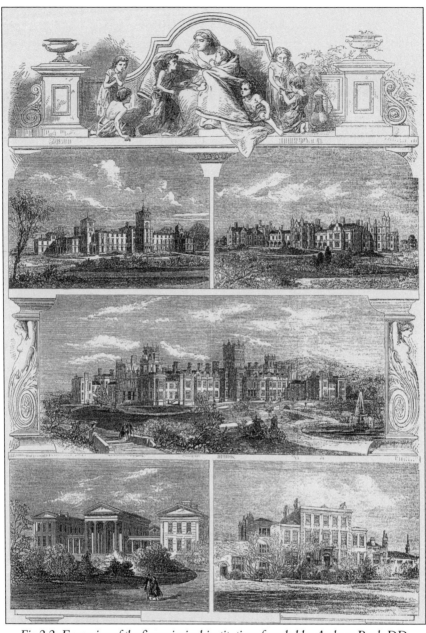

Fig 2.2: Engraving of the five principal institutions founded by Andrew Reed, DD.
(Illustrated London News *1862: 40 (15 March): 270).*

The Asylum for	*The Infant Orphan Asylum*
Fatherless Children (Reedham)	*(Wanstead)*

The Idiot Asylum (Earlswood)

The London Orphan	*Royal Hospital for*
Asylum (Clapton)	*Incurables (Putney)*

Table 2.1: The five Charities founded by the Revd. Andrew Reed D.D.

	Date of foundation
1. The (East) London Orphan Asylum, Clapton, (later, The Watford and Royal British Orphan School)	1813
2. The Infant Orphan Asylum, Wanstead (later The [Royal] Infant Orphanage)	1827
3. The Asylum for Fatherless Children, Reedham (The Reedham Orphanage) at Coulsdon, near Croydon	1843
4. The Idiot Asylum, Earlswood (The Royal Earlswood Institution for Mental Defectives)	1847
5. The Royal Hospital for Incurables, Putney (RHI) (now the Royal Hospital for Neuro-disability)	1854

Watford, and in 1936, it housed 470 children and had an annual income of £24,000.

In July 1827, Reed founded the second of his great charities – the *Infant Orphan Asylum* for fatherless children *under seven years of age.* The original (temporary) premises were situated in Hackney Road, the second in Dalston, and the definitive one, to meet increasing demands, at Wanstead; the first stone of this new asylum was laid by Prince Albert (1819-61), the Prince Consort, in June 1841. When the governors decided that the Church of England's catechism be made compulsory there, Reed resigned from the Board, but nevertheless continued to support the Charity. In 1936, it was known as the Royal Infant Orphanage with an occupation of 340 children, and an annual income of £20,000.

In 1843, he founded his third public charity – an *infant orphan asylum;* 1200*l* (£) was rapidly raised, and houses at Richmond, Hackney Road, and Stamford Hill (in North London) were successfully used before a definitive estate (on which an orphanage [Reedham] was built) was bought at Coulsdon, near Croydon. This position is important, because Reed had visions of establishing the *permanent* home of RHI on, or near, this site (Chapter 7). In 1936, the number of 'inmates' was 300 and the annual income £19,000.

Reed's fourth charity was an *Asylum for Idiots*, housed initially at Highgate Hill, and subsequently at Earlswood, Surrey. It was opened in October 1847, and a branch for the eastern counties was later established at Essex Hall, Colchester. In 1859, this became the Eastern Counties Idiot Asylum (later the Royal Eastern Counties Ltd for the 'Mental Defective'). In 1852, the Earlswood estate (near Redhill) was purchased and the new asylum with accommodation for 400 inmates was also opened by the Prince Consort in 1855. In 1936 its turnover was £45,000 and that of its subsidiary (with accommodation for 1,500 inmates) £70,000.

Reed's fifth (and last) great philanthropic venture was begun in July 1854 (Chapter 1) – the *Royal Hospital for Incurables,* which forms the *raison d'être* of this book. The prime object of this project was to care for 'inmates' of metropolitan hospitals who were discharged as 'hopelessly incurable', with no shelter in view but the workhouse.

Apart from these five charities, Reed was largely responsible for two other public institutions. One was Hackney Grammar School (1829); the other, the East London Savings Bank (1837) which he founded to assist in counteracting *improvidence* which he believed to be an important underlying factor behind the vices of the poor. It has been estimated that the overall cost of the asylums which Reed founded amounted to some 129,320*l* (£).[4] It is of interest that four of these Charities (all except the Asylum for Idiots at Earlswood) remain extant to this day – 150 years later!

Reed – the man

Reed was described by one obituarist as a 'staunch Voluntary and an almost rigid Independent, though not what is called a "political Dissenter",' and perhaps not since the days of John Howard (1726?-90) had an individual been associated with so many 'works of universal philanthropy'. He was always aware of the importance of toleration, with the Dissenter, Roman Catholic, or Jew. In questions such as Public Education, Slavery, Church Rates and Free Trade, he was a strong partisan from the standpoint of religion. Reed was wholeheartedly opposed to the monopoly in bread which the Corn Laws, which were in force in 1840, maintained. In addition to the eminent men already mentioned, the Dukes of York (1763-1827) and Wellington (1769-1852) were apparently to be numbered among his 'most earnest advisors and supporters'.[5]

Although described as highly intelligent, Reed was, apparently, 'cold to strangers' and sometimes 'insensitive to others' views' but overall he must have possessed a powerful presence as the Duke of Wellington recalled at an anniversary dinner of the *London Orphan Asylum*:

> I have not been to a public dinner for some years, and I had resolved that, as age and infirmities are creeping upon me, I would go no more; but I am here tonight at the request of *that great man* [my italics] whose wishes are to me law and whose entreaties I felt as a command it was impossible to resist.[6]

In addition to their portrait, the RHN possesses a splendidly sculptured bust of Reed (fig 2.3). There is mention of several other portraits in the RHI Board minutes. In 1892, one was presented to the hospital by one of his sons, Dr Martin Reed; this, however, required a good deal of attention, and was offered to 'some other of the Institutions founded by the late Dr Andrew Reed'. Later, a portrait was sent to the RHI by the Reverend Martin Reed, but this was apparently offered to, and accepted by, the *Infant Orphan Asylum*.[7]

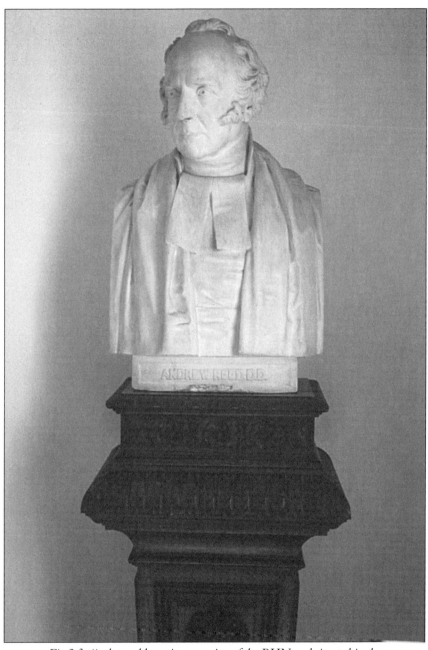

*Fig 2.3: Sculptured bust, in possession of the RHN and situated in the
main entrance hall.*

References and Notes

1. Anonymous, 'Revd. Dr Andrew Reed', *Gentleman's Magazine* 1862 (April): 510-12; A. Reed, C. Reed (eds), *Memoirs of the Life and Philanthropic Labours of Andrew Reed, D.D., with Selections from his Journals* (2nd Edn. London 1863); W.B. Lowther, 'Reed, Andrew (1787-1862)', in S. Lee (ed)., *Dictionary of National Biography* (London: Smith, Elder & Co. 1909): 16: 831-2; L. French, *The Royal Hospital & Home for Incurables, Putney, & its founder* (London: the Royal Hospital 1936): 40; C.H. Irwin, *Andrew Reed: philanthropist* (London: The Religious Tract Society, undated): 32.

2. G.C. Boase, 'Reed, Sir Charles (1819-81)', in: S. Lee (ed), *Dictionary of National Biography* (London: Smith, Elder & Co. 1909); 16: 832-4.

3. Board minutes. Book 4: 138-41, 157; Book 7: 166; Book 10: 400.

4. Op.cit. See note 1 above: Reed & Reed, 13-28, Irwin; Anonymous, 'The life-work of a modern philanthropist', *Ill. London News* 1862; 264-70.

5. Op.cit. See note 1 above, Anonymous.

6. Op.cit. See note 1 above, French 16-18.

7. Op.cit. See note 3 above. Book 18: 109; Book 20: 517-7; Book 21: 203.

CHAPTER 3

The original rules and constitution (1854), and the rôle of women in the Charity

THE **CONSTITUTION** of the Charity (incorporating the Rules) seems to have been drafted by Reed himself in 1854. These drafts had been submitted to the third of the provisional meetings (Chapter 1), and after discussion were 'adopted' for submission to the General Meeting (held on 31 July). These rules (which were amended at the fifth Annual Meeting, also held at the London Tavern, on 30 November 1859), were duly read by Reed himself at the 1854 General Meeting, when they were formally adopted:

1. That the name of the Charity be *The Royal Hospital.*
2. That the *Object* be to give permanent relief to such persons as are hopelessly disqualified for the duties of life, by *Disease, Accident,* or *Deformity.*
3. That the *Design,* therefore, is, not to interfere with the action of existing charities, but to take action precisely when *their action ceases.*

   It will not provide for temporary affliction which is excellently supplied by our great hospitals, but for that which is *permanent* and *continuous,* for which there is now *no provision.* It will not deal with the hopeful case, but with the *hopeless,* and provide, in a hospital, a final home for such as would otherwise be the *rejected* and *outcast of mankind.*
4. That the *Design* shall be carried out on the broad principle of Christian kindness and liberality, in the hope of uniting all the good for the good of all who really need help, in the spirit of that wisdom and love, which 'cometh down from above', and which is 'the bond of perfectness', to the exclusion of all party and sectarian influences whatever.
5. That the charity does not exist to relieve any case for which provision is found elsewhere. *That, therefore, it does not formally receive the lunatic, the blind, the deaf and dumb, the idiot, the consumptive, the victim of fever or smallpox, &c* [my italics], but not withstanding this declaration, they will not endure that any case of hopeless *affliction* shall remain without protection, or without a home.
6. The *Methods* of relief will be various, and somewhat discretional. *The mere pauper case will not be eligible, as the law of the land sufficiently provides for the wants of that class* [my italics].

   Those who need only *partial relief,* and first aid and comfort in the bosom of their families, will be treated as *extra-patients* [see below], without breaking up the endearments of private life. They will enjoy a monthly allowance, and the benefit of medical visitation and attendance.

Such as have survived their friends, and need *total relief,* and have exhausted their own means under their affliction, will be received to the full benefits of *A Home.*

Every case will be accepted as incurable, but will be treated by the best medical science *hopefully,* and should the means be happily successful, the benefited party will be required to leave the foundation.

Cases that can offer *Payment,* either for themselves, or by their immediate relatives, will be received on *No Other Terms,* and the rate of payment will be determined by the ability of the party, and the accommodation actually required.

7. The *Elections* [which obviously took up a great deal of time at subsequent Board meetings] are to occur annually, or oftener, to be regulated by the Board in respect to the *number* of applicants, and the means placed at their disposal.

No case shall be eligible for the election list during its *minority,* except it shall be in a state of orphanhood, and without means of support.

In *special instances* of urgency and destitution, a case may have prompt admission or relief, subject to the ensuing election.

In *very special cases* in which *three-fourths* of the Board shall agree, there shall be power to act absolutely and to place an applicant on the foundation, without the intervention of an election, such case or cases from time to time to be reported to the Annual Meeting.

The *two preceding* provisions are meant chiefly to apply to such cases as have had the temporary benefit of the general hospitals, and are commended for more permanent care to this hospital by the Medical Officers as likely to find a *partial* or *complete* cure.

Provision shall be made to accommodate cases of hopeless affliction *for Life,* where the parties insisted in their welfare may secure comfort and protection for them, to the latest day of their suffering.

The *Extra-patients* are to be received by election, and can only have relief *subject* to the ensuing election, and on the evident urgency of the case.

That the election cases are taken for life, but should any cases, by the combined influence of medical skill and of domestic comfort, be happily restored to the enjoyment of useful health, it shall be competent to the Board, under recorded medical testimony, to dismiss such patients.

8. That before any case, whether Election or Payment, is deemed eligible, it shall be subject to careful inquiry, and professional examination, the

result of which inquiry must be, that the case is judged to be beyond the *likelihood of cure.*

9. That although the *incurable* and *hopeless* case alone is eligible for the benefits of this Charity, the Board are to regard it as their most sacred duty, to use all likely means, professional and otherwise, to restore it to health and the duties of life.

10. That if it shall appear that the election of any case has been affected by false representations, such election shall be declared void.

11. That each case may enjoy *six* elections and no more, and over that time it may accumulate the votes to its own advantage.

12. That all persons subscribing five guineas at one time, or half-a-guinea annually, shall be governors of the institution.

13. That the right of voting at elections shall increase in the same proportion as the subscriptions, and that all persons subscribing thirty guineas at one time, or three guineas annually, shall have a right to attend the sittings of the Board, and shall receive the regular notices, on an intimation being made to the Board to that effect.

14. That all ministers preaching on behalf of this Charity, shall be constituted life governors.

15. That an executor paying a legacy of £100 shall be a governor for life, and that, if it exceeds that sum, all the executors shall have the same privilege.

16. That there be a general annual meeting of the Society, when a report, domestic and financial, on the state of the Charity, shall be made, and the officers chosen.

17. That no such meeting shall be an authorized one, unless publicly advertised, and notice given to the members, and that no rule affecting the *constitution* can be allowed or withdrawn without *special notice.*

18. That the appointment of the Board of Directors, the Treasurer, and the Secretary, rest with the meeting, and that they be chosen annually and act gratuitously.

19. That the Board shall consist of not less than twenty-four persons, and that three of them in rotation, be ineligible for re-election for one year.

20. That the Treasurer and Secretary are ex officio, members of the Board.

21. That the appointment and dismissal of all servants and officers, not declared to be in the nomination of the general meeting, rest with the Board of Directors.

(The *amended* rules ran to 22 (I-XXII) but the direction of the Charity was not significantly altered.) Subsequent Annual Meetings approved a number of minor changes to the rules.[1]

Following a subsequent Board Meeting held on 31 October 1854, the first minute book contains several *Bye-laws* of the new institution.

1. That the Cases be classed in the election List as Extra-patients, and Home patients, and that the arrangement rest with discretion of the Board.
2. That the Elections do occur half-yearly, in the months of November and June.
3. That the First Election occur on Monday, 27th November, and that six patients be chosen.
4. That the Payment cases [also minuted on 11th January 1855] range as follows:-

   The *reduced* payment shall be £25 per annum, and shall apply to those who cannot pay a larger sum. Such cases as are thus benefited must therefore reveal their circumstances to the judgement of the Board.

   The full and proper payment shall be £50 per annum; circumstances then would not come into consideration, unless it should appear that they were really affluent.

   Such cases as may require separate attendance, and superior and private accommodation will be expected to pay a higher sum at the discretion of the Board.

   Cases taken for life to be open to the discretion of the Board; £500 being taken as an average; the payment may vary above and below that sum, according to circumstances.
5. All the payments are to be made in advance.
6. No case can be accepted, which by noise or violence would disturb the peace of the family.
7. That the maximum allowance of the Extra cases be one guinea per month with the requisite medical attendance.[2]

It should be noted therefore that the original constitution of the institution excluded all 'paupers' (who, it was assumed – rightly or wrongly – were cared for by the state or the local municipality), as well as those with one of several *specific* diagnoses, e.g. tuberculosis, 'fever', smallpox and a wide range of psychiatric disorders. As Alvey has concluded, Reed had clearly formed concrete ideas about what sort of hospital he wanted. There were essentially three categories of patient: (i) those who were chronically bed-ridden, (ii) those who to some extent could help themselves, and (iii) those active enough for 'almshouse' accommodation (with some privacy) – but excluding all those mentioned in clauses 5 and 6 of the Constitution.[3] Admission was largely dependent therefore on the influence/wealth of the members of the Board of Directors; in fact, 'influence' from a member of the Board carried a great deal of weight, and was of paramount importance in gaining acceptance, either as a 'Home' or an 'Extra' patient.

What sort of person, therefore, was deemed suitable to become an inmate?

A later minute states: '… as a rule, the older persons, and such as have enjoyed a condition of health and have led an active and useful life, are preferred.' The question as to whether blindness alone was sufficient grounds for election to the RHI was debated as early as 1863; it was resolved 'That while blindness alone is not, as a rule, to be regarded as a qualification for the benefits of this Charity, this Board considers itself at liberty, upon a case.' In 1877 the ambiguity of the term 'mere pauper' in Rule III of the amended version was emphasised, and a motion that the rule be amended to indicate that 'any person having received parochial relief shall be ineligible' was carried. In 1913, the Board ruled that '"Poorer" should be deleted from "Poorer middle classes" when referring to the class for which the benefits of this Hospital are intended.'[4]

Later Changes to the Rules
In early 1859, a sub-committee under the chairmanship of Viscount Raynham was set up, 'to examine and revise the constitution of the Charity and amend the rules as at present existing'. In June of that year, a number of alterations were made to the rules, the most significant being 'That the Board consider the question of the disposal of the [Coulsdon] estate, and whether it will be desirable to build upon it.'[5]

Later, Rule III was again changed, so that only: … 'idiots, persons of unsound mind, and those who have been afflicted from birth, or who have received parochial relief' were excluded. Under Rule XVI of the amended version 'under 30 years of age' was substituted. Rule XXXII (sic), which related to the acceptance (or otherwise) of donations and investments was also modified.[6]

Fig 3.1 gives an example of a much later change (in 1936) to two by-laws – nos. 40 and 42.

Medical Testimonial
In October 1854, many of the most eminent physicians and surgeons in London (many of them 'household names') signed a 'Medical Testimonial'; they strongly supported the foundation of this Charity which they believed to be an essential addition to the *General* Hospitals of London. Furthermore, it would not interfere in any way with the existing hospitals, and would provide 'a Refuge for Incurable Persons whose Former Station in Life unfits them for the Workhouse'. The 39 signatories were:

SIR JAMES CLARK, BART., MD, FRS, Physician in Ordinary to HER MAJESTY.

A. WHYTE BARCLAY, MD, Physician to the Chelsea, Belgrave, and Brompton Dispensary.

Royal Hospital and Home for Incurables, Putney.

(Incorporated by Royal Charter.)

A SPECIAL GENERAL MEETING

WILL BE HELD AT 11.30 A.M.,

AT THE

SOUTHERN HOUSE, CANNON STREET STATION, E.C.4,

On Friday, 29th May, 1936.

Sir EDWARD MACLAGAN, K.C.S.I., K.C.I.E.,

in the Chair.

The following alterations in the Bye-laws, having been made by the Board of Management, are placed before the Meeting for adoption, namely :—

Present Bye-Law.	New Bye-Law.
40. The Board may nominate for election to a pension or admission to the Hospital and Home duly qualified applicants for relief. The amount of any pensions shall not exceed £25 per annum.	40. The Board may nominate for election to a pension or admission to the Hospital and Home duly qualified applicants for relief.
42. Candidates may remain on the list until elected and during that time may accumulate their votes, subject to the following provision, that is to say, if after ten consecutive elections a candidate shall not have registered 400 votes, the name of such candidate shall be removed from the list. Subject and without prejudice to the discretion hereinbefore given to the Board as to the admission of candidates the name of any candidate who shall have become of unsound mind or an inmate of a lunatic asylum or parish infirmary shall forthwith be removed from the list of candidates.	42. Candidates may remain on the list until elected, and during that time may accumulate their votes, but no candidate may be elected for admission or pension until he or she shall have polled a minimum number of votes to be prescribed by the Board from time to time. If a candidate, after a number of Elections to be prescribed by the Board from time to time shall not have registered the prescribed number of votes, his or her name shall be removed from the list. Subject and without prejudice to the discretion hereinbefore given to the Board as to the admission of candidates the name of any candidate who shall have become of unsound mind or an inmate of a lunatic asylum or parish infirmary shall forthwith be removed from the list of candidates.

City Offices : Bond Court House, Walbrook, E.C.4.

CHARLES CUTTING,
Secretary.

Fig. 3.1: Notice of a Special General Meeting (in 1936) to change Bye-laws 40 and 42.

THOMAS A. BARKER, MD, Physician to St Thomas's Hospital.

GEORGE H. BARLOW, MD, Physician to Guy's Hospital.

JAMES R. BENNETT, MD, Physician to St Thomas's Hospital.

ARCHIBALD BILLING, MD, Late Senior Physician to the London Hospital.

JOHN BIRKETT, FRCS, Surgeon to Guy's Hospital.

JOHN CONOLLY, MD, DCL, Consulting Physician to the Middlesex Lunatic Asylum.

JOHN T. CONQUEST, MD, Physician to the City of London Lying-in Hospital.

MERVYN A.M. CRAWFORD, MD, Physician to the Middlesex Hospital.

CAMPBELL DE MORGAN, FRCS, Surgeon to the Middlesex Hospital.

FREDERICK J. FARRE, MD, Assistant Physician to St Bartholomew's Hospital.

WILLIAM FERGUSSON, FRCS, Surgeon to King's College Hospital.

SAMUEL O. HABERSHON, MD, Assistant Physician to Guy's Hospital.

F. SEYMOUR HADEN, FRCS, Consulting Surgeon to the Chapel Royal Fund.

CHARLES HAWKINS, FRCS, Consulting Surgeon to Queen Charlotte's Hospital.

MITCHELL HENRY, FRCS, Surgeon to the Middlesex hospital.

PRESCOTT HEWETT, FRCS, Assistant Surgeon to St George's Hospital, and Professor of Anatomy and Surgery to the Royal College of Surgeons of England.

WILLIAM J. LITTLE, MD, Senior Physician to the London Hospital.

JAMES LUKE, FRCS, FRS, Senior Surgeon to the London Hospital, and President of the Royal College of Surgeons.

GILBERT MACKMURDO, FRCS, Surgeon to St Thomas's Hospital.

EDMUND A. PARKES, MD, Physician to University College Hospital.

RICHARD PARTRIDGE, FRCS, Surgeon to King's College Hospital.

THOMAS B. PEACOCK, MD, Assistant Physician to St Thomas's Hospital.

RICHARD QUAIN, FRCS, Surgeon to University College Hospital.

CHARLES B. RADCLIFFE, MD, Physician to the Westminster Hospital.

FRANCIS H. RAMSBOTHAM, MD, Obstetric Physician to the London Hospital.

WILLIAM SHARPEY, MD, FRS, Professor of Anatomy and Physician to University College.

ALEXANDER SHAW, FRCS, Surgeon to the Middlesex Hospital.

FRANCIS SIBSON, MD, FRS, Physician to St Mary's Hospital.

EDWARD H. SIEVEKING, MD, Physician to St Mary's Hospital.

THOMAS H. SILVESTER, MD, Physician to the Clapham General Dispensary.

SAMUEL SOLLY, FRCS, FRS, Surgeon to St Thomas's Hospital.

ALEXANDER P. STEWART, MD, Assistant Physician to the Middlesex Hospital.

ROBERT B. TODD, MD, Physician to King's College Hospital.

ALEXANDER TWEEDIE, MD, FRS, Physician to the London Fever Hospital.

WALTER H. WALSHE, MD, Physician to University College Hospital.

THOMAS WATSON, MD, Consulting Physician to King's College Hospital.

T. SPENCER WELLS, FRCS, Surgeon to the Samaritan Hospital.[7]

A Managerial rôle for women?

In the early days of the Charity, women were not allowed as in most other institutions, to do anything in a managerial capacity. Today, almost half of the Board of Management are women. Indeed, until widespread criticism of the management of the RHI (Chapter 14) there were not even Lady Visitors!

Lady Visitors

It was probably a scathing report from the House of Lords Select Committee that influenced the Board to give way on the matter of Lady Visitors (whose rôle was to 'visit the Hospital at any time') [Chapter 14]. The 1897-8 *Annual Report* stated:

> The Board have for some time been impressed with the desirability of securing the aid of ladies in the internal management of the Hospital.

They were to be seven in number, subscribers, *not* connected with the members of the Board, and answerable to the House-Committee.[8]

Women on the Board of Management?

The Board of Management was however, a very different matter. In 1893, the eligibility (or otherwise) of Lady Board members was apparently raised in a conversation between Rücker (the Chairman) and Freshfield (the RHI legal adviser); the ultimate decision, then, was that the 'point was [not] one that pressed for a decision'![9] The initial 'rocking of the boat' of the all-male hierarchy came about in 1898, i.e. nearly half a century after foundation of the RHI. Miss Georgiana Hill gave notice (in May 1898) that she intended recommending 'the addition of ladies to the Board of Management' at the 1898 AGM. Later that month, the Secretary (Andrew) received a letter from Freshfield concerning this matter:

31 Old Jewry, E.C.
24th May 1898

My dear Sir,

I have considered the question arising on the proposed admission of ladies on the Board of the [RHI] and of the Ladies Committee which has been formed. I will give you now my opinion on the matter as it stands as regards the admission of women on the Board.

If a woman, a Governor, is elected at a General Meeting of the Governors to serve on the Board she is properly elected and the Governors cannot exclude her. If they do, the remedy is probably in the hands of the subscribers at the next General Meeting, namely, that they will elect an entirely new Board of Management and a Board pledged to the admission of ladies. No notice need be given of this other than the ordinary notice if in fact a notice is required when a person not on the Board of Managers is to be put forward.

On the other point it occurs to me that the better course will be to inform Miss Hill of what has been done in the appointment of Lady Visitors to the Hospital and she should be asked whether in the face of what has happened she is now prepared to withdraw the motion, notice of which she has given. If she does withdraw it the question drops. If she refuses to withdraw it the following considerations arise. The notice which Miss Hill has at present given is this, that it is desirable that ladies should be admitted to the Board. This is merely courting an expression of opinion by the general body of Subscribers at a General Meeting. It does not of itself put ladies on the Board, nor does it authorise the Board to place any particular number of women there. The women if they are to be elected must be elected by the subscribers in the ordinary way. If this were done I assume that Miss Hill would thereupon bring forward the name of some Governor to be elected on the Board. If she were elected the Board would be called upon under Rule II to increase the number of the Board so as to admit the ladies elected. If they don't do so I presume that a Special General Meeting would be called to consider the conduct of the Board and at the next General Meeting the whole of the existing Board might or might not fail to secure re-election. The other alternative of course is that the Subscribers would consider themselves injured and might discontinue their subscriptions.

This is how the matter stands. It sounds a little complicated, but it is really quite simple.

Yours faithfully
William Freshfield

F. Andrew Esq.

It seems clear, therefore, that the 'establishment' was at that time fundamentally hostile to the idea of women on the Board. As a result of this letter from Freshfield, the Board were in agreement that the Secretary 'be instructed to write to Miss Hill informing her of the appointment of Lady Visitors to the Hospital'.[10]

But it is clear that Miss Hill was not to be put off by this ploy, and her proposed motion was:

> That in view of the fact that by far the larger proportion of the Inmates of the [RHI] are women [Chapter 13], it is desirable that women should be added to the Board of Management.

The draft 1897-8 Annual Report stated:

> The Board cannot commend such a resolution to the Meeting, and they hope Miss Hill will withdraw it ...
>
> ... For, whatever may be said for such a motion in theory, the lady herself would possibly be unprepared to meet the responsibilities, some of them of a legal character, and others requiring delicacy of treatment that arise in the multitudinous matters coming under the notice of the Board.[11]

But the President (of the RHI), Lord Northampton,[12] refused to add his signature to the report:

> 51 Lennox Gardens, S.W.
> 14th Nov: 1898.
>
> Dear Mr Andrew,
>
> I start tomorrow (Tuesday) for my winter abroad, and, therefore, have no time to really go into the matter about which you write.
>
> I am bound, however, to state that, as a general principle, I think it best there should be one or two ladies on the Board of Management of such an Institution as the [RHI].
>
> The fact that there are Lady Visitors seems to me to have no bearing on the case. I should be sorry therefore to sign the circular which the Board of Management proposed to issue, although I am ready to confess that they probably know more on the subject than I do myself.
>
> Yours very truly
>
> Northampton

'The Secretary [told the Board] that he had informed the Treasurer of Northampton's refusal to sign the circular, and asked him if he [the Treasurer] were willing to sign it with only the countersignature of the Secretary.' Allcroft had replied by telegram in the affirmative. The Secretary was therefore 'instructed to commence the issue of the circulars at once'. They were sent to the subscribers and a number of replies were soon received: in favour of Miss Hill's resolution [were] 15; against it 186. Miss Hill evidently went ahead and moved her resolution at the AGM, but it was 'negatived by a large majority'.[13]

In April 1899, a letter from Mrs Bernard Shaw was read to the Board, in which she withdrew her annual subscription of 10 guineas 'unless, as proposed at the last Annual Meeting ... women were added to the Board'.[14]

In July 1899 a letter was tabled at a Special Board Meeting:

14th July 1899.

Dear Sir,

... It is hoped that every Member of the Board will make a point of attending this Meeting, as the issue involved in the consideration of Miss Hill's Motion is a very important one.

Yours very truly

F. Andrew

Secy.

The Chairman (Allcroft) told the meeting that he had specially invited the Marquess of Northampton, President of the Hospital, to attend the Meeting but he read a reply from the Marquess expressing his regret at not being able to do so.

The Secretary (Andrew) then read a copy of his letter to Messrs Freshfields & Williams asking for their further opinion and advice, 'as desired at the Meeting on the 13th inst'. Their reply was as follows:

31 Old Jewry E.C.
19th July 1899.

Dear Sir,

We are of opinion that Subscribers cannot vote by proxy under the Regulations as they stand. 'The two well known methods of voting in this country are by a show of hands and a poll'. There is a Common Law right to a poll in the absence of any regulation to the contrary but no Common Law right to vote by proxy. At Meetings where proxies are available it must be so by virtue of special provision in the Constitution.

We are further of opinion that the question of the admission of women to the Board is a question of management, and management is by the regulations committed to the Board. The Board have been advised that women are eligible but the expediency of electing them is a matter on which the Board are entitled to have an opinion of their own in the interest of the Charity and on which in our opinion they are entitled to ascertain the wishes of the Subscribers in any manner at a reasonable cost to the Charity, and at the same time if they think fit to express their own view as a guide to the subscribers. We think a circular may properly in the discretion of the Board be sent out and at the cost of the Charity.

We are, &c.

Freshfields & Williams

The minute continued: 'It was Moved by the Capt Webbe, seconded by Mr Ellis and carried unanimously "That a circular be prepared, to be issued with the next Voting paper, informing the Subscribers of Miss Hill's intention and inviting them to attend the Meeting and give their support to the Board, such circular to be signed by the Treasurer and Secretary. Should Miss Hill again renew her Motion for the Annual General Meeting in November 1900 it was resolved that it be met by a resolution, that Miss Hill be not heard.' A draft of the suggested circular was read and approved; it was as follows:

The Royal Hospital for Incurables
106 Queen Victoria Street E.C.
November 1899.

Annual General Meeting
Cannon Street Hotel
Friday 24th November 1899
At eleven o'clock

Important Notice

The Board beg to inform the Governors that Miss Georgiana Hill has given notice that she will on this occasion renew the Motion which was negatived by a considerable majority at the last Annual General Meeting (25 November 1898) ... The Board then remarked that such a step [i.e. ladies on the Committee of Management] was unnecessary and undesirable seeing that a Committee of Ladies appointed by the Board already existed. This view was shared by the Lady Visitors themselves, who know well the Inmates and their needs.

The Board are still of the same opinion, nor do they see what good can possibly come of an annual discussion upon a subject on which the Governors have already expressed an opinion.

The Board gratefully acknowledge the assistance given from the first by Ladies in protecting the interests of the Institution and the well being of its Inmates and Pensioners; but it does not appear that the need has yet arisen for placing the burden of Management in their hands.

The Board have had many proofs of the confidence of the Subscribers; and they trust their friends will again attend the Meeting and support them, so as to stop an uncalled for and expensive agitation.[15]

Georgiana Hill again wrote to the Board about this matter on 21 January 1901, and a letter of acknowledgement was duly sent.[16] But at a Board meeting on 26 September of that year, a letter from the President (still the Marquess of Northampton) was read: he 'had been asked [he wrote] to take such steps as were considered necessary to have placed on the list for election as members of the Board at the annual meeting the name of a lady.' 'It was resolved [by the Board] to reply that the suggestion had already been defeated by overwhelming majorities at two annual meetings, and that the Board were unanimously against the proposal and that the present Ladies' Visiting Committee was considered sufficient.'[17]

At a subsequent meeting a further letter from Northampton was read, asking 'what notice was necessary to give in proposing a member of the Board and as to the mode of election'. It was resolved in reply 'that the Board nominated & elected. The same being confirmed at the [AGM]. Further that hitherto it had been the rule to give a years notice of any motion – affecting the constitution &c.' Later (at the same meeting) it was pointed out that the President himself was *not* a member of the Board – either by election or in an ex-officio capacity! It was therefore resolved (by the Board) that 'all presidents be members of the Board ex officio'. On 30 October, 'It was resolved to reply [to the President] that the Board did not propose to place any hindrance in the way of the lady being proposed – neither would they insist upon a year's notice of motion being given.'[18]

On 20 November: 'The Board had received a letter from Mrs Casher [which was duly read] suggesting advertising the fact that there was a movement to place a lady on the Board against the wishes of the Board.' Mrs Casher was the wife of a Brixton clergyman who had served on the Board between 1874 and 1892. The Board 'resolved to take no such steps'. A letter from the President was also read 'stating that he did not propose to take any personal action in reference to the suggestion of Ladies on the Board.' However, there was a great deal going on 'behind the scenes', and prior to the AGM of 1901, a circular (fig 3.2) was distributed to *all* subscribers, requesting that they attend, and furthermore support the Board of Management. Miss Hill's proposition was therefore once again overwhelmingly defeated.[19]

The matter seems to have ended amicably, for in October of that year:

> The Ladies Visiting Committee [perhaps surprisingly] offered to assist the Board in any way in their power in placing the subject of Miss Georgiana Hill's motion before the [AGM].

In February 1904, it was resolved that 'the Secretary be permitted to organize a Ladies' Association for the financial benefit of the Institution.[20] The far more serious matter was, of course, that involving ladies *on the Board*. A further letter was read (to the Board) from Georgiana Hill – on 26 March 1914; she stated that 'she must withdraw her subscription … until ladies are permitted to serve on the Board of Management.' A similar letter of withdrawal of her contribution had been received from Mrs Theodora Williams 'unless at the next Annual Meeting women are given places on the Board.' The Secretary was directed to reply to both letters indicating that the Board had no intention of altering 'the decision already arrived at …'[21]

In December 1919, the Chairman (T.W. Wickham) told the Board that he had received a letter, with reference to a resolution from the Ladies' Visiting Committee, that that committee ought to be 'phased out'. The letter continued, 'The members of the Ladies' Visiting Committee are, with one exception, sure that the co-operation of women on the Board would not only be in accordance with public opinion, but also an advantage to the Hospital.' In

The Royal Hospital for Incurables,

PUTNEY HEATH.

IMPORTANT NOTICE *re* ANNUAL GENERAL MEETING,

November 29th, 1901, at Cannon Street Hotel, at 11 a.m.

TO THE SUBSCRIBERS . . .

THE BOARD OF MANAGEMENT beg to call attention to the following reply to the circular issued by a self-constituted "Reform Committee," of which Miss E. W. FYFE is Chairwoman *pro tem.*, and Miss GEORGIANA HILL is Hon. Secretary.

That LORD TWEEDMOUTH, at the last Annual Dinner, in replying to the letters his lordship had received—presumably from members of the above Reform Committee—expressed himself in favour of ladies being added to the Board. This opinion was endorsed by the President, and so far as can be ascertained, was shared by one other person out of over one hundred guests. The Board—apart from the President—are unanimously opposed to the proposal.

The Select Committee of the House of Lords issued their report without either visiting the Hospital or interviewing any inmate or member of the Staff there. **They did not recommend that ladies should be added to the Board, but that a Ladies' Committee should be appointed**—a suggestion which the Board have since carried out. The Board note that no mention is made of the existence of this Committee of Lady Visitors in the circular referred to, the members of which enjoy the same privileges as the Board of Management in visiting the Institution. They make a regular report to, and when necessary, confer with the latter body. One member of this Committee is also a duly appointed Visitor under the poor law of a large workhouse in London.

The fourth paragraph is certainly misleading. It speaks of "a very pronounced feeling among the subscribers that it is desirable to add women to the Board of Management." The Board can only point out that at two Annual General Meetings held during the past three years the proposal has been fully discussed and rejected by overwhelming majorities— so much so that Miss HILL, when asked by the Chairman if it was necessary to make a count, replied in the negative.

The Board therefore urge the presence of Subscribers on November 29th next, and in doing so they desire to thank all who in the past have so heartily supported them in resisting an unnecessary innovation into what has proved hitherto to be a successful management.

Issued by Order of the Board,

W. DAVID NEWTON, *Secretary.*

October 30th, 1901.

Offices : 106, QUEEN VICTORIA STREET, E.C.

Fig 3.2: Circular letter sent (in 1901) to all subscribers in a successful attempt to prevent women being elected to the Board of Management of the RHI.

a reply, the Chairman indicated that the Board regretted their decision, but was glad 'the ladies are willing to continue as Visitors to the Hospital'. He also extended to the Members of the Ladies' Visiting Committee an invitation to attend a House Committee meeting to 'talk things over'. Wickham followed this by writing a letter thanking the members of the Ladies' Visiting Committee for all of their work for the RHHI over the years. Instead there were to be: 'Authorised Visitors'.[22]

In July 1920, the Board approved, in a letter written by Miss Thorne, of the names of three ladies willing to act as Authorised Visitors – Mrs Hitch, Miss Robinson and Miss Archdale. The Chairman wrote that it was highly desirable that they should be Annual Subscribers, because if they were not, they were *not* Governors of the Institution. In addition, Mrs Browning was also apparently acceptable to the Board.[23]

A solution at last

It was not therefore until 1928 that this matter was resolved. After a prolonged discussion, Sir Edward Maclagan (a future Chairman of the Board) proposed, and Newton seconded, 'That the Board of Management should arrange for the submission at the next [AGM] of the names of two ladies for election to the Board'. The motion was carried, although Major Goff dissented! It was further agreed to inform a deputation from the 'Authorised Lady Visitors' (who were expected to attend the AGM), of this resolution. At the next meeting, the Chairman (W.F. Clerke) began by clarifying the existing position with regard to ladies on the Board. It was then moved by the chairman, seconded by Mr Potter, and carried 'that Miss Thorne (or Miss Ellis) be invited to join the Board'. Another proposal was that Miss Denny (or Mrs Arnold) be asked to join the Board. Mrs Arnold was the daughter of Mr & Mrs Lesslie who had presented a new organ for the Assembly Room in 1911. It was agreed 'to authorise the House Committee to approach other suitable ladies if the four mentioned decline to accept office'. The Chairman then signed a letter to Miss Thorne (and the secretary was 'instructed to frame a similar letter to the other ladies if it is necessary'). The letter ran:

Dear Miss Thorne,

At today's meeting of the Board it was proposed, seconded and carried that you be invited to join the Governing Body of this Institution. If you consent to this, as we all hope will be the case, you would be elected a member of the Board and of the House Committee. The latter body, as you know, meet every Wednesday down at the Hospital and transact the bulk of the work, and it is at the House Committees that your colleagues on the Board would be especially glad to see you. You would be quite welcome at the monthly meetings of the Board in the City, though there is no real need for your attendance at such meetings unless perfectly convenient to you.

The Board are very anxious that you should allow yourself to be elected. Beginnings are always difficult and we realise that, with your long and practical knowledge of the working of our Institution, you would be a great help in establishing, as it were, the influence of Ladies on our Board and House Committee.

Kindest regards,

Yours sincerely,
W.F. Clerke

Chairman.

P.S.: If quite convenient to you, Mr Newton and I would call at your house on Monday and discuss the subject of this letter with you, rather than that you should send a negative reply without waiting to hear our personal views.'[24]

Miss Thorne and Mrs Arnold were duly elected to the Board at the AGM of 1928. A third – Mrs Hitch – was elected in 1932. There had therefore been a complete change of heart, and from thenceforth, women have been welcomed to the Board and especially the House Committee.[25]

At a Board meeting in February 1935, two ladies – Mrs Pendarves and Miss Thorne – were appointed to the Finance Committee.[26] Thus, the ladies had truly entered the male-dominated citadel!

References and Notes

1. Board minutes. Book 1: 4-5; 19-27; 30; *See also: Constitution [and] Minutes of General Meetings, The Amended Rules:* 38-52; Anonymous, *The Royal Hospital for Incurables, designed for the permanent care and comfort of those who by Disease, Accident, or Deformity, are hopelessly disqualified for the duties of life* (London: Royal Hospital for Incurables, 1868): 229.
2. Op.cit. See note 1 above (Board minutes) Book 1:37-9; Op.cit. See note 1 above: (Anonymous).
3. N. Alvey, 'The Royal Hospital and Home, Putney', *Local historian*, 1994: 15-26.
4. Op.cit. See note 1 above (Board minutes) Book 4: 343, 347-8; Book 11: 309, 316, 338, 432; Book 20: 206; Book 24: 69.
5. Ibid. Book 2: 194-5, 242-3.
6. Ibid. Book 22: 174, 188-9.
7. Op.cit. See note 1 above: Anonymous: 11-14.
8. Annual RHI Report 1897-8: 10.
9. Op.cit. See note 1 above (Board minutes) Book 19: 17.
10. Ibid. Book 21: 51, 64-6, 69-70.
11. Op.cit. See note 8 above: 11.
12. **William George Spencer Scott Compton** KG, the fifth Marquess of

Northampton (1851-1913) was educated at Eton and Trinity College, Cambridge. Following service in the diplomatic corps, he became private secretary to Earl Cowper, and from 1889-97 was MP for the Barnsley Division of Yorkshire. He had acceded to the Marquisate on the death of his father on 11 September 1897. On the resignation of the Earl of Aberdeen from the Presidency – on his appointment as Governor-General of the Dominion of Canada – the Board had agreed (in May 1894) to invite HRH the Duke of York to accept the office, but he was unable 'to accede to the wishes of the Board', and it was then that the Rt. Hon. Earl Compton, MP was invited; his letter of acceptance was read to the Board in June 1894, *See:* Board minutes (Book 19: 134, 138-9, 140, 154-6).

13. Op.cit. See note 1 above (Board minutes), Book 21: 177-8: 181; Annual RHI Report 1898-9: 9.
14. Ibid: 303. **Charlotte Frances Payne-Townshend** (1857-1943), daughter of an Irish barrister, had married George Bernard Shaw (1856-1950), the distinguished playwright, in 1898.
15. Op.cit. See note 1 above (Board minutes), Book 21: 372-6.
16. Ibid. Book 22: 304, 332, 405.
17. Ibid: 418-9.
18. Ibid: 411, 413, 416.
19. Ibid: 426.
20. Ibid. Book 23: 94.
21. Ibid. Book 24: 119-20.
22. Ibid: 405-6, 410-2, 424.
23. Ibid: 459, 487.
24. Ibid: Book 25: 438-9, 444-7; Book 26: 120.
25. Anonymous, 'Women as hospital managers: Safe sphere of activity' *Daily Telegraph* 1 December 1928; Anonymous, '"It's the melancholy face that gets stung by the bee": income down – still optimistic; what the Royal Hospital for Incurables needs', *City Press* 7 December 1928.
26. Op.cit. See note 1 above (Board minutes), Book 25: 274.

CHAPTER 4

The first patients at the RHI

FROM WHAT WERE THE early patients suffering? This chapter summarises the 100 earliest 'applicants' (table 4.1) for admission to this pioneer hospital – nearly half being deemed acceptable for either 'Home' or 'Extra' patient care. Although they were drawn from all parts of the country, the vast majority came from London – especially the East End. There were a number of causes for rejection under the 'election' procedure, although most were excluded by a simple lack of votes; others were 'minors' (i.e. under 21 years old) (nos 11, 36 and 89), and some 'paupers' (nos 5, 38, 61 and 76) – who would not have been acceptable under the terms of the constitution (chapter 3). Others (e.g. no 25) were 'excluded from the benefits of the Charity on the ground of immorality'!

The first of the Royal Hospital's *case books* contains details of the first 500 cases who 'presented' to the Board of Directors of that Institution. Patients were, in the early days, divided into 'home' patients (who thus became 'inmates' at the Charity's house at Carshalton), or 'extra' patients (they lived outside the hospital premises, and were cared for by a friend or relation) (Chapter 3). In the case of the latter category, the RHI paid a 'pension' which contributed to their upkeep. The 'extra' patients were initially granted 12 guineas a year, but in 1860 this was raised to £20=00, but without free medicine.

All patients (or their sponsors) were given the choice as to how they might ideally receive assistance from the RHI. The two options were by 'election' (which depended on gaining a sufficient number of votes from the subscribers, or by 'payment' of £50 in the first few years and £25 thereafter (Chapter 3). The majority (84) of the first 100 applicants applied for admission by *election*, while only a minority (11 males and 5 females) preferred payment – either in full or part. The system of election was a complex one. (For a full list of subscribers together with the voting rights of each one, the reader is referred to: Anonymous. *The Royal Hospital for Incurables designed for the permanent care and comfort of those who by Disease, Accident, or Deformity are hopelessly disqualified for the duties of life* (London: Royal Hospital for Incurables 1868: 55-229).

'Reduced payment' usually involved paying £25 per annum (nos 39, 80, 82, 83, 86 and 96). Other patients who had applied to be admitted 'by payment on [the] lowest scale' (nos 43 and 66) were accepted as *home* patients but all had to contribute £25 per annum. Several others (cases 89, 94 and 98) who applied for admission by payment at the 'lowest scale' were however, rejected. No 66 was compelled to make 'a subscription of £10=10 annually'. Another candidate (no

Table 4.1 – Details of the first 100 patients who applied for admission to the RHI (1854-55)

No.*	Sex	Date of Birth (nineteenth century unless stated)	Diagnosis	Duration of illness (yr)	Date presented (nineteenth century)	Category+
1	M	15 8 35	'Nervous disorder'	From birth	12 10 54	H
2†	F	18 8 05	Chronic bronchitis	2 (?)	"	E
3	F	17 10 25	'Paralysis'	From birth	"	H
4	M	15 4 14	'Affection of the liver and nervous disease'	11	"	H
5	M	25 12 16	'Paralysis'	3	"	H
6	M	14 12 32	'Idiocy'	From infancy	"	H
7	M	?12 **1774**	'Deprived of the use of limbs, thro' accident'	30	"	E
8	F	16 12 19	Epilepsy	18	"	H
9	F	23 6 31	'Nervous debility'	4	"	H
10	M	26 2 27	'Idiocy'	From birth	"	H
11	M	17 2 42	'Arms taken off by a machine'	1	"	–
12	F	23 7 17	Consumption	7	"	E
13	F	25 6 **1798**	Rheumatism	21	"	H
14	M	22 7 09	'Paralysis'	4½	26 10 54	H
15	M	24 10 04	'Disease of the lower extremities'	6	"	E
16	M	27 6 33	'Idiocy'	From birth	31 10 54	H
17	M	13 11 **1787**	'Broken thigh; dislocated hip; rupture'	2	"	E
18	M	14 3 10	Chronic rheumatism	12	"	H (elected as E)
19	M	26 2 26	Rheumatic gout	4	"	E
20	M	6 9 33	'Spinal affection'	17	"	E
21	F	8 12 23	'Disease of the bladder'	10	"	E
22	M	7 4 24	'Paralysis'	From birth	"	E
23†	F	11 6 15	Consumption	1	"	E
24	M	7 10 21	'Imbecility'	From birth	9 11 54	H
25	M	31 10 22	'Crippled, and withered in every limb'	From birth	"	E

No.*	Sex	Date of Birth (nineteenth century unless stated)	Diagnosis	Duration of illness (yr)	Date presented (nineteenth century)	Category+
26	M	7 5 07	'Broken leg and arm'	9	9 11 54	H
27	M	2 4 13	Chronic rheumatism	7	"	E
28	F	24 5 04	'Paralysis'	3	"	H
29	F	17 12 16	'Paralysis'	1	"	E
30	F	25 2 19	'Affection of the spine'	20	"	H
31†	F	'1810'	Consumption	2	"	H
32	F	20 3 1790	Hernia, Chronic rheumatism	10	"	E
33	F	'1797'	Total blindness	6	"	E
34	F	10 9 27	'Hysteria, partial paralysis'	4	23 11 54	H
35	M	20 5 09	Blindness, almost total	3	"	H
36	F	13 7 38	Paraphlegia [sic]	1	14 12 54	H
37	F	17 2 33	Dislocated hip	15	"	E
38	F	'1780'	Asthma & fits	9	11 1 55	E
39	M	18 3 25	Dysentery	3	"	H
40	M	19 6 14	'Paralysis'	7½	14 12 54	E
41	M	? 11 1787	Epilepsy, Paraphlegia [sic]	2¼	25 1 55	E
42	F	26 6 33	Contraction, caused by a severe burn	11	"	E
43	M	24 5 31	Epilepsy	4	8 2 55	H
44	M	7 4 1792	Rheumatism	10	"	E
45	F	16 12 01	'Ovarian disease'	6	"	E
46	M	12 11 1792	Nearly total blindness	3	14 12 54	E
47	F	14 10 1794	'General debility & loss of speech'	3	8 2 55	E
48	F	10 11 18	'A complete cripple'	From birth	22 2 55	E
49	F	17 2 02	'Affection of the spine'	25	"	H
50	F	28 7 16	'Paralysis'	37	11 1 55	H
51	F	'1784'	'Abscess in utero, with partial blindness'	–	25 1 55	H
52	F	25 7 20	'Curvature of the spine'	4	8 2 55	E
53	F	'1826'	Chronic articular rheumatism	11	8 3 55	H
54	F	'1822'	Epilepsy	8	"	E

No.*	Sex	Date of Birth (nineteenth century unless stated)	Diagnosis	Duration of illness (yr)	Date presented (nineteenth century)	Category+
55	M	21 6 **1799**	Blindness, nearly total	3	22 3 55	E
56	F	'About 1831'	'Incurable idiocy'	From birth	12 4 55	H
57	M	14 3 33	'Injury to the spine'	1¼	"	E
58	F	18 2 21	'Paralysis, and partial imbecility'	From infancy	"	H
59	F	21 9 14	'General debility and subject to nervous excitement'	10	"	H
60	M	**'1791'**	'Paralysis & Dropsy'	10	"	H
61	F	18 6 24	'Idiocy'	From infancy	10 5 55	H
62	M	17 12 19	Chronic asthma	14	"	E
63	M	22 6 06	Chronic bronchitis	4	"	E
64	F	11 7 **1795**	'Cancer'	(3 months)	"	E
65	F	11 4 **1797**	'Paralysis of the right side'	1	"	E
66	M	24 11 29	Epilepsy	(from 10 years of age)	"	H
67	F	18 12 14	'Neuralgia'	11	"	H
68	F	11 9 **1792**	'Compound fracture of the leg'	(since 20 1 53)	"	E
69	F	**'1796'**	Chronic rheumatism	12½	7 6 55	H
70	F	4 9 **1783**	'Diseased bone of the foot'	1½	"	E
71	F	2 5 35	Epilepsy	From infancy	10 5 55	H
72	M	3 11 09	'Injury of leg, and diseased ankle'	3	28 6 55	H
73	F	'1802'	Serofula	42	"	H
74	F	? 12 01	'Curvature of the spine; the extremities paralysed'	Almost from infancy	7 6 55	H
75	M	29 4 01	'Paralysis'	2½	28 6 55	E
76	F	**'1799'**	'Broken arm and collar bone'	(5 weeks)	12 7 55	H/E
77	F	'1810'	'Spinal affection & lumbar abscess'	2	28 6 55	H
78	M	20 9 32	'Idiocy'	From birth	"	H
79	M	25 10 29	'Paralysis & contraction of the limbs'	(from the age of 2 years)	12 7 55	H

No.*	Sex	Date of Birth (nineteenth century unless stated)	Diagnosis	Duration of illness (yr)	Date presented (nineteenth century)	Category+
80	M	2 10 34	'Spasmodic affection of muscles and nerves'	(from birth)	9 8 55	H
81	M	31 12 36	Epilepsy	5	"	H
82	M	31 5 09	'Paralysis, and disease of the liver'	8	"	H
83	M	23 10 34	Epilepsy	13	23 8 55	H
84	F	3 5 13	Epilepsy	7	10 5 55	H
85	M	3 7 30	'Disease of brain, paralysis, blindness'	5	13 9 55	E
86	F	(49 years)	'Paralysis'	(3 months)	27 9 55	H
87	M	–	'Mental imbecility'	(from infancy)	9 8 55	H
88	M	30 4 **1790**	'Softening of the brain'	2	"	E
89	M	16 7 42	Epilepsy	3	23 8 55	H
90	M	3 2 **1790**	Rheumatic fever, and its sequences	4	27 9 55	H
91	M	16 10 24	Phthisis	5	11 10 55	E
92	F	12 12 34	'Idiocy'	(from infancy)	13 9 55	H/E
93	M	28 5 **1791**	'Paralysis'	13	11 10 55	H
94	M	3 1 20	Consolidation of the right lung, etc	4³/₄	8 11 55	E
95	F	(48 years)	'Internal ulcer'	9	22 11 55	E
96	F	22 3 28	'Affection of the lungs'	>20	13 12 55	H
97	F	**'1782'**	Chronic rheumatism	4	25 10 55	H
98	M	7 1 **1789**	'Paralysis'	6	29 11 55	H
99	F	(about 48 yr)	'Stone cancer'	5	13 12 55	E
100	F	(age 57 yr)	Melancholia	11	"	H

*The numbers of those accepted are in bold. +H = home patient; E = extra-patient.
† Died before decision taken.

97) was accepted on a 'reduced scale', with the annual donation being £15. No 81 applied for admission by payment of £50=00 per annum; although this was accepted, and he entered the hospital, he was withdrawn by his father at Christmas 1856! It is clear therefore, that if they chose not to be *elected,* patients were expected to pay their way! It is also clear from minute books 1 & 2 that a very careful watch was kept over payments; if the appropriate sum was not

immediately forthcoming the patient was removed from the hospital. Incidentally, the number seeking admission by the latter (paying) 'route' increased significantly towards the end of the first 100 'applications'.

Table 4.1 gives details of these first 100 of the 500 individuals considered for benevolence from the RHI. Several died whilst awaiting the election, while others did so shortly after admission – as a result of advanced disease. The distribution of the sexes was approximately equal in the 'presentations' (applications): 49 males and 51 females of mean age 37.2 (12-80) and 42.5 (16-75) years respectively. Twenty males (13 'home' and 7 'extra'), and 22 females (17 'home' and 5 'extra') were 'accepted'. There was a wide range of diagnoses; however, chronic neurological disease predominated – a good deal dating from birth (or infancy). It should be appreciated that many medical diagnoses in the mid-nineteenth century are suspect using present clinical standards (criteria).

It seems probable that 'birth injury' accounted for some (and probably most) of the cases debilitated from birth. A few suffered from the long-term effects of accidents. 'Rheumatism' accounted for a minority. There is scant evidence of malignant disease although here again the accuracy of diagnosis in the mid-nineteenth century was obviously far from that of today (using sophisticated technological methods). It is perhaps surprising (in view of the initial constitution and rules of the RHI) that tuberculosis (not then universally considered a communicable disease) was acceptable – consumption (three cases), phthisis and scrofula; 'curvature' or 'affection' of the spine might account for several more.[1] The mean length of survival (after 'presentation') of three of these cases was short, death being recorded in a very short space of time.

It is now impossible to deduce whether multiple sclerosis (MS) accounted for any of these early admissions. This disease was first described by the London pathologist Robert Hooper (1773-1835) in *The Morbid Anatomy of the Human Brain*, published in 1828. In 1840, Jean Cruveilhier (1791-1874), professor of pathological anatomy at Paris, also documented it. Later in the nineteenth century, Jean Martin Charcot (1825-93) noted the characteristic lesions in 1868, and Walter Moxon (1836-86) did likewise in Britain in 1875. The index of awareness of this disease would therefore have been low in the mid-nineteenth century.[2]

References and Notes

1. R.P. Cotton, *The nature, symptoms, and treatment of consumption* (London: John Churchill, 1852): 5-11. *See also:* C.T. Williams, Old and new views on the treatment of consumption: The Harveian Oration delivered on 18 October 1911 (London: RCP).
2. A. Sebastian, *A dictionary of the History of Medicine* (London: the Parthenon Publishing Group 1999): 523. *See also:* W. Moxon, 'Eight cases of insular scelerosis of the brain and spinal cord', *Guy's Hospital Reports* 1875, 20: 437-80.

CHAPTER 5

Medical care, and the management of infectious disease

OBVIOUSLY, ONE OF THE first requirements of the fledgling establishment was medical cover, for although the patients were not, on the whole, *acutely* ill, there were sufficient medical reasons for their hospitalisation (Chapter 4). At a Board meeting on 12 October 1854, Reed (the founder) announced that 'Dr Little [fig 5.1] had consented to act as [the first] Medical Examiner'.[1] It should be noted that in line with most voluntary hospitals of this era, there was a medical officer (usually, but not always, resident), as well as *Visiting* Physicians and Surgeons who made less frequent appearances.

The importance of satisfactory *medical* cover for the hospital was again raised in May 1855: 'Dr Reed stated that his attention had been turned to procuring for the Hospital a Medical Staff, and that he had at length procured the honorary services of the following gentlemen:

'As [Visiting] Consulting Physician, William Munk Esq., M.D. [fig 5.2]
As [Visiting] Consulting Surgeon, James Luke Esq., F.R.C.S. [fig 5.3].[2]

The minutes of a Board meeting held on 14 February 1856 recorded two further events regarding medical matters:

(i) That the services of G. Bottomley [FRCS, of Croydon who had visited the Hospital professionally 'for some time'] be accepted as gratuitous, and that [£30 annually] be allowed for medicine and sundry charges', [and]

(ii) ... since Mr Bottomley's attendance, Dr Little's visits had been discontinued'; he would however still 'receive a fee of three guineas for each visit.

Bottomley's term as 'Honorary Surgeon to the Charity' came to an end with the removal of the establishment from Carshalton to Putney in mid-1857 (Chapter 1); he was then made a Life Governor.[3]

At a later meeting (10 June 1856), the following was minuted: '... Prescott Hewett Esq. [at that time assistant surgeon to St George's Hospital] had consented to add his name to the Medical Testimonial.'[4] The name of Seymour Haden was also added to the list of (Visiting) Medical Officers of the Charity at the Second Annual Meeting held on 27 November 1856.[5]

At a meeting a year later (12 November 1857) it was reported that 'Dr [J.J.] Paul had offered himself as [the first] medical officer of the hospital ...'. After examination of his testimonials, he was duly appointed Honorary Medical Officer, and 'allowed thirty pounds per annum to cover the expense of needful

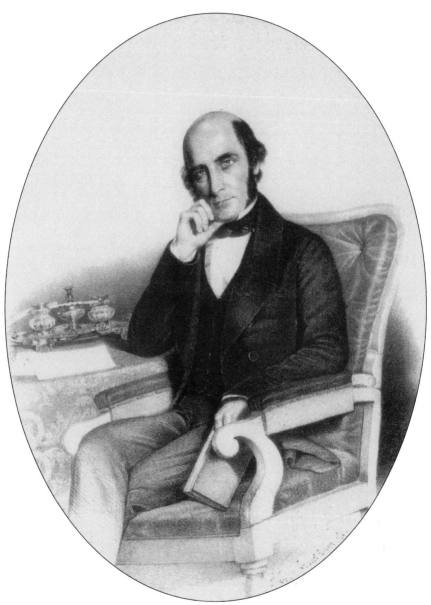

Fig 5.1: Dr William J. Little, FRCP (portrait by Shapper – dated 1854)
(reproduced with permission, The Wellcome Library, London).

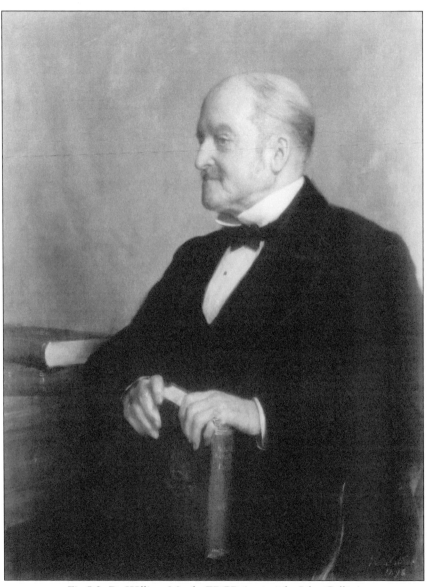

Fig 5.2: Dr William Munk, FRCP (portrait by John Collier)
(reproduced with permission, The Royal College of Physicians).

drugs and medicine'. In May 1858, a minute stated that it was proposed to grant '£50 annually to cover the cost of drugs'; Paul however requested £60, which the Committee declined. However, he seems to have been very persistent with this request – which was repeatedly rejected by the Board.[6]

At a meeting on 28 April 1859, the 'Matron reported that Dr [John] Conolly had visited the case of Baber [one of the Inmates], and had spoken of her as decidedly insane, but that a written certificate should be given.' Conolly's role was to give an outside *specialist* opinion; he was not on the staff of the RHI.[7]

It will by now be clear to the reader that there were, in the early days of the RHI, as in most other instituttutions, three categories of medical carers: (i) the (non-resident) medical officer – who was expected to pay at least one call at the hospital daily; (ii) consultant physicians or surgeons – who advised on all aspects of *in-patient* care; and (iii) medical practitioners around the country who looked after the *out-patients* (or pensioners).

Medical Officers

Dr Paul (see above) was the first *medical officer* of the RHI (see above). The arrangement whereby the medical officer was expected to supply his own drugs (a system which was in operation in the workhouses) today seems anomalous, and there is little doubt that it caused problems then. Whether he was content with his lot is impossible to say; however, he seems to have been very conscious of his salary, and made repeated requests to the Board for an increase. In February 1861, the Board (probably reluctantly) agreed to an increase to '£60 a year'. An early minute states that the Board resolved 'That the Secretary be requested to confer with the Medical Officer … and inquire whether the Board were required to supply his prescription …'.[8]

A minute of a Board meeting held in August 1861 contains a somewhat sobering entry; a patient had written to a subscriber – namely Mr Wright of Canonbury … stating that 'she had not been able to procure any medicine when much in need of it'; although Dr Paul had seen her, he had not prescribed any medicine, so she had had to purchase her own – which had cost, since her admission in June, £2.10 – and as a result she intended 'to quit the hospital'. The Board resolved 'That, having received, with much regret, complaints from subscribers and friends of the patients respecting the medical attendance and oversight of the hospital, consider it advisable to release Dr Paul from his engagement, and hereby request the Secretary to inform him that he will not be required to continue his services after the 1st day of October next.'[9] As a result of this unfortunate incident, a *new* medical officer was required forthwith. The following month there had been three applications – from Messrs Abercrombie, Cream and Ridge – and on 26 September, the second of those was appointed at £60 annually, this to include 'needful drugs' which would be both 'provided and dispensed' by him. Cream

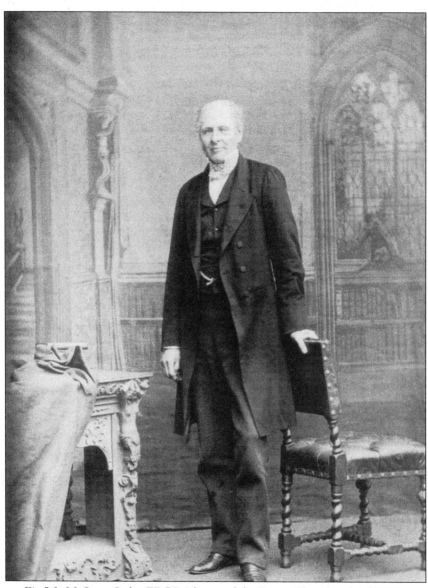

Fig 5.3: Mr James Luke, FRCS (photograph by Ernest Edwards – dated 1867).
(Reproduced with permission, The Wellcome Library, London.)

seems to have proved an overall success. There is for example mention of his services in 1864; he had expressed an opinion (and Dr Little agreed) that one of the in-patients was insane (she was duly dispatched to Camberwell House), and also that '... cases of Hysteria and Epilepsy and merely functional derangement should *not* [my italics] be admitted into the Institution.'[10]

Later that year, a Board minute reads: 'That a request had been considered from Dr Cream that in future Drugs be supplied by the Institution instead of himself as hitherto ...'.

The following year, Cream complained to the Board that Mrs Turner (who had recently been engaged as Head Nurse) '... was inefficient, and also insolent in her behaviour'. As a result she was given 'one month's notice to quit', and a Mrs Lilley was appointed in her stead. Of major concern, however, was the fact that the Board received complaints concerning the behaviour (unspecified) of a senior member of the nursing staff and Cream; the conclusion seems to have been, that 'Madame Goldschmidt [Jenny Lind (1821-87), had the] intention to get both Dr Cream and Mrs Bellringer [the matron] out'! In December 1863, a minute states: '... it was resolved [by the House Committee] to speak to the Medical Officer ... on the frequency of his visits to the Hospital, and the making up of the Stimulant Book.' In September 1865 the Board agreed to increase Cream's salary to '£80 a year' on condition that he visited the Hospital daily ('between the hours of 11 and one or after five daily'); in addition, he was expected to 'dispense the medicines of the Establishment as at present'. In November, his salary was again raised to '£100 a year'. However, it was reported in January 1866 that 'Cream had not complied with the rules laid down for his guidance'. The Board did not 'recommend his dismissal at that time', but a month later it reported its 'unanimous dissatisfaction at Dr. Cream's neglect of the Rules laid down for his guidance'. He duly resigned and his duties ended 'on Wednesday, the 28th Inst'.[11]

A Special Board meeting was immediately called to appoint a *new* medical officer: 'The following Gentlemen attended as Candidates, viz. Henry Usher, M.B., Edwd. Sutcliff, M.D., John W. George M.R.C.S., Theodore Bloomenthal, M.D., J.H. Todd Cinnor [sic] M.R.C.S., Charles Henry Grover, M.R.C.S., J.J. Barrett, M.D., T.J. Woodhouse, M.D., W.C. Tucker, M.D. Applications were also presented from Mr C.H. Payne, of Wimbledon, and C.M. Kempe of New Shoreham.' After three rounds of voting (by show of hands), Woodhouse was duly appointed, at £100 a year. Woodhouse 'promised compliance with [the rules] and thanked the Board for the appointment.' Like his predecessors, he was soon to request an increase in salary, and in late 1868, this was raised to £125 per annum.

It was agreed in September 1870, in response to a request from Woodhouse, that 'it was desirable to raise [his salary] to £150 from Christmas next'. And in January 1876, the Board resolved that his salary ' be raised from £175 to £200 per annum, from Christmas 1875'. This increase was due to length of service, an increase in the number of 'inmates', and the fact that three years had elapsed since his last increase.

Some years later, '... in view of the long services, rendered with kindness and efficiency by Dr Woodhouse [whose wife had recently died], [the House Committee] recommended to the Board [who unanimously endorsed it] to advance his salary from £320 to £325 a year.' Various *locum tenens* were recruited from time to time, to 'cover' this popular and most successful medical officer. For example, in early 1892 Dr Grün (see below) deputised; later that year Dr Baker did likewise (while Woodhouse was reported absent on account of serious illness), and while he was ill and away Dr Gay (see below) of Putney deputised. It was resolved in December 1901, 'that [in view of ill-health] Dr Woodhouse be asked to retire [on a] pension of one hundred and seventy pounds per annum'. Woodhouse agreed to this and the position of medical officer was thus advertised in *The Times, Lancet, BMJ* and *Boro. News.* Woodhouse's death was announced in June 1902.[12]

There were, this time, no fewer than 88 applications for the position, but the Board were able to reduce this to eight. At a Special Meeting held later in January, this was further reduced to three, all of whom, Dickinson, Gay and Jewell, were to be interviewed. Dr Gay [who had already undertaken a spell as locum tenens] was elected, at a salary of £250 per annum. Appendix 3 gives *rules* for the Medical Officer in 1902 (i.e. when Gay was appointed); the salary then was £250.[13]

Dr John Gay served as medical officer to the RHI for a period of over thirty years, from 1901 to 1932. His salary was increased from £250 to £300 a year from 1 January 1912. All was not plain sailing however, for he was criticised in a letter (dated 25 July 1912) for allowing Dr Middleton of Bournemouth to treat 'some patients in this Hospital'. The letter, signed by the Secretary (Cutting) continued: '... the Committee desire, in all cases, to be consulted before any medical men not associated with the Hospital are allowed to treat our patients.' In December 1920, he was granted £50 'in view of the high cost of living'. It was agreed in 1928 to advance his salary from £300 a year to £350. This was part of a 'package' to raise the salaries of all 'servants' of the Institution. Gay was compelled to retire in October 1932 on account of advancing years. An honorarium of £500 was awarded in 'recognition of his long service as Medical Officer'.[14] The death of Gay was reported to a meeting of the Board held on 25 April 1935. The post was duly advertised in the *Lancet* and *BMJ*. Four candidates were interviewed; Dr Geoffrey Duckworth MRCP (Lond) MRCS who was 33 years old was elected, at a starting salary of '£300 a year'.[15]

The next medical officer was Dr Winton; his contract was not renewed by the Board in 1946. Following his departure on 31 March 1947, the post was advertised 'at a salary of £450 a year, the hours of attendance [being] from

11 a.m. to 1 p.m. daily'. Of five candidates, Dr J. Badenoch was ultimately appointed as the 'most suitable', but the announcement was delayed because it was felt that some members of the Board might be opposed to her gender. After one year, her salary was raised to £600 to bring it roughly into line with the BMA's recommendations which had been approved by the Minister of Health. Dr Badenoch resigned in November 1952 'for personal reasons', and on 26 January 1953, Dr Verna Kendall of 123 Home Park Road, Wimbledon Park, SW19 was appointed part-time Medical officer ... with effect from 1 February 1953.[16]

Pay was to increase further over the years, and in 1960 the salary of Dr Verna Kendall (who had been appointed in 1952) was raised by £50 to £1,075 per annum, for '5 notional half-days per week'. In November 1962, the Board approved a recommendation of the Medical Committee that Dr Maureen A. Tudor be appointed part-time to assist Dr Kendall, at £645 per annum. At the same meeting, the Board approved an increase to £1,290 per annum in Dr Kendall's remuneration with effect from 1 October 1962.[17]

Consultant physicians/surgeons

In the early days of the Charity, the consultant staff were paid on the basis of visits; it was not until 1952 (i.e. after the Charity had been in existence for over a hundred years) that Lord Amulree (a member of the Board) suggested that fees payable to the consultant staff should be on the basis of an honorarium.[18] Dr Little (see above), who was also the senior physician to the (Royal) London Hospital, seems from the outset to have taken a keen personal interest in medical condition(s) at the RHI. For example, the following letter, addressed to the Committee and dated 20 August 1860, was written from 34 Brook Street, Grosvenor Square W:

Gentlemen, [he began]

I beg to report that I visited the Asylum on three occasions, July 5, 13, and Aug. 1 and examined the whole of the Inmates, and have conferred with Dr. Paul [the medical officer] on the subjects hereafter mentioned. The general condition of the Establishment appears to be satisfactory, the patients generally as happy as their condition permits, with a small amount of incidental sickness.

I carefully examined the condition of Sarah Plumley, as to her removal to a Lunatic Asylum, and am of opinion that she labors under Congenital imbecility, neither dangerous to herself nor to others, incurable, and consequently not requiring removal to a Lunatic Asylum. I particularly examined also Kesiah [sic] Grant, who is affected with paralysis of the most important muscles of both arms of sixteen years' standing, quite incurable, and incapable of earning her livelihood, Being however, in good bodily health, able to walk about, she appears to me a fit subject for out-door pension, rather than in-patient.

Having as before stated, carefully examined every inmate, I am led to the opinion that there are several of whom it cannot be said that they are *hopelessly disqualified* [my italics] for the duties of life.

Little then mentioned six patients by name and continued:

Several might do something for an existence out of the house, when not too much sympathized with by mistaken friends.

My attention was also directed to the large number of inmates habitually taking wine, brandy or gin in addition to the allowance of malt liquor [see below]. 46 female patients divide between them *Daily* 21 glasses of wine, $1/2$ (?) pint of Brandy (8oz.) 4oz. of Gin; while 26 male patients divide between them 4oz. of Gin only. [There are frequent references in the early minutes of the need to order supplies of alcoholic beverages (see below), e.g., in October 1860 'The Sub. Secretary was instructed to order 6 doz. of Port, and the same quantity of Sherry (the latter to be a little fuller-bodied than the last) of Messrs. Tower, Lawson and Trowell']. The females which consume the principal part of the alcoholic beverages are of the class of hysterical hypochondrical and nervous cases.

I am of opinion that the progress of their diseases will not be materially affected by the use of abstinence from the quantity of wine and spirits they consume. It simply makes them 'feel comfortable'. Dr. Paul and I are of the opinion that, during the five or six finer months of the year, wine and spirits may generally be discontinued in the Asylum, it being left to the Visiting Medical Officer to prescribe it from time to time in such cases as he deems fit. I would suggest that, like as at the London Hospital, with which I am connected [he was the Senior Physician there], the Medical Officer should be requested at frequent periods (once a fortnight for example) to sign a book in which daily consumption of wine is requested, as a means of attracting his attention to the actual consumption.

Considerable expense has been incurred with visits to London for the purpose of Galvanism [see below]. I would recommend that Dr. Paul be requested to name to the Committee the cases in which he thinks Galvanism has decidedly proved beneficial, and that its use should be discontinued in the remaining cases.

As a means of more efficiently guarding against the admission of unsuitable cases, I would suggest that all applicants for admission should be examined before reception into Asylum [this was subsequently done] by a medical officer in London appointed by the Board. The possibility of rejection after election would ensure, in country cases and London cases not examined by authority of the Board due discrimination as to eligibility. It is quite certain that the Inmates of our Asylum do not represent, as a body, a fair sample of the distressing cases which continually pass through the hands of Physicians and Surgeons as Incurable Cases.

Dr Little emphasised the point (which he had made in his report – see above) that 'many of the cases were not of the class proposed to be relieved by the Institution, not being, strictly speaking, incurable.' He suggested (and the Board agreed with him) that he (and Cream) draw up a series of questions, which should appear on the form of application, and he felt that those individuals who were not 'totally disqualified for the duties of life' should be rejected.[19]

At this time too, the possibility of sending patients to 'the Sea Bathing Infirmary at Margate' was an option – but this course of action was left to the medical officer, Dr Paul.[20]

Designation of Consultant Staff

Meanwhile, a good deal of dissatisfaction was growing about the actual *designation* of the consultant medical staff. At a meeting of the Board held in July 1861 for example, a letter from Munk (see above) was read and the subsequent discussion served to clarify the position of the medical staff of the RHI: When asked to serve as an honorary medical officer, he wrote, he had consented to act as 'consulting physician' but in the present hospital report he was styled as 'physician', a change 'made without his knowledge'. It was explained by the Sub-Secretary that when Mr Haden had been appointed 'visiting surgeon', Dr Reed 'with the assistance of Dr. Little' had 'adopted the present arrangement of the medical staff'. The meeting subsequently resolved that Dr Little and Dr Munk be henceforth styled *'consulting physicians'*, Mr Luke *'consulting surgeon'*, and Mr Haden *'visiting surgeon'*. A later 'outburst' came in March 1862; a letter from Haden was read 'complaining that his title had been altered to *visiting surgeon* [my italics] and requesting that he might be styled 'visitor'. This was accepted by the Board, with the caveat that 'no slight' had been intended![21]

Future consultants and their contributions

Dr Cream, the second medical officer of the institution (see above) felt in early 1864, that it would be desirable to add an 'operating surgeon' to the honorary staff; he suggested Mr Bernard Brodhurst of St George's Hospital. The Secretary was directed to confer with Mr Luke, who agreed, and a letter of acceptance from Brodhurst was read to the Board at a subsequent meeting.[22]

The matter of urgent removal of *insane* patients (Drs Little and Paul, and the matron were involved) was the subject of recurring debate by the Board.

With the exception of Little, there are few references in the early minute books to the consultant staff playing an active rôle in patient care! However in October 1862, the Board was informed 'that Dr Munk had seen one of the patients and had given his opinion,' but he suggested that Dr Robert Lee should also see her. This was agreed! In early 1860, because Little was away, Dr C. Handfield Jones was requested to see a patient suffering from a 'protracted attack of ague'; for this he received 'a guinea for his trouble'.[23] In August 1872 a House Committee minute states: '... Dr Munk has paid a second visit to the Hospital [and made a verbal report to the effect] that he considered the general tone of the patients much improved; that he saw no necessity for going again with the question of stimulants [see below], ... and that he advised a rest of say six weeks for the Head Nurse, Mrs Chapman, whose services he strongly recommended the C^{ee} to retain. [He] had also seen several cases of special illness to which his attention had been directed.'

When Dr Munk died in 1899, he was replaced by Dr (later Sir James) Goodhart. The other founding Consultant Physician (Little) had by this time also died. The Board was told in November 1899, that inquiry at the RCP had revealed that Dr Little had died in 1894 (i.e. five years before)! In February 1876, Dr Peacock expressed 'his willingness to be one of the Consulting Physicians of the Hospital'; the following month the offer of this appointment was confirmed by the Board, unanimously, and rapidly accepted. The appointment was also announced in the *Annual Report* for 1875-76.[24]

Luke, the original Consultant Surgeon to the RHI, died in 1880. A further loss from the Hon. Medical Staff was the first Medical Officer for Seaside House (Chapter 10); the death of Dr Edgar Duke was recorded in the RHI *Annual Report* for 1897-98; he was succeeded by Dr William Herbert Davies.[25]

It was not always easy, however, to recruit Consultants to the RHI. In February 1890, for example, Dr Philip Pye-Smith was invited by the Board to accept the position of Honorary Consulting Physician; however, he declined, and 'the Secretary … asked for an interview with the hope of [his] reconsidering the matter.' In October 1881 the Board resolved: 'That Mr [later Sir] Prescott G. Hewett FRCS, FRS [1812-91] be invited to accept the office of Honorary Consulting Surgeon to the Institution.' He had signed the medical testimonial list in 1854 (Chapter 3) but this honour too also was declined.[26]

The senior medical staff in 1916 are listed in an RHI publication. As in former days, they continued to be of exceptionally high calibre. The consulting physicians were Sir James Goodhart, Bt. (who had succeeded Munk – see above), and (Sir) E. Farquar Buzzard. The consulting Surgeon was Sir George Makins, and the Opthalmic Surgeon Sir Arnold Lawson.[27]

In November 1912, Dr Belfrage (who had joined the Board in 1911 and died in June 1950) suggested the appointment of an Assistant Consulting Physician (with 'knowledge of nervous ailments') until Goodhart's resignation was received; he died in June 1916. This was agreed. Dr Belfrage also drew the Board's attention to a letter in *The Times* in October written by Dr E.J. Grün (see above); Belfrage wanted to know when Grün had worked at the RHI, and 'if necessary to follow this up with a disclaimer …'. A new Consulting Surgeon – Lt. Col. Percy Sargent DSO, FRCS (of St Thomas's Hospital and the National Hospital, Queen Square) was proposed by Sir George Makins in July 1919.[28]

A letter from H.E. Farquar Buzzard to Dr Gay (dated 13 March 1923) is of interest; this indicated that one of the inmates who had been labelled 'an incurable heart case' did *not* have mitral stenosis or, in fact, any other form of organic heart disease. Nevertheless, she was described by Buzzard, as a 'poor feeble creature close on 60 years of age' and was allowed to stay in the Hospital.[29]

Dr A.H. Douthwaite first attended a Board meeting on 11 June 1931; the Chairman (Turton Wright) informed him that 'the House Committee had recently had under discussion the desirability of making certain that everything is being done that is possible for our patients, especially those suffering from rheumatoid arthritis.' Douthwaite replied that in advanced cases, only palliative care was available but ' he undertook to visit the Hospital and to see some of the cases, when he would be in a position to make up his mind as to whether he could suggest anything to do good.' The meeting immediately decided to appoint Douthwaite to the honorary consulting staff, and Dr Belfrage 'undertook to introduce [him] to Dr Gay, and to see a number of the rheumatoid arthritic cases.' Douthwaite subsequently made four visits to the RHI 'when he examined a very large number of patients suffering from rheumatoid arthritis' for which he was paid thirty guineas.'[30]

Although the Board agreed on 22 November 1934 *not* to appoint a Consulting Pathologist, they did agree to the appointment of a Consulting Neurologist (Dr James Collier) and an Opthalmic Surgeon (Mr Gerard G. Penman), to succeed Sir Arnold Lawson. However, the premature death of Collier was recorded on 28 February 1935 and at a subsequent meeting, Dr D.E. Denny-Brown (see above) was appointed in his place.

The death of Sir Percy Sargent was reported to a Board meeting held in January 1933 and at the next meeting (in February) it was agreed to invite Mr Charles Max Page to succeed him. In 1960, Mr G.G. Penman, MD, FRCS, the Ophthalmic Surgeon, resigned owing to the fact that he 'was taking up residence outside the London area', and Dr N.S. Plummer, MD, FRCP was appointed consulting Physician.[31]

In 1948, Dr H.E Allen was appointed as Consulting Radiologist to the Home, and in 1949 it was agreed that Dr F.S. Cooksey OBE, MD, Director of the Department of Physical medicine at King's College Hospital, be invited to join the Consulting Staff & Medical Committee. This meant that ultimately a Department of Physical Medicine would be set up, and although this was approved in principle by the Board in 1963, the project, which was costly, was put 'on hold' as it was not known at that time 'what compensation will be paid by the Wandsworth Borough Council under the compulsory purchase order' (Chapter 18).

Care of the out-patients (Pensioners)

The out-patients (i.e. those receiving a pension from the RHI but living elsewhere) were distributed around the country; therefore, they had to be cared for by *local* practitioners. In the minutes are numerous references to them, together with the fact they were paid by the RHI. Only a few examples will be given, from the early days of the institution.

A minute dated 9 January 1862 refers to: 'An arrangement ... agreed to with

Mr McKay, surgeon, of 22, Hereford Place, Commercial Road, for attendance on [one of the out-patients]. 1/6 to be charged for each visit when medicine was supplied.' A Dr Smith had attended one of the pensioners; he claimed that her medicine(s) had cost 30s. per month, and suggested that the Board might prefer to have it dispensed by a chemist! Five guineas were allocated to Allchin to attend a case, but a previous minute states that the same practitioner had attended two out-patients for which he was 'charging only the cost of [the] drugs'. Another minute recorded that since Allchin (a surgeon) had attended an out-patient without requesting a fee, he 'be constituted an honorary life governor ...'. It was agreed in October 1863 'that Dr. Osbourne continue to attend a pensioner for another year ... Fee for the year £5-5-'. And on 11 April 1867, 'letters [were presented] from Messrs Wetherell and Kirby consenting to attend [two patients] respectively for £5.5. a year.'

Some, however, demanded higher fees: medical attendance (for one pensioner) amounted for example, to £12.12s. a year, the regular medical attendant being a Dr Williams of Sudbury. And at a Board meeting in June 1861, a letter from Dr H.G. Wright (1828-69) stated that he had 'arranged to receive [an outpatient into the Samaritan Hospital] in order to perform an operation which, it was hoped, would be of benefit to her.' Use was also made of eminent medical personnel; for example on one occasion a minute reads: '... it was Resolved [by the Board] "That permission be given to Mr Walker to attend Mr [C.E.] Brown-Séquard [FRS, 1817-94] at the Hospital for Epilepsy".'

Gratuitous medical advice (see above) seems to have been commonplace. Thus, a surgeon, Mr H.T. Berry, MRCS of 19 Tysoe Street attended one of the patients at no charge, while another was similarly treated by Mr Harris of Hackney. Early in the history of the RHI the matter of *gratuitous* attendance by medical gentlemen' had been discussed by the Board;[32] although it was suggested 'according to them the privilege of life or annual membership', this course of action was considered 'on the whole, inadvisable'.[33] Of interest, is an entry in the minute book for 23 July 1861; a letter from one of the out-patients was read indicating that he had been 'advised to emigrate to the colonies for the benefit of his health' and that he would therefore 'sail for New Zealand in September'.[34]

A letter was presented from an out-patient '... asking an allowance for a doctor's bill beyond the sum of £2 annually granted.' And another entry with respect to 'an annual arrangement' for medical attendance was minuted in September 1869. A third states '... Mr Lynch had agreed to attend [a] patient at the rate of 30/- a year.'

In December 1869: 'It was agreed to pay Mr Freeman of Highgate £1-5-0 for medical attendance [on a deceased out-patient of the Hospital].' At a later meeting it was 'agreed to pay the balance of his acct. £1-15' as well as 'a sum of 18/- for medicine supplied by a chemist to the late Pensioner.' 'Mr Wickham reported that he had arranged with Mr Frank Wm Cooper of Leytonstone to attend (an out-patient] at the yearly fee of £5.' Yet another entry refers to 'an acct. [for] £10-19-0 from Messrs Pearse & Barrett, surgeons, 3 Tavistock Sq., of which £3-14-0 was for a period of four months.' In a follow-up it was stated that 'numerous visits had been paid and much medicine required in very serious illness' and as a result this bill should be paid but to propose to the surgeons that they continue attending to the case 'at a yearly fee of £7-7', which they agreed to do. Mr Frank Cooper was willing (according to a minute in July) to 'renew the arrangement [i.e. to look after an out-patient] upon the same terms [£5-5 a year].'

Medical Matters involving 'inmates'

In December 1878, Allingham, Surgeon (whose fee was £3-3-0) was called in to see one of the inmates 'who had been dangerously ill'. And in January 1880, Mr George Lawson, FRCS (1831-1903), oculist, visited the Hospital, saw 13 cases, and operated on one, advised operations in two other cases, and ordered spectacles in three cases. His fee was £5.5s.0d. A consultation regarding an 'inmate' with Dr Symes Thompson was organised in August 1892. Sometime later, in November 1900, Lawson was nominated as Honorary Surgeon to the RHI, to replace the late Bernard E. Brodhurst, Esq., FRCS. This appointment was accepted. Lawson was later requested to see one of the divisional nurses on account of a 'tumour in the breast'.[35]

Dr [John] Langdon-Down was called in to 'report as to the mental condition of [one of the inmates]'. Although he recorded that 'her mind was [not] affected in any way,' he found that 'she surreptitiously [imported] Bromide of Potassium to the House for the purpose of procuring sleep.' Whilst there, Dr Woodhouse asked him to give an opinion on three other inmates. Clearly the Board would have liked to dismiss the patient initially seen by Langdon-Down for 'improper behaviour', but a plea on her behalf by the Revd. Richard Glover, DD proved successful; a 'further trial' was thus agreed. For this work, he was paid £5.5s.0d.[36]

In April 1881 '... at the request of Woodhouse, Sir Joseph Fayrer, FRS [the doyen of the Indian Medical Service was] called in to see [an "inmate" whose diagnosis is not recorded and] and had given general advice, and approved the present treatment.'[37]

In February 1883, the Board was approached by the Middlesex Hospital for a donation 'in consideration of Medical care and maintenance of two inmates ...'. Messrs. Freshfields and Williams (the legal advisers) considered that the Board was under an obligation to do so, and 'Thirty Guineas' were therefore donated.[38]

Galvanism

In the 1850s and 1860s there was a great vogue for galvanic treatment, especially of neuro-psychiatric disease. The Italian physician Luigi Galvani (1737-98) had demonstrated the presence and conduction of electricity in 1791; he believed that muscles and nerves generated electricity, most of his evidence emanating from the stimulation of frogs' legs *in vitro*. This discovery led to the introduction of the galvanometer, the earliest of which was constructed by Ludwig Ferdinand von Helmholtz (1821-94) in 1836. Following this, improved models of the instrument rapidly followed, and paved the way for the electrocardiograph.

Little seems overall to have been somewhat sceptical of this new form of 'treatment'; the major protagonist was Paul (the medical officer). At a meeting in late November 1859, 'A letter was read from Dr Paul stating the necessity, in his opinion, for a galvanic apparatus at the hospital' because he knew of 'several patients who ... would be benefited by its use.' At the same meeting a further letter (from a Mr Thistleton) on this subject was read; he would, he wrote, treat patients 'by means of his galvanic apparatus at his own Residence [for] one guinea per week per patient.' The meeting resolved that Dr Little should be consulted. Little's report was read to the Board in late January 1860; he felt that magnetism would benefit only eight patients (five of them suffering from hysteria) but that if they *were* sent to Thisleton for treatment, Dr Paul should accompany them! In February 1860 the Matron reported that two patients so treated were 'much improved'. At a meeting on 28 February 1861 however, the Board resolved: 'That Mr. Allen having offered his services to process Margaret Tillotson's admission into the Hospital for Epilepsy, this Committee recommend the Board to place her, if consenting, for two months in that Institution.'[39]

'Stimulants'

Alcohol is of course not a *stimulant* but a depressant of central nervous activity; owing to the fact however that it lessens inhibitions, it has for long been considered a stimulant! Dr Little, as we have seen already (in Chapter 1), was of the opinion that alcoholic beverages were being too freely used at the RHI. He subsequently wrote, and advised on this topic. Both he and Dr Cream met the Board on 28 November 1861 and recommended (with acceptance) 'That the habitual use of wine and spirits by the patients be discontinued, and that these articles be supplied only when ordered by the medical officer, and that the orders shall require renewal from week to week.' They also agreed to a recommendation (which was also accepted by the Board) 'That in place of the various kinds of ale now used in the Institution ... one kind only, of the strength of common porter, be used as at the London Hospital.' In response to comments made by the doctors, it was also resolved at the same meeting 'That no food be supplied to any of the patients, except at the regular hours appointed for meals, unless ordered by the medical officer.'

Despite these restrictions, the Board decided in August 1859 that 'ten dozen of Port Wine be laid in ...', and at a later meeting it was agreed that '10 doz. Port and 3 doz. Sherry' should, in addition, be ordered. In January 1860 the ordering of a further supply of wine was agreed. It was stated at that meeting that the wine consumption was 23 glasses per day! Attention was also drawn to a recent admission 'who appeared addicted to the undue use of spirits'. Reed, however, felt that in conjunction with Little and Paul, they should 'carefully ... regulate the use of [wine and spirits]'.

Later, on 14 March 1867, the Board considered: 'That the attention of Dr. Woodhouse [should be] directed to the great increase in the Consumption of Stimulants, and that a reduction had been promised.' Concern about high consumption continued, however, but by 23 December of that year it was minuted: 'That the rate of Consumption of stimulants had much diminished ...'![40]

Post-mortem examinations at the RHI
In October 1886, Dr Graham Balfour (see Chapter 11), by then a member of the Board, indicated to the Board that he intended bringing the following motion to a subsequent meeting: 'To rescind the resolution of March 1866 prohibiting post mortem examinations.' At the November meeting, the 'motion was put and carried, the numbers being – For 3, Against 2.' Therefore, from that time medical officers 'would be permitted in doubtful and exceptional cases, with the assistance of medical men, and with the consent of friends to carry out post-mortems.'[41]

Other matters
In 1947, the Hospital was to experience a 'shake-up' in its medical facilities. Dr Copeman recommended, in a letter which was circulated to all Board members, that: (i) methods by which patients' records are kept should be revised, (ii) a portable x-ray apparatus should be installed, and (iii) a clinical laboratory should be set up. In the event, the matter was shelved until the Hospital's future with regard to the NHS Act was resolved (Chapter 15). A sub-committee was set up to consider these proposals (which were accepted) and also to consider 'The King's Fund's suggestion of the formation of a Medical Comm'.[42]

Infectious Disease at the RHI
Infection superimposed on the underlying condition was a constant problem facing the medical staff at the RHI. Most was of a trivial nature, and the Board minutes record frequent reports by the medical officers. However, there were several instances of specific disease entities being involved, and the following outlines some of them.

Tuberculosis

Infection by *Mycobacterium tuberculosis* was extremely common in the nineteenth century. Two interviews (with microscopic demonstrations) involving Dr Grün, who had worked with Robert Koch[43] in Berlin are recorded; Koch had recently developed a controversial 'new method of treatment for consumption [with tuberculin], lupus &c'. Grün was apparently desirous of being appointed Honorary Assistant Medical Officer to the RHI (see above), but this honour had previously been declined by the Board. He treated a volunteer (with 'an early supply of the lymph' – 'tuberculin') for which he was reimbursed to cover his expenses, £2.10s.0d.

Also on the subject of tuberculosis, the Board was asked (in March 1896) to 'make a grant to enable …, a former nurse [of the RHI], to remain at the Hospital for Consumption at Ventnor [Isle of Wight].' This request was, interestingly, declined.[44]

Smallpox

Although vaccination had been introduced by Edward Jenner (1749-1823) in 1796, this viral disease remained common in nineteenth century Britain. In January 1871 '… the Night Attendant [of the RHI] … died, at his home in Putney of Smallpox.' In order to 'obviate as much as possible, the possibility of contagion' two measures (which were not abandoned until March) were immediately adopted: 'First, the suspension of visits by the relatives and friends of the inmates [and] second, the temporary prohibition to Inmates and officials to leave the Premises.' In February the minutes of the House Committee state: 'That Dr Woodhouse had commenced a general vaccination of the Inmates and Officials [numbering in all 150].' These measures were presumably effective, for no further cases were reported in this outbreak.

Six years later, in January 1877, another smallpox epidemic was reported, and the Committee 'ordered the vaccination of all the officials, and as many Inmates as possible …'. Later that month '206 Inmates and Officials had been vaccinated', but six Inmates and two Officials were apparently 'unwilling to be vaccinated'. Munk (who was an authority on this viral infection) apparently 'declined to advise [on precautionary measures] saying that they were matters that rested entirely with the Comm^ee.'[45]

Cholera

The RHI was not founded until the last of the three great cholera epidemics (1853-54) in London, the first being in 1831-2. Therefore, this was *not* a major problem facing the Medical Officers of the RHI; however, in September 1893, the supply of fish from Grimsby was discontinued on account of a suspicion of 'cholera in that port'.[46]

Leprosy

On 24 July 1919, a *Special Report* was read about one of the pensioners, who had been elected in May 1876; he was 'now 71 years old, blind and [the minute claimed] was suffering from leprosy'. It is of interest that this is the sole case of this chronic disabling disease – which until relatively recently was *incurable* – to be found in the records of the RHHI![47]

Influenza

The debilitated inmates of the RHI were clearly a 'sitting target' for an influenza outbreak. In January 1893, a minute records 33 cases among 'inmates', and seven involving female staff.[48]

References and Notes

1. Board minutes. Book 1: 34; **William John Little,** FRCP (1810-94) was born in the East End of London, and educated at St Margaret's (near Dover) and the Jesuit College of St Omer, France. After serving as apprentice to an apothecary in East London, he studied at the London Hospital, qualifying in 1830. Little began his medical career in general practice in London, but deciding to become a physician, proceeded to Berlin and obtained the MD there in1837. He contracted poliomyelitis as a child and this left him with a talipes equino-varus-like deformity, which was operated upon, with success, in Berlin. He had also been one of the first physicians to use intravenous saline injections in cases of cholera (in 1832); in the 1848-9 outbreak in London, he advocated the addition of wine to the infusion! In 1839 Little settled into consulting practice in London. Between then and his resignation in 1863 he pursued hospital medicine (becoming a full, and ultimately the senior, physician at the London Hospital); between 1839 and 1844 he had worked at the Orthopaedic Institution (later the Royal Orthopaedic Hospital) – which he founded. Little also served at the Royal Orphan Asylum (Wanstead), and the Asylum for Idiots (Reigate). His greatest literary contribution was *Treatment of Deformities in the Human Frame* (1853). *See also: Munk's Roll* 4: 249; *Lancet* 1894; **ii:** 168-9; *BMJ* 1894; **ii:** 106.

2. Op.cit. See note 1 above (Board minutes) Book 1: 69; **William Munk,** FRCP (1816-98) received his medical education at University College, London, and graduated MD (Leyden) in 1837. Following a post (in morbid anatomy) at St Thomas's Hospital, as well as several honorary appointments (including this one at the RHI), he had been appointed physician to the Smallpox Hospital, initially at St Pancras and later at Highgate (from 1853-93) where he became a leading authority on that disease. He also apparently made a passionate plea for the more liberal use of narcotics and analgesics for the relief of pain in incurable disease. At the Royal College of Physicians (RCP), Munk held the office of Harveian Librarian from 1857 until 1898;

the first two volumes of his invaluable *Roll of the Royal College of Physicians* (*Munk's Roll*) appeared in 1861. He published a new edition (the original was written in 1827) of *The Gold-Headed Cane* in 1884. He also published a book on *Euthanasia* (1887) as well as on the lives of two presidents of the RCP – John Ayrton Paris (1857) and Henry Halford (1895). Munk also served as Senior Censor and Vice-President (1889); *See also: Munk's Roll* 1826-1925 4: 75-6; *Lancet* 1898: **ii:** 1818; *Times, Lond.* 21 December 1898: 6; *BMJ* 1898; **ii:** 1914; *Dictionary of National Biography* Suppl. 1084-5; **(Sir) James Luke,** FRCS, FRS (1799-1881) was one of the original 300 Fellows of the Royal College of Surgeons (RCS). Born at Exeter, he was educated at Blundell's School, and articled to John Andrews of the London Hospital. Luke attended lectures given by Abernethy (at St Bartholomew's Hospital) and Astley Cooper (at Guy's), and was appointed Lecturer on Anatomy in 1823, and two years later, on surgery. He was subsequently elected Assistant Surgeon (1827) Surgeon (1833), and consulting Surgeon (1861). At the RCS, Luke was a Member of Council (1846-66), Vice-President (1851, 1852, 1860, and 1861), and President (1853, 1862); he was also Hunterian Orator for 1852. As well as being Honorary Surgeon to the RHI, he was Surgeon to the Marine Society, St Luke's Mental Hospital, and the West of England Insurance Company. Luke was innovative in the surgery of strangulated hernia, and was greatly interested in the treatment of cleft palate. *See also: Plarr's Lives of Fellows of the Royal College of Surgeons of England* 1930, 1: 740-1; *Lancet* 1881, **ii:** 360; *BMJ* 1881, **ii:** 420; S.D. Clippingdale, *Lond. Hosp Gaz* 1913-14, 20: 8.

3. Op.cit. See note 1 above (Board minutes): 133, 323. **George Bottomley** FRCS (? – 1868) was born at Halifax, Yorkshire; orphaned at four years of age, he was brought up by his maternal grandfather, a retired Army Surgeon practising at Croydon. After qualifying from St Thomas's/Guy's in 1811, he entered into partnership with his grandfather. He was a staunch member of the National Association (which sought to elevate the position of general practitioners, and to establish a separate college). He also took a prominent role in the local affairs of the BMA. *See also: Plarr's Lives* 1930; I: 119; *BMJ* 1868, **ii:** 404.

4. Op.cit. See note 1 above (Board minutes): 144. **(Sir) Prescott Gardner Hewett, Bt.,** FRCS, FRS (1812-91) was educated largely in Paris – learning anatomy and later surgery – where he 'acquired a perfect mastery of French'. At first he intended becoming a professional artist, but later 'became inspired with a love for the surgical profession'. On return to England he entered St George's (qualifying in 1836), where, largely due to the influence of Sir Benjamin Brodie, he was appointed (probably in 1840) Demonstrator of Anatomy and Curator of the Museum. In 1845, he was made Lecturer on Anatomy; he was appointed Assistant Surgeon (1848),

full Surgeon (1861), and Consulting Surgeon (1875) successively. In 1863, Hewett was elected President of the Pathological Society of London, and in 1873 President of the Clinical Society; at the RCS, he was Vice-President (1874 and 1875) and President (1876). He was also appointed Surgeon-Extraordinary to Queen Victoria (1867), Sergeant-Surgeon Extraordinary (1877), and Sergeant-Surgeon (1884); in 1867, he was appointed Surgeon to the Prince of Wales (later King Edward VII). His numerous papers covered such diverse topics as hernia, aneurism, injuries of the head, and pyaemia. Hewett's collection of water-colour sketches was presented to the nation after his death. *See also: Plarr's Lives* 1930, 1: 530-1; *Lancet* 1891, **ii**: 1459-60; *BMJ* 1891, **ii**: 21 & 1361; D. Power. *Dictionary of National Biography* Suppl: 842-3; *Trans R Med Chirurg Soc* 1892, 75; *St George's Hosp Gaz* 1895, 3.

5. Op.cit. See note 1 above (Board minutes): 238, 2nd Annual Meeting; **(Sir) Francis Seymour Haden** FRCS (1818-1910) was educated at Derby School, Christ's Hospital, and University College Hospital, London, qualifying in medicine in 1842; he later studied at the Sorbonne in Paris and at Grenoble. He also lectured on anatomy at the Military Hospital, and between 1843 and 1844 travelled in Italy. Between 1851 and 1957 he was Honorary Surgeon to the Department of Science and Art. Haden was Consulting Surgeon to the Chapel Royal, and was described as 'one of the principal movers' in the foundation of the RHI. He was later a Vice-President of the Obstetric Society. A considerable artist, in 1847 he married the half-sister of McNeill Whistler (1834-1903); in 1880 he founded the (Royal) Society of Painter-Etchers of which was president at the time of his death; *See also:* Anonymous, *Times, Lond.* 2 June 1910: 12; *Lancet* 1910, **i**: 1653-4; *BMJ* 1910, **i**: 1449-50; *Plarr's Lives* 1930, 1: 486; A.M. Hine in *Dictionary of National Biography* 1901-11, 2: 180-2.

6. Op.cit. See note 1 above (Board minutes): 375, Book 2: 16, 63, 96. **James Johnstone Paul** (? – 1866) had qualified at Dublin. He obtained the LRCS (Edinburgh) in 1835, and the MD degree of St Andrews in 1849. Following service in the Royal Navy (he became Assistant Surgeon at the Royal Hospital, Greenwich, and served for seven years on the 'coast of Africa', and two in the Mediterranean) he subsequently became Medical Officer to the RHI and the Royal Victoria Patriotic Asylum, Wandsworth Common.

7. Op.cit. See note 1 above (Board minutes). Book 2: 220. **John Conolly** FRCP (1794-1866) was a distinguished authority on 'the insane'. After four years' service with the Cambridgeshire militia, he took up medicine and graduated MD (Edinburgh). Following general practice at Lewes, Chichester and Stratford-on-Avon (for five years) he took up practice in London in 1827 and became Professor of the Practice of Medicine at University College. Not unduly successful, he spent the following eight years at Warwick as inspecting physician to the county asylums. In 1839,

after a year in Birmingham, he took charge of the Middlesex Asylum at Hanwell and made a permanent mark in 'the history of the treatment of the insane'. As a result of his success, 'insanity came to be studied [according to one obituarist] as a disease and not a crime'. Conolly wrote extensively, and gave the Croonian lectures (on mania) at the RCP in 1848-49; *See also: Munk's Roll* 4: 33-4; *Lancet* 1866, **i**; *BMJ* 1866: **i**: 288-9; N. Conolly, *Dictionary of National Biography*, 4: 951-4.

8. Op.cit. See note 1 above (Board minutes). Book 3: 316.

9. Ibid: 434-5. Book 2: 420.

10. Ibid. Book 4: 3, Book 5: 313. **R. Chevallier Cream** had qualified (MD [Edin], LSA, and LRCS Ed) in 1837 having studied medicine at Edinburgh and Paris. Before being appointed to the RHI he had worked at the Suffolk General Hospital, Bury St Edmund's. *See also: Medical Directory* 1861: 413.

11. Ibid: 129-30, 355, 448-9, 456-7; Book 6: 40, 67, 81, 115, 127, 157.

12. Ibid: 153-4. Book 7: 430, 448; Book 8: 350, 364; Book 18: 35-6. **Thomas James Woodhouse** FRCS (1834-1902) received his medical training at St Thomas's Hospital, and after qualification in 1857 worked at Hackney and Fulham. He obtained the FRCS in 1860. For 36 years (from 1887), he served the RHI. His hobbies were: archaeology and book collecting. *See also: Plarr's Lives* 1930; 2: 544.

13. Op.cit. See note 1 above (Board minutes): 34: Book 19: 1, 3; Book 22: 429-30, 433-4, 443-4, 471, 475; Book 24: 18, 24-5, 478; Book 25: 471; Book 26: 280-1. **John Gay** (1862-1935) of 119, Upper Richmond Road, Putney, SW obtained the MRCS and LRCP in 1884 and 1887 respectively; in 1892, he obtained the DPH (England). He later moved to 137 Upper Richmond Road. Gay received his medical training at St Bartholomew's, Paris and Dublin, and was a House Surgeon at the former, following which he became Resident Clinical Assistant at the City of London Hospital for Diseases of the Chest. Gay was a member of several medical societies. His published work included a short paper on blood-letting (*Lancet* 1891; **i**: 1148). *See also: Medical Directory* 1893: 168; Anonymous, 'Death of Dr John Gay: medical officer of Royal Hospital and Home for Incurables: former alderman of Wandsworth Borough Council, *Wandsworth Borough News* April 1935.

14. Ibid. (Board minutes). Book 26: 232, 236-7.

15. Ibid. 239-40, 243.

16. Ibid. Book 27: 236, 237, 241, 245-6, 278, 449, 457.

17. Ibid. Book 28: 191, 282.

18. Ibid. Book 27: 450-1.

19. Ibid. Book 3: 144-7.

20. Ibid: 150, 157.

21. Ibid: 420, 430; Book 4: 175-6.

22. Ibid. Book 5: 165, 190. **Bernard Edward Brodhurst** FRCS (1822-1900)

had a very distinguished surgical career. He qualified from the (Royal) London Hospital in 1844, and immediately afterwards spent time in Paris, Vienna, Prague, Berlin, Pavia, Pisa, Florence and Rome. In the last city, he attended, in 1848, to wounded and sick (malaria was rampant) soldiers during a siege. Returning to London, he became Surgeon to the Royal Orthopaedic Hospital (1852), and Assistant Surgeon to St George's Hospital (1862). For many years he had the 'chief orthopaedic practice in England'. He was also a prolific writer on orthopaedic surgery. *See also: Plarr's Lives* 1, 142-4; *BMJ* 1900, **i:** 548; *Med Circular* 1852; **i:** 375; *Prov Med J* 1893, 12: 169.

23. Op.cit. See note 1 above (Board minutes). Book 2: 280-1, 289-290, 432; Book 4: 200-1. **Robert Lee** FRCP, FRS (1793-1877) received his medical training in Edinburgh. He later studied in Paris, and moving to London began practice as an obstetric physician; however, following a severe illness he changed tack and became domestic physician to the family of Prince Woronzow. On return to England he was appointed to the chair of midwifery at St George's Hospital, London. Lee was Harveian Orator at the RCP in 1864. *See also: Munk's Roll*, 3: 266-9. **Charles Montague Handfield-Jones** FRCP, FRS (1855-1920) was a consultant physician at St Mary's Hospital, London. *See also: Munk's Roll*, 4: 421.

24. Op.cit. See note 1 above (Board minutes). Book 9: 236; Book 21: 205; *RHI Annual Report* 1898-9: 2. **Sir James Frederic Goodhart,** Bt, FRCP (1845-1916) was educated at Epsom College, and Guy's Hospital, qualifying in 1868. After house-appointments (at Guy's and the Evelina Hospital for Children), he proceeded to Aberdeen, graduating there in 1871. He returned to Guy's and became Assistant in Pathology at the RCS. Goodhart was elected Assistant Physician to Guy's in 1877, Curator of the museum (1882), Lecturer on Pathology (1884), and subsequently Physician (1887). He also became physician to the Evelina Hospital in 1888. At the RCP, he was Censor, and delivered the Bradshaw Lecture (1885) and the Harveian Oration (1912). *See also:* Anonymous, *Lancet* 1916, **i:** 1144-6; *BMJ* 1916, **i:** 805-7; *Munk's Roll* 4: 274-5; *Guy's Hosp Rep* 1921, 71: 377; Op.cit (See note 1 above (Board minutes), Book 11: 33, 42, 54, 201-2; Book 21: 435. **Thomas Bevill Peacock,** FRCP (1812-82) was initially apprenticed to a Darlington surgeon; he then attended University College, London and St George's Hospital, qualifying in 1835. He made two voyages to Ceylon as a ship's surgeon and then studied in Paris. After appointments at Chester and Edinburgh (where he obtained the MD degree), he moved to London, being appointed Physician to the Aldersgate Street Dispensary and to the Royal Free Hospital. He then founded (and became a physician at) the Liverpool Street Hospital (later, the City of London Hospital for Diseases of the Chest). He was elected Assistant (1849) and subsequently (1860) full physician to St. Thomas's Hospital; he was a staunch supporter of the

School of Nursing there. At the RCP, Peacock was Censor and Croonian Lecturer (1865). He was a founder (and ultimately president) of the Pathological Society. Peacock, who had 'joined in the declaration given in 1854' died in 1882. *See also: Lancet* 1882; **i**: 1013-4; *Dictionary of National Biography* 15: 588-9; *Med-Chir Trans* 1883, 66: 20; *Munk's Roll 4*: 61-2; *St Thomas's Hosp Rep* 1882, 11: 179; op.cit. see note 1 above (RHI Annual Report 1881-2) Board minutes, Book 14: 75.

25. Op.cit. See note 1 above (Board minutes). Book 13: 367; RHI Annual Report 1897-98.

26. Op.cit. See note 1 above (Board minutes): 260. **Philip Henry Pye-Smith, FRCP, FRS (1840-1914)** was educated at Mill Hill School, University College London and Guy's Hospital, graduating with the MB degree in 1863; he then studied at Paris, Berlin & Vienna. Most of his career was spent at Guy's: Lecturer on Physiology (1873), full Physician (1883), and Lecturer in Medicine (1884). At the RCP, he was a Censor, Lumleian Lecturer and Harveian Orator (1893). He also became Vice-Chancellor of London University. *See also: Lancet* 1914, **i**: 1578-9; *BMJ* 1914, **i**: 1215-6; *Munk's Roll 4*: 185-6, Book 13: 353, 366.

27. **(Sir) Edward Farquhar Buzzard,** Bt, KCVO, FRCP (1871-1945) was Physician to St Thomas's Hospital, and the National Hospital for the Paralysed and Epileptic. Between 1928 and 1943 he held the Regius Chair of Medicine at Oxford. Educated at Charterhouse, Magdalen College, Oxford (he gained a blue at football), and St Thomas's Hospital, Buzzard graduated BM, BCh in 1898. At the RCP, Buzzard was Goulstonian Lecturer (1907) and Harveian Orator (1941) as well as Senior Censor. He was appointed Physician-Extraordinary to King George V in 1924, and then Physician-in-Ordinary (1932) and Extra Physician (1937) to King George VI. He wrote *Pathology of the Nervous System* (1921) and contributed to articles in Allbutt's *System of Medicine*. *See also: Munk's Roll,* 4: 473-4; *Lancet* 1945, ii: 864-5; *Times, Lond.* 19 December 1945: 8; *BMJ* 1945, ii: 943-4; *Manchester Guardian* 19 December 1945; W.J. Bishop, *Dictionary of National Biography* 1941-50: 124-126; *St Thomas's Hospital Gazette* 1946; H. Cairns *Nature* 1946, 157: 218-9. **Sir Arnold Lawson** KBE, FRCS (1867-1947) was educated at Merchant Taylors' School and the Middlesex Hospital, qualifying in 1891. He subsequently became Consulting Ophthalmic Surgeon to the Middlesex and Royal London Ophthalmic Hospitals and Ophthalmic Consultant to the Royal Navy. His father had been Surgeon Oculist to Queen Victoria. Lawson was appointed Ophthalmic Surgeon to the RHI in 1901. His publications included several works (mostly edited) on eye disease. *See also: Times, Lond.* 1947, 21 & 24 January: 9, 7; *BMJ* 1947, **i**: 161, 870; *Lancet* 1847; **i**: 198; *Plarr's Lives* (1930-51): 472-4; *Br J Ophthal* 1947, 31: 251-4; Op.cit. See note 1 above (Board

minutes), Book 22: 451; Book 23: 65. **Sir George Henry Makins** GCMG, FRCS (1853-1933) was educated at King's Collegiate School, Gloucester, and St Thomas's Hospital – where he was House Physician to J.S. Bristowe. In 1879, he spent some months at Halle and Vienna after which he returned to St Thomas's, becoming Resident Assistant Surgeon. In 1885 he was elected surgical registrar, in 1887 Assistant Surgeon and 1898 Surgeon. He was also Assistant Surgeon at the Evelina Hospital, and in 1900 he was appointed Lecturer on Anatomy. Makins also saw service in South Africa (in the Boer War), France and India and attained the rank of Major-General. Makins was appointed Visiting Surgeon to the RHI in 1901. At the RCS, he was an examiner, Vice-President (1912 & 13) and President (1917-20). He also delivered the Bradshaw Lecture, and was Hunterian Orator. He published several papers on various aspects of surgery. *See also: Times, Lond.* 3 November 1933: 166; *Lancet* 1933, **ii**: 1122, 1178 and 1237; *BMJ* 1933, **ii**: 897; *Plarr's Lives* (1930-51): 523-6. Op.cit. See note 1 above (Board minutes), Book 22: 456.

28. Op.cit. See note 1 above (Board minutes). Book 4: 101; Book 5: 134, 229, 321, 467; Book 27: 353.

29. Ibid. Book 25: 106-7.

30. Ibid: Book 26: 93-4, 106-7. **Arthur Henry Douthwaite** FRCP (1896-1974), the son of a medical missionary, was born in China. During the Great War (1914-18), he was a Civilian POW in Germany (where he was on holiday at the outbreak of hostilities). In 1921 he graduated from Guy's Hospital, and undertook several junior appointments there. However, he developed a tuberculous pleural effusion, was advised to live on the south coast, and spent five years as a general practitioner in Worthing. In 1927, he was appointed to the consultant staff of Guy's as a general physician, his major interests lying in gastroenterology and therapeutics. At the RCP, Douthwaite was Senior Censor and Croonian lecturer in 1956. He was also President of the Medical Society of London, the Section of Medicine of the RSM, and the British Society of Gastroenterology. *See also:* Anonymous, *Lancet* 1974, **ii**: 848-9; Anonymous, *BMJ* 1974, **4**: 50; Anonymous, *Munk's Roll* 6: 154-5.

31. Op.cit. See note 1 above (Board minutes), Book 26: 262-3, 272-3, 277. **James Stansfield Collier** FRCP *1870-1935) was educated at the City and Guilds Institute and St Mary's Hospital, London. After junior appointments at his teaching hospital and the National Hospital for the Paralysed and Epileptic, he subsequently became Assistant Physician and Full Physician to the latter institution in 1902 and 1921, respectively. He also became a physician, in 1908, to St George's Hospital, London. At the RCP, he was Lumleian (1928) and Fitzpatrick (1931-2) lecturer and Harveian Orator (1934); he was also Senior Censor. *See also: Lancet* 1935, **i**:

403-4, 464-5; *BMJ* 1935: **i**: 392-3; *Munk's Roll 4:* 446. **Gerard Giles Penman,** FRCS (1899-1982) was born in South Africa, and educated at Sherborne School, Pembroke College, Cambridge, and St Thomas's Hospital, London. He became Opthalmic Surgeon to the Royal Northern Hospital for Sick Children, Moorfields Eye Hospital and the RHI. He published several important papers on ophthalmological matters. He retired prematurely on the grounds of ill-health but lived to the age of 83 years. *See also: Lancet* 1982; **ii**: 1289; *Plarr's Lives* 1974-82: 315-6; Op.cit. See note 1 above (Board minutes) Book 27: 350-1. **Derek Ernest Denny-Brown,** OBE, FRCP (1901-81) was born in New Zealand. He received his education at New Plymouth High School, Otago University, and Magdalen College, Oxford. He held junior appointments at the National Hospital, Queen Square and Guy's Hospital, and in 1935 was appointed Physician both at Queen Square and St Bartholomew's, London. In 1939, Denny-Brown was appointed Director of the Neurological Unit at the Boston City Hospital. During the Second World War (1939-45) he served with the British Army and in 1946 he became James Jackson Putnam Professor of Neurology at Harvard University. From 1972-3, he was Fogarty International Scholar at the National Institutes of Health, Bethesda, Maryland. At the RCP, he was Goulstonian (1937) and Croonian (1960) lecturer. *See also: Times, Lond.* 1981, 28 April, op.cit. See note 1 above (Board minutes) Book 27; 166, 168; Book 28: 191, 197. *Lancet* 1981, **i**: 116; *BMJ* 1981, 282: 2146; *Munk's Roll 7:* 146-8, **Norman Swift Plummer,** FRCP (1907-78) was born in South Africa and received his education there, and at Guy's Hospital. He became a physician to Charing Cross Hospital in 1935. During the second world war (1939-45) he served in the Middle East with the rank of Brigadier. After the war, he returned to Charing Cross and also the London Chest Hospital; he was also a Consultant Physician to Bromley and Edenbridge Hospitals. His original research centred on mycotic infections of the respiratory tract. At the RCP, he became Senior Censor and Vice-President. *See also: Times, Lond.* 1978, 13 April, 20; *Lancet* 1978, **i**: 946; *BMJ* 1978, **ii**: 284; *Munk's Roll 7:* 474-5.

32. **Henry Thomas Berry** qualified MRCS, LSA in 1842. He was subsequently a member of the Guy's Physicians' Society. *See also*: *Medical Directory* 1860: 103.

33. Op.cit. See note 1 above (Board minutes): Book 2: 390; Book 3: 259; Book 4: 243.

34. Ibid. Book 5: 51.

35. Ibid. Book 12: 172, 451; Book 18: 205; Book 19: 11; Book 22: 226, 244.

36. **John Langdon Haydon Langdon-Down** FRCP (1828-96) was born and educated in Cornwall; at the age of 14 he was apprenticed to a local practitioner. He initially entered the laboratory of the Pharmaceutical Society,

London and after a spell of ill-health decided to return to medicine and graduated at the London Hospital in 1858; he later became Medical Tutor and Lecturer on comparative anatomy there. He was appointed Medical Superintendent of the Earlswood Asylum for Idiots (where he stayed for ten years) and in 1859 Assistant Physician to the London Hospital. Becoming an authority on mental deficiency he founded a home for mentally deficient children of the wealthier classes at Normansfield. *See also*: Anonymous, *Lancet* 1896, **ii**: 1104-5; Anonymous, *BMJ* 1896, **ii**: 1170-1; Anonymous, *Munk's Roll 4*: 171-2; O.C. Ward, *John Langdon Down 1828-1896: a caring pioneer* (London: RSM Press 1998): Op.cit. See note 1 above (Board minutes), Book 19: 236, 242, 246, 251-2.

37. Ibid. Book 13: 240. **Sir Joseph Fayrer,** Bt, KCSI, FRCP, FRS (1824-1907) received his schooling in Liverpool and after serving as a midshipman in the West Indian Mail Steam-Packet Service (which took him to the West Indies and South America) qualified in medicine in 1847 from Charing Cross Hospital – where a fellow student was T.H. Huxley (1825-95). He spent most of his active career in India and became an authority on snake-bite. He then served on the Medical Board of the India Office, and at the RCP gave the Croonian lectures in 1882. *See also:* Anonymous *Munk's Roll 4*: 201-3; Anonymous *Lancet* 1907, **i**: 1530-4; Anonymous *BMJ* 1907, **i**: 1277-81; *Dictionary of National Biography*. (1901-1911, vol 2): 15; J. Fayrer, *Recollections of my life* (1900, Edinburgh: Blackwood): 508.

38. Op.cit. See note 1 above (Board minutes), Book 8: 56, 129, 136, 210, 257, 428, 436-7, 443, 450; Book 10: 162; Book 14: 141; Book 16: 157.

39. Ibid: Book 2: 335-6, 378, 299; Book 3: 315-6.

40. Ibid: Book 4: 48-9, 63-5, 293, 372; Book 6: 478; Book 7: 11, 230.

41. Ibid. Book 15: 372, 383-4, 394, 415.

42. Ibid. Book 27: 248, 252-3, 274.

43. Robert Koch (1843-1910) was one of the founders of the 'germ theory' of disease. His first bacterial work was on anthrax, and he began his widely known work on tuberculosis in 1881; the following year he demonstrated *Mycobacterium tuberculosis*. He also discovered the causative agents of diphtheria and cholera.

44. Op.cit. See note 1 above (Board minutes), Book 17: 263-4; Book 20: 78; Book 24: 58; G.A. Rooke, J.L. Stanford, 'The Koch phenomenon and the immunopathology of tuberculosis', *Curr Top Microbiol Immunol*. 1996, 215, 239-62. *See also: Times, Lond*. 1912, October.

45. Op.cit. See note 1 above (Board minutes), Book 8: 431, 440, 446, 453; Book 11: 238, 245,

46. Ibid. Book 18: 456.

47. Ibid. Book 24: 387.

48. Ibid. Book 18: 34.

CHAPTER 6

Advice from Florence Nightingale, and others, on the proposed new hospital at Coulsdon, Surrey – in 1861

THE READER SHOULD be left in no doubt: it was Reed's intention (since 1854) to provide a definitive site for the RHI at Coulsdon (South of Croydon), in close proximity to the 'fatherless' asylum. So confident was he of achieving his ambition that he sought the views of several of the most eminent authorities on hospital design. Therefore (the Secretary) Andrew wrote to (amongst others) Florence Nightingale (1820-1910) [fig 6.1] and T. Roger Smith (1830-1903), an eminent hospital architect.[1] Unfortunately for Reed, there were, amongst the Board of Directors, several who were totally opposed to the Coulsdon site – as we shall see in Chapter 7.

In the mid-nineteenth century, the miasmatic theory concerning the transmission of infection still held sway; although opposed by the contagionists, this theory held that bad air was the vehicle by which most diseases were conveyed. It was not until much later in the century that the 'germ-theory' of disease became widely (but not universally) accepted – largely as a result of researches by Louis Pasteur (1822-95) in France, Robert Koch (1843-1910) in Germany, and Joseph (later Lord) Lister (1827-1912) in Britain. Thus satisfactory sanitation and ventilation in hospitals was deemed of paramount importance in the *prevention* of disease.[2]

Florence Nightingale had, at the time of the correspondence cited in this chapter, been back in England for about five years after her much-publicised spell at the Barrack Hospital, Scutari, during the Crimean War (1854-56). She was (and remained all of her life) a miasmatist. Whilst in Turkey, she had been faced with enormous morbidity and mortality, which she later appreciated (due largely to the interpretation of mortality rates by William Farr, an eminent statistician)[3] had been caused by the appalling hygiene/sanitation in her hospital. Realisation of this possibly had an adverse effect on her health which affected her thereafter.[4] Although best known for her activities in nurse-training (Sidney Herbert [later first Baron Herbert of Lea – 1810-61] had founded the Nightingale Fund for nurse-training during her sojourn in Turkey – when she was held in very high public esteem and possessed the 'lady of the lamp' image), her major interests from then onwards were centred on hospital design, ventilation and sanitation dominating the scenario. In particular, she

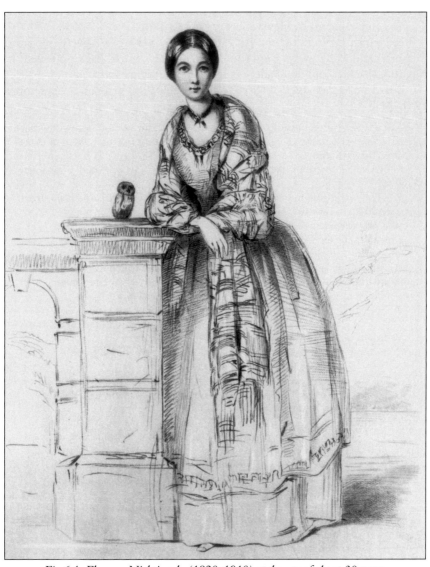

*Fig 6.1: Florence Nightingale (1820-1910) at the age of about 30 years.
Lithograph by Athena F. Hall after a sketch by her sister Parthenope (later Lady Verney)
(reproduced by permission of the Wellcome Library, London).*

became totally opposed to the corridor plan; and was a very strong advocate of the 'pavilion plan' – which was by no means her invention, but which achieved its zenith with the building of the *new* St Thomas's Hospital, on the southern Thames embankment by Henry Currey (1820-1900).[5]

Reed's plan for building the RHI in a country setting, relatively free from miasmas and well away from the 'Great Wen', must have appealed to Nightingale. In a reply to Andrew's letter of 26 August (written on behalf of the Board of Management), she wrote (from Hampstead) on 4 September 1861.* [Fig 6.2]

> … To answer your questions first, i.e. as well as I can without knowing your selected site – upon the character of which, of course, every requirement of cubic space &c must depend.
>
> 1. "A single room for <u>one</u> Patient" cannot have less that 2500 cub. ft. or about 150 sq. ft.
>
> 2.3 For every Patient, where the No. exceeds 8, I should give 1500 cub. ft. or about 100 sq. ft. It matters not whether they have a "day-room" or not.
>
> 4. For "day-rooms" 600 cub. ft. for each Patient or about 50 sq. ft.
>
> I regret to see the word "Corridor" used. A "Corridor", if it means a long room with windows on one side, can rarely be kept healthy.
>
> As you do <u>not</u> "include" the "list" of "maladies" under which the Patients suffer nor any indication of the proposed site, (which however I take for granted is in the country as it ought to be,) I can but add a few general hints.
>
> 1. <u>Superficial area signifies a great deal more than cubic space.</u>
>   Indeed a height of above 17 ft is actually, in my opinion prejudicial. But a height under [?] ft. ~~must not be either~~ is certainly so.
> 2. In a <u>very</u> airy site, the "1500" c^c=ft" I prescribe might be lowered to 1200 c^c=ft. <u>But only in large wards.</u>
> 3. All the wards & day rooms should be ventilated & warmed on the new principales [sic] of the "Barrack & Hospital" Improvement Commission.
> 4. Of course it is not intended that <u>any one</u> at all should sleep in the Day Rooms.
> 5. I have given my reasons (in all my published books) for objecting to "wards of from 3-8 beds" & for preferring "wards of from 20-32 beds". Privacy does not extend beyond the bed on each side the Patient [sic]. And if he has one bed on each side of him, he may as well have ten.
>
>   Whereas Nursing, in any sense of the word, is impossible in the smaller wards, women fit to be Head Nurses are not, alas, so common. And one such can easily over=look 32 beds in the same ward – cannot possibly overlook them in "wards of from 3-8 beds".
>
>   In like manner, I would only assign single rooms to "noisy" or "offensive" Patients or to such as require absolute quiet and a <u>constant</u> watcher.
>
>   I do not presume to say more. Because I do not know the characters of your Patients – nor your requirements.

---

*(fig 6.2) These two unpublished letters were 'discovered' amongst some 'old minutes' by the Secretary (Brig. R.M. Villiers) in 1953 (*Board Minutes*. Book 27: 468).

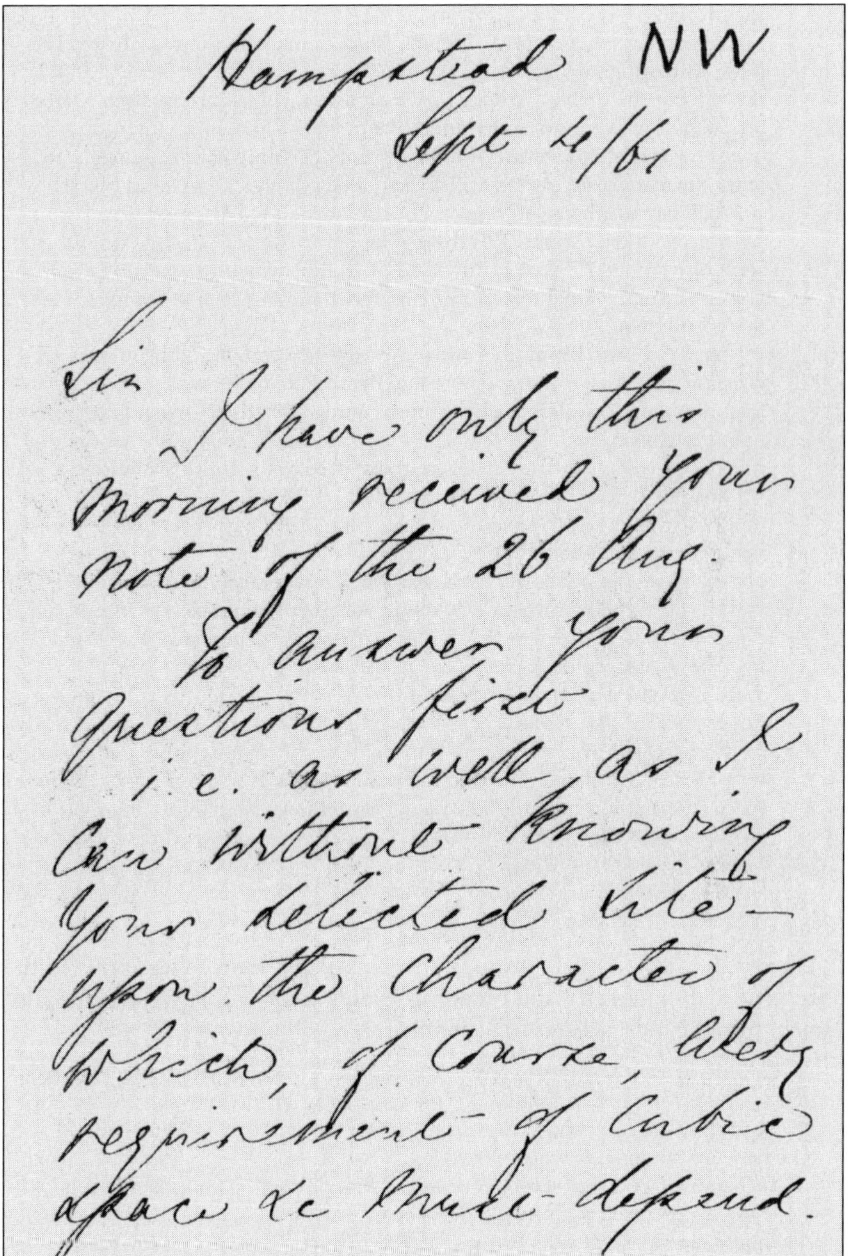

Hampstead NW
Sept 4/61

Sir
 I have only this
morning received your
note of the 26 Aug.
 To answer your
questions first
 i.e. as well as I
can without knowing
your selected site —
upon the character of
which, of course, likely
requirement of Cubic
space &c must depend.

Fig. 6.2: First page of Florence Nightingale's letter to Andrew (Secretary of the RHI) dated 4 September 1861.

I will only add:

1. I have had large experience among both Patients who go into Hospital & those who ordinarily do not.

2. Among the "Incurables" whom I have nursed, there has always been a large proportion who required that kind of nursing which, in my opinion, can only be given in large wards – & who would certainly have been neglected in the smaller wards, each of which cannot be put under one Head Nurse.

   I shall be most happy to render any assistance in looking over plans, or in answering any questions. But it must be before the 12th of this month, or after November 1st. And in my state of health, which may terminate my power of work at any moment, you are much more certain of having me ~~aft~~ this month than in November.

   I shall be very happy to contribute towards your building if it is on principles conducive, in my opinion, to the welfare of the sick.

3. In some <u>new</u> Convalescent Institutions abroad, wards of 3 or 4 have been found to answer, with Day & Exercise Rooms. But as soon as the Convalescents became <u>Patients</u> they had to be transferred to the Infirmary Wards.

   I imagine that some of your "Incurables" are like the "Convalescents", in the sense that they don't require the Nursing of <u>Patients</u>. For such I should not object to the 3-bed wards & should think 3 or 4 better than 8 bed-wards. For such I should not object to single rooms, except on account of expence.

   But, for those who require <u>Nursing</u>, whether "Incurables", Operations, Accidents, or "Sick", every year only confirms my experience that from 20 to 32 bed wards are the best.

4. The material of your Walls & Ceilings & of your floors is of immense importance.

5. As a <u>general</u> rule, Hospl^s cut up into small wards, require more cub. space than Hospl^s with large wards. In a certain sense, a Patient profits by all the space (the air) in his ward. E.g. An "offensive" case does more mischief in an 8-bed ward than in a 32-bed ward. Popularly, it is supposed to be just the reverse.

   Yours faithfully,
   Florence Nightingale[6]

Clearly, Andrew replied promptly to this letter (enclosing some of the details she had requested), and Nightingale duly wrote a follow-up letter (also written from Hampstead) on 10 September:

… The list of Patients you have enclosed rather confirms me in what I have stated – but is too small in number for me to come to any definite conclusion.

I should require to know the numbers for whom you intend to build – whether equal for men & women &c &c –

One curious fact comes out of your list of "Candidates". "As Home Patients" – that there are two men to thirty women.

I should classify such cases as those in the List into one large & several small wards. But, as I say, the numbers are too few to judge.

It is certainly impossible to put an Aneurism of the Aorta into the same ward with an Epilepsy case.

I am not aware whether your "Outpatients" tally with what we call "Out Patients" at General Hospitals, or whether they are cases waiting to come in.

I think the List bears out the remarks I have made, on the whole – and shews that more than ordinary care is requisite in arranging the details of the plans.

If you desire me to look at them, I should prefer seeing the rough draft plans first, in order to avoid expensive alterations afterwards.

Your site is well chosen. The gravelly soil about Croydon is good. But it requires to be very carefully drained & for your Hospital to be well raised ...[7]

A letter from Nightingale (presumably one of those transcribed above), on the question of space, was read to a Board meeting on 12 September 1861.

T. Roger Smith FRIBA also responded to a letter (the first page of which is missing) from Andrew (also written on behalf of the Board of Management), and offered this advice:

... provide about 1200 cubic feet of space for each person expected to occupy the same.

The best written authorities are, I believe Miss Nightingale's "Notes on Hospitals" and the recently published "Report of the Commission appointed for improving the Sanitary condition of Barracks and Hospitals".

The medical staffs of the Middlesex and King's College Hospital have also paid attention to the subject. I would further suggest that you could do well to apply to the authorities of the Consumption Hospital [*Hospital for Consumption and Diseases of the Chest, Brompton, which had been founded in 1841*]. ... of fresh air – but it is <u>impossible</u> to obtain such a supply without injurious drafts should ample cubic space not be provided.

I need not add that the ~~suggested~~ amount of space here suggested would require a very much larger superficial area than nine square feet by day and twenty five square "feet by night" as specified on P. 2 of the printed instructions.

I trust the committee will not think it obtrusive if I suggest that on this point the best living authority without doubt is Miss Nightingale and that her opinion and that of the two eminent men who framed the Sanitary Commission in the Crimea – Dr Sutherland and Mr Robert Rawlinson ought to be asked if the Committee feel in any doubt.

I shall be very much obliged if you will forward me the plan and sections of the ground. It will be possible, if I am furnished with that to make some progress with my design while awaiting the decision of the Committee as to the actual size of wards.

I am Sir

Your ob[t] servant

T. Roger Smith[8]

There was thus at this time great concern about the volume of air available to each patient. Figures for four *general* hospitals in London in 1869 provide comparative statistics. At University College, St Mary's, the Middlesex and St George's Hospitals, the figures given were 1300 (approx), 1400->2000 (approx), <1481 (average 1014), and 1000 cu.ft. per bed, respectively. It was claimed that at the latter institution the figure would be up to 2000 cu.ft. per bed in the new wards.[9]

In the light of the comments of Nightingale and Smith, the Building Committee's recommendation was that: '1,000 cubic ft. should be allowed for bed-room, and 400 for day-room accommodation, for each patient.' And on 24 October 1861 the Board resolved: 'That the designs for the New Hospital be not exhibited till the Board have fully considered them.' A meeting was especially summoned for 'the inspection of the drawings' on 26 November.[10]

At a Board meeting in January 1862, a letter was read from H. Bonham Carter, Esq., Secretary of the Nightingale Fund: 'Miss Nightingale was willing to examine the rough drawings of the selected plans, before their final settlement, although her health would not allow of her doing so at present.'[11]

References and Notes

  1. **Florence Nightingale** OM (1820-1910) became in her lifetime the doyen of the nursing profession. Soon after the outbreak of the Crimean war, she accepted an invitation from Sidney Herbert (Secretary for War) to take a group of nurses to Scutari. Although she revolutionised conditions at the Barrack Hospital, the morbidity and mortality rates remained exceptionally high. On return to England she took a great interest in hospital design, and became the figurehead of the School of Nursing at St Thomas's Hospital London. *See also:* E.T. Cook. *The life of Florence Nightingale* (2 vols) (London, Macmillan & Co. 1913), 507 & 510; Z. Cope, *Florence Nightingale and the doctors* (London: Museum Press 1958) 163; F.B. Smith, *Florence Nightingale: reputation and power* (London: Croom Helm 1982) 216; W.J. Bishop, S. Goldie, *A bio-bibliography of Florence Nightingale*, (London: Dawsons of Pall Mall 1962): 160; C. Woodham-Smith, *Florence Nightingale 1820-1910* (London: Constable 1982) 615; S.M. Goldie (ed) *'I have done my duty': Florence Nightingale in the Crimean War 1854-1856* (Manchester: Manchester University Press 1987) 326; H. Small, *Florence Nightingale: avenging angel* (London: Constable 1998) 221; B.M. Dossey, *Florence Nightingale: mystic, visionary, healer* (Springhouse, Pennsylvania: Springhouse Corporation 1999), 440; G.C. Cook, A.J. Webb, 'Reactions from the medical and nursing professions to Nightingale's "reforms" of nurse training in the late 19th century', *Postgrad Med J* 2001, 78: 118-123. **Thomas Roger Smith** FRIBA (1830-1903) was an eminent Victorian architect. He designed several hospitals, including the North London Hospital for Consumption at Hampstead (1880), The Sanatorium at Reedham (1883), and also many of the laboratories at University College London (1892). He was made district surveyor under the Metropolitan Board of Works for Southwark and North Lambeth, and later of West Wandsworth.
  2. H. Richardson (ed). 'Historical context, & General Hospitals', *English*

Hospitals 1660-1948: a survey of their architecture, and design (Swindon: Royal Commission of the Historical Monuments of England 1998): 1-43; C. Stevenson, *Medicine and magnificence: British hospital and asylum architecture, 1660-1815* (London: Yale University Press 2000): 312; G.C. Cook, 'Henry Currey (1820-1900): leading Victoria hospital architect, and early exponent of the "pavilion principle"', *Postgrad Med J* 2002, 78: 352-9.

3. **William Farr** CB, MD, FRS (1807-83) was an eminent Victorian statistician. He studied medicine in Paris, and became commissioner of the 1871 census. Farr was President of the Statistical Society in 1871 and 1872. *See also:* G.C. Cook, A.J. Webb, 'William Farr's influence on Florence Nightingale', *J. med. Biog.* 2001, 9: 122.

4. Op.cit. See note 1 above (Small).

5. **Sidney Herbert** (1810-61) was the second son of the eleventh Earl of Pembroke. He became secretary to the Board of Control (1834-5), Secretary to the Admiralty (1841-5), and War Secretary (1845-6, 1852-5, and 1859-60). He led a movement for medical reform in the army and education of officers. Herbert was created a peer in 1860; Op.cit. See note 3 above (Cook).

6. F. Nightingale to F. Andrew 4 September 1861: 13 [Royal Hospital for Neuro-disability archive]. Board minutes. Book 4: 3.

7. F. Nightingale to F. Andrew 10 September 1861: 4: Royal Hospital for Neuro-disability archive.

8. T. Roger Smith to F. Andrew 1861 [Royal Hospital for Neuro-disability archive]; F. Nightingale, *Notes on hospitals: being two papers read before the National Association for the Promotion of Social Science, at Liverpool, in October 1858 with evidence given to the Royal Commission on the state of the Army in 1857* (London: John W. Parker and Son, 1859): 108; J.J. Frederick. *Record of Recommendations regarding Sanitary Improvements in Barracks and Hospitals together with the Actual Improvements carried out during the last 50 years, 1899.* **John Sutherland** (1808-91) was educated in Edinburgh where he obtained the MD degree. He became a promoter of sanitary science, and was a close confident of Florence Nightingale. He was despatched to the Crimea by Viscount Palmerston (1784-1865) to investigate the condition of the troops there. In 1848, he was appointed an inspector under the first Board of Health. **Robert Rawlinson** Kt., KCB (1810-98) was a civil engineer, who early in his career had worked with Robert Stephenson. He became an Inspector under the Public Health Act of 1848. In 1855, he had headed the sanitary commission sent by the government to the Crimea.

9. Four letters addressed to S.K. Cook (Secretary to the Seamen's Hospital Society [SHS]). 1869: [SHS archive].

10. Board minutes. Book 4. 21, 73, 80.

11. Ibid: 126.

CHAPTER 7

Fierce controversy surrounding the Coulsdon site

As WAS MADE CLEAR in Chapter 6, Reed (the founder of the RHI) had, from the outset, a virtual obsession that the RHI should be situated at Coulsdon – in close proximity to the Reedham Orphanage (formerly the Asylum for Fatherless Children), which was one of the five Charities instigated by him (Chapter 2). However, not all of the Board of Directors agreed with him, and ultimately West Hill (Chapter 8) 'won the day' as the definitive 'home' of the institution!

In the late 1850s and early 1860s, Board meetings were dominated by the future of the Coulsdon estate, which had been purchased by the RHI in 1855 for £2,500 (Chapter 1). A minute dated January 1858 records: 'Dr Reed stated that the Assignment for the Coulsdon Estate had not been engrossed as he was anxious first to obtain Mr Moore's name as a trustee.' At the same meeting it was resolved 'That a further sum of £500 be paid towards defraying the cost of the Estate.' And in July it was resolved: 'That the Board of the New Asylum be informed in writing that [they] are prepared to complete the purchase of the Estate, and that steps be taken for the execution of the deeds.' In reply to a question from Mr Hall, 'Dr Reed explained that owing to [a] delay in obtaining the signatures of persons not in town [the deeds] were not yet in the hands of the Board.'[1] Therefore considerable delay ensued in the execution of a formal deed of conveyance.

By December of that year, searching questions were being asked (again by Hall) about 'the whole matter of the land and building' at Coulsdon (there was clearly already a great deal of unease amongst the Board members, and the overall impression was that Reed was attempting to 'steam-roller' the strategy through); however, 'after a full consideration of the value & position of the estate and the terms of the assignment' the matter was dropped for the time being. At a meeting of the Board in June the following year (1859), it was resolved 'That the state of the Coulsdon Estate is undesirable for the purposes of this Hospital [it was felt that the Coulsdon site on the bleak North Downs was unsuitable for chronic invalids], and that it is inexpedient to erect a permanent Building upon it.' As a result, in August 1859, 'The Sub-Secretary reported [to the Board] that Mr Fiennes [felt] obliged to withdraw his subscription & to relinquish his seat at the Board.'[2]

Following this, the matter was again shelved until 1860, when in February this same resolution was formally carried by the Board. Reed protested however, that the last two annual meetings (of 1858 and 59) had 'adopted a report *approving* [my italics] the site'! After a great deal of discussion, the Board considered that there should be an in-depth 're-consideration of the matter', and discussion devolved on 'the water-supply, the soil, the aspect and position of the land, the general climate, and … accessibility to visitors'. The motion was carried – 9 for, and 8 against. A month later a motion was put 'that [this] Resolution of [the] Board, … affecting the erection of a Building on the Coulsdon Estate, be rescinded'; this was defeated: 10 votes for and 19 against. And at the same meeting it was resolved unanimously, 'That a Committee be appointed to report to a special meeting of the Board, on the present position of the hospital in reference to the Coulsdon Estate, and that it consist of: Mr Jones, [Mr] Moore, Dr Reed, Mr Sherson, [Mr] Taylor, [Mr] Vining [and] Mr Alderman Wise.'[3]

The *Special* Board meeting was duly convened in April 1860 to discuss the whole future of the Coulsdon site, a matter which was to consume a huge amount of time thereafter. A report from the Committee appointed to look into the matter was presented, and it was resolved: 'That the opinion of Counsel be taken upon the legal position [difficulties were clearly envisaged] of the Charity in reference to the Coulsdon Estate the property of this institution.' An amendment was added: 'That a Committee of nine be appointed [a subsequent resolution, which was also carried, named Messrs Moore, Sherson, Taylor, Vining, Jones, Wright, Hall, Osbourne and Allen] to deal with the circumstances in which the Charity is placed in reference to the Coulsdon Estate, and to obtain legal advice to assist them and this Committee on the subject, and report to this Board at a future meeting to be held at the earliest possible period.' Both resolutions were carried!

The point at issue seems to have been that the sale of the land to the RHI had been solely on condition that it was used for the erection of a 'Hospital for Incurables and such other buildings as may be thought desirable for the purposes of that charity …'. After a great deal of discussion, which highlighted the legal problems in the conveyance document dated 14 September 1858, the following resolution was carried unanimously: 'That the Committee apply for an interview with the Board of the Asylum for Fatherless Children at their earliest convenience.' This joint meeting subsequently took place, when it was decided that 'the Warehousemen and Clerks' Schools would relieve the Hospital of the land at Coulsdon, if the Fatherless Board would grant [the necessary] licence.' In the event, there was disagreement between the 'teams' and the 'Board of the Fatherless' proved *not* particularly helpful. This left the RHI Board in a difficult position; it was the overall wish of the Committee to dispose of the Coulsdon estate but there was little or no co-operation from the 'opposing' camp.[4]

History of the RHI's involvement with the Coulsdon site

A '*Statement*' in November 1860 (presumably prepared for the Annual Meeting of that year) gave a summary of the *history* of the Coulsdon venture up to that date: '[it] is situated about four miles from Croydon, towards Brighton, [and] was purchased in 1855, as a site for the Hospital at a cost of £2500. It consists of 20 acres of hill-side land, adjoining the like quantity in part of which the home of the Fatherless Children has been erected ...'. This narrative continued: 'The Estate was originally selected by a small number of the board, at a time when the nature of the diseases from which many of the objects of the charity suffer was not and [could not] then be ascertained, and when, as is believed, it was not intended to admit persons subject to Tubercular disease [tuberculosis].' Owing to lack of funds for building purposes 'very little attention was paid to the subject, until about June 1859 [when] enquiries were made respecting its eligibility as a site for the Hospital ...'.

This matter was formalised on 30 June when a resolution was carried that '... the site of the Coulsdon Estate is undesirable for the purposes of this Hospital ...' [see above]. Following this, discussion took place and it was decided amongst other things to seek 'medical opinion'. Then in February 1860, the reasons for rejecting this site were clearly summarised:

1. The situation is too high and exposed for several classes of the Patients, especially those who suffer from pulmonary affections. One third of the House [in-] patients are afflicted with pulmonary and tubercular diseases.
2. The situation is unsheltered by Trees, the surface of the ground is irregular, and the approach to the premises steep and difficult, whilst the capacity of the patients for physical exertion is exceedingly small, they require more than ordinary facilities for out-door recreation.
3. The distance from London and Croydon is inconvenient, the means of approach expensive, and there is an absence of accommodation for the friends and relatives of the Patients who may visit them, there being no lodgings to be obtained within a distance of four miles, whilst much of the comfort of the Patients arises from the visits of their friends and relatives, and much of the success of the Hospital depends on the opportunities which Ladies and other Visitors may have in uniting with the Committee in alleviating the sufferings of that large family of *incurables* for which the Home is to be provided.

At this stage, the question (of the future of the estate) was deemed to have been settled 'unless the subscribers at their next, or some subsequent meeting should otherwise decide'. Although under serious consideration, the building of a permanent Hospital was not imminent; this site had to be disposed of in order to raise sufficient funds for a definitive venue! The Committee were of the overall opinion that 'a site of 5 or 6 acres would be ample for the wants of the Institution – that it should be in some place easily accessible from London – and near a Town or Village where accommodation for Visitors may be easily obtained – in a healthy situation [Chapter 6], as far as possible from exposure to extremes of temperature and climate – with a good supply of water – and with a level or slightly undulating surface.' It was hoped that 'a licence from the Trustees and Committee of 'the Fatherless' would enable the Trustees of the Hospital to sell the Estate.' This would [the *Statement* declared] 'avert the necessity for any application to the Court of Chancery.'[5]

Attempts to dispose of the Coulsdon Estate

A Board meeting in June 1860 had resolved 'That the Board have not taken any steps to erect a Dwelling for the inmates of the Hospital, in consequence of their decision *not* [my italics] to build on the Coulsdon Estate, and their efforts to dispose of that property *not* [my italics] having hitherto been successful.' An amendment was however, put 'That the decision of the Board not to build on the Coulsdon Estate adopted on the 9th. Feby., 1860 having been in opposition to the instructions of the General Meeting of November 30, 1859 and though carried by a majority of one was carried under protest as a question with which the Board was not competent to deal.' Although this amendment was rejected (by 4 to 7), the resolution itself was carried (8 to 3).

In early July, a complete lack of progress had been made on disposal of the Coulsdon Estate, and another *Special* meeting was arranged later that month. This resolved (the motion was put by Charles Reed): 'That having regard to the circumstance that the case presented to Mr Gifford [the RHI's Counsel], and upon which his opinion is founded, is not a fair, accurate, and complete statement of the facts of the case, – and seeing that the Special Committee, in bringing their Report, wisely abstain from recommending any further action upon so insecure a basis: – and seeing that this Board are divided upon this question: – this Board does not hesitate to declare that it will not sanction the further promotion of a course which the Fatherless Asylum are advised that they have not the legal power to assent to, and which must occasion a needless waste of money – must be injurious to the best interests of the charities, and could prove a source of regret to any persons who have instituted or occasioned it. That a subscription be now opened to defray the law costs incurred in this case up to the present time, that the members of the Board not now present be invited to contribute to the same, with a view to maintain the funds of the Royal Hospital sacred to the cause of the charity.' An amendment was put 'That insomuch as the object of the Board in referring the case to Counsel was to ascertain their exact legal position, and whilst they maintain that all essential matter has been embodied in the case referred to him, this Board, in order to put an end to all questions as to the completeness of the case

Hereby Resolves 'To submit the case to Mr. Gifford, with all the omitted minutes, quoted and referred to by Mr Reed.'

Both the amendment (9 to 5) and the substantive resolution (9 to 5) were carried. The Sub-Secretary was directed 'to draw up and submit to the Board, any minutes relating to the Coulsdon Estate not in the case, with a view to their being added to the case, and the whole referred to Mr Gifford for a fresh opinion'. This motion was carried unanimously.[6]

A difference of opinion

At another *Special* General Meeting held in November 1860 it was formally resolved (unanimously) 'that it is undesirable to adopt the Coulsdon Estate, as a site for the Hospital'; and a month later 'The Finance Committee were requested to ascertain as soon as possible the legal liabilities of the charity so far as the matter of the Coulsdon Estate was concerned.' It is clear that whilst their fundamental feelings lay in the incurables movement, a significant proportion of the Board did not approve of the Coulsdon site, and at a further meeting that month, there were a number of formal resignations.

At a Board meeting, also in November 1860 '... the Committee ... passed the following resolution "That the opinion obtained [on the Coulsdon Estate] be submitted to the Committee of Management with a recommendation that the question of abandoning the Coulsdon Estate as a site for the Hospital be submitted to the Subscribers to the Charity at the next or some subsequent General Meeting".' This resolution was adopted.[7]

A 'stormy' Annual Meeting

There was therefore a stalemate, and neither the RHI nor 'the Fatherless Asylum' were likely to win their case without legal intervention. This led to the resignation of those who did *not* support Reed and his fellow enthusiasts for the Coulsdon site; therefore the Chairman, two Vice-Presidents and nearly a dozen members of the Board, including the Treasurer, resigned.

The RHI *Annual Report* for 1860 stated: 'In respect of the Coulsdon Estate, the Board have to report that having come to a resolution that the site is not eligible for building the Hospital, they will refer the whole matter ... to a Special General Meeting ...[8]

The *sixth* Annual Meeting (and 13th election) of the RHI was held at the London Tavern on 28 November 1860. This proved to be unlike previous Annual Meetings and was dominated by matters relating to 'building upon the Coulsdon property'. Lord Raynham, who should have chaired the proceedings, was of course absent. Shortly afterwards, 'Mr Osborne, Col Cust, Mr Hall, Mr Jenkin Jones & Mr Moore, severally withdrew their names [from the Board of Management] and the meeting received their resignation.' This was followed by a series of 'Medical Testimonials', all of them *in favour* of building on the Coulsdon site; matters ranged from the quality of Coulsdon water, to the atmosphere, altitude, absence of miasmas, terrain and distance (and accessibility) from London. The contributors to these testimonials were: Professor Thomas Way (of 15 Welbeck St), George Bottomley (Surgeon to the London and Brighton Railway); Dr T. Carpenter MD (late House Surgeon to St Thomas's Hospital); Edward Westall FRCS (Surgeon of Croydon); Dr Rose (Honorary Physician to the Fatherless Asylum), another from George Bottomley (designated this time as 'Surgeon of Croydon'), and Dr W. Little MD (Physician to the Royal Hospital). Their 'testimonials' were dated from 30 June 1859 to 20 June 1860. There can be little doubt that the proceedings had been orchestrated by Andrew Reed and his supporters – all of whom remained totally in favour of building on the Coulsdon site.

The final communication at this Annual Meeting was from Mr James Bacon, QC of Lincoln's Inn, who addressed (in a letter dated 1 November 1860) the legality (or otherwise) of not using the land – which was owned by the 'Trustees of the Fatherless' – as well as by those of the RHI. Both had to agree the sale of the land. He did *not*, he continued, 'concur [with] Mr Gifford's opinion on a case laid before him on behalf of the Hospital.' 'The expenditure of money upon property by the Hospital Trustees, and the several other circumstances which took place prior to the time at which it was suggested that the site was undesirable for the purposes of the Hospital must, in my opinion, have an important bearing upon the case.' He continued, '... upon the whole I am unable to bring my mind to the conclusion that a Court of Law would order the Deed to be altered by expunging the Clauses which are now objected to.' He concluded his lengthy communication: '... I cannot forbear from by-pressing [sic] the opinion that it would prove a source of great dissatisfaction and regret to all the friends of both charities to find their benevolent intentions frustrated or impeded as they must be if a litigation should ensure, whatever may be the result of that litigation.'[9]

Formation of a 'rival' institution (the British Home for Incurables)

A further insight into the serious rift at the RHI – which resulted in the foundation of the *British Home for Incurables* (BHI) – is to be found in the following minute, some years later:

> The Secy. [of the RHI] reported that he had received a contribution of £1000 from Mr James Peek – [' a gentleman associated with Dr Andrew Reed in the institution of the Charity, in 1854' – Chapter 1], of Torquay, and presented the correspondence resulting in the gift viz 1st a letter from Mr Peek, referring to an interview he had had with the late Dr Andrew Reed two or three years prior to the formation [of the RHI] in relation to a Pension Fund for the relief of necessitous incurable persons above the pauper class, and promising £1000 to such an object. When this Charity was Instituted, Mr Peek kept his gift in

abeyance, paying the interest to the Hospital; and *at the time of the 'Split', as Mr Peek termed the rupture which led to the Institution of the British Home for Incurables* [my italics], he gave the money to that Charity.

Peek was now willing to donate £1000 in accordance with his original proposal, on the understanding that it be invested, and the interest applied to a Fund for the payment of Out Pensioners. 2nd a letter from the Secy. thanking Mr Peek for his offer, and pointing out that no separate fund for Pensioners existed, and suggesting that Mr Peek should allow the interest of his money to be applied to the general fund out of which pensioners were paid. 3rd a letter from Mr Peek, consenting to this arrangement & enclosing a cheque for £1000 – 4th letter from the Secy. of acknowledgement and thanks.[10]

Shortly after the *mass* resignation from the Board of the RHI (see above), Viscount Raynham (who had been Chairman of the RHI) chaired a meeting at the offices of the National Mercantile Life Assurance Society (27 Poultry, EC) on Thursday 21 March 1861 in order to found an Institution to be named 'The British Home for Incurables', 'for the relief of Incurable Cases of disease, accident, or deformity, subject to rules and regulations to be framed thereafter.' This was moved by Mr George Moore and seconded by Mr S. Anderson. At that meeting were a group of men (as well as Raynham) who had formerly been members of Reed's Committee at the RHI, including Osborne, Jones, Anderson, P. Wright, S. Anderson, Sherson, Moore, Vining, Hall, Taylor, Cust, and Brady; Sherson (who was replaced at the April meeting by Osborne, owing to the fact that he had accepted 'an appointment in connection with the Grand Exhibition for 1862 …') and Jones were elected Joint Honorary Secretaries, and Cust and Moore 'Treasurers to the Institution'. A nucleus for a Provisional Committee was formed at that meeting, and this ultimately consisted of 27 gentlemen who were named at the Inaugural Meeting held on 20 July at the Mansion House – with the Lord Mayor presiding. The rules and constitution were agreed and published in the first *Annual Report* (1861) of the BHI.

At that meeting also, the 4th Marquis Townshend was elected 'first President of the Institution', and nine Vice-Presidents, including the Archbishop of Canterbury (John Bird Sumner [1780-1862]), the Bishops of London and Winchester, the Lord Mayor and the Viscount Raynham MP, were also elected. The Board of Management was 27 strong. Various committees were soon set in motion; these included: General purposes, By-law, Advertising, Finance, Matron, House and furnishing, Concert, and Dinner Committees. [Table 7.1 gives details of the original physicians and surgeons of the BHI].

Obviously a building to accommodate the newly-formed Charity was an urgent priority, and the following year, Jones stated at a Board meeting that an auctioneer 'had mentioned to him that the British Orphan Asylum, Clapham

Table 7.1: Original physicians and surgeons of the British Home for Incurables (BHI)

Benjamin Guy Babington FRCP, FRS (1794-1866) was appointed Consulting Physician to the BHI in 1861. He had been educated at Charterhouse, Haileybury and Guy's Hospital. His father was William Babington FRCP, physician to Guy's Hospital, whom he followed by being elected assistant (1837) and subsequently full physician (1840-55) at that hospital. In his early days, he saw service in the Royal Navy and Indian Civil Service. An interest in organic chemistry fitted him to assist Astley Cooper and Richard Bright in their investigation of renal disease. He founded the Epidemiological Society, of which he subsequently became president. At the RCP, he was a censor and Croonian Lecturer (1841). *See also: Dictionary of National Biography* 1: 783-4; *Lancet* 1866, **i**: 445; *Munk's Roll* 4: 3-4; *Proc Med-Chir Soc* 1867: 5: 249-50; *Al Cantab* I: 106.

George Cursham FRCP (1795-1871) was appointed physician to the BHI in 1861. He had qualified with the LSA diploma in 1816, and the Paris MD degree in 1828. He was also a physician to the Hospital for Consumption, Brompton and the Female Orphans' Asylum. Cursham subsequently became a provincial inspector of anatomy. *See also: Lancet* 1871, **ii**: 489-90; *Munk's Roll* 4: 34; *Med Chir Proc* 1872, 7: 39.

Sir William Fergusson, Bt. FRCS, FRS (1808-77) was appointed consulting surgeon to the BHI in 1861. He had been educated at Lochmaben High School and Edinburgh University, where he was a pupil of the celebrated anatomist Robert Knox. Fergusson was elected surgeon to the Edinburgh Royal Dispensary (1831), and shared with James Syme the best surgical practice in Scotland. In 1840, he was appointed Professor of Surgery at Kings' College Hospital, London and did not resign until 1870. At the RCS, Fergusson was a member of Council (1861-77), vice-president (1869), president (1870) and Hunterian Orator (1871). In 1849, he was appointed Surgeon in Ordinary to Prince Albert, and in 1855 Surgeon Extraordinary to Queen Victoria; in 1867 he was elevated to Sergeant-Surgeon. He was also President of the Pathological Society (1859-60), and the BMA (1873). *See also: Dictionary of National Biography* 6: 1229-1231; *Lancet* 1877, **i**: 255-8; *BMJ* 1877, **i**: 240-2; *Plarr's Lives* **i**: 398-9; *Middlesex Hosp J* 1912, 16: 122; *Med Times Gazette* 1877, **i**: 186-9.

Shortly after its foundation, **Stephen Henry Ward** FRCP (1819-80) (*Munk's Roll* 4: 189-90; *Med Times and Gazette* 1880) joined the staff of the BHI as a physician, and **Charles Ray** MRCS (1886) (*Medical Directory* 1886: 234) as a surgeon. Ward had been educated in Hackney and the London Hospital; his principal appointments were at the *Dreadnought* Hospital Greenwich (on the third of the Seamen's Hospital Society's hospital-ships) (1859) and the City of London Hospital for Diseases of the Chest (1864). He also became president of the Hunterian Society. Ray was a graduate of St Bartholomew's Hospital; he qualified in 1836, and obtained the MD (Pisa) in 1838. The 1865 Annual Report of the BHI also includes the name of a Visiting Surgeon – **Edward Tayloe,** MRCS (?-1890); he had qualified in 1837 at University College Hospital, London (*Medical Directory* 1890; **i**: 304).

Rise, was about to be disposed of'. The 30-year unexpired lease, according to Jones, 'might be purchased for the sum of £2500 subject to a ground rent of £20 per annum'. This became the property of the BHI in early 1863 and remained the 'Home' for this Institution until the new premises were opened in 1894.[11]

The first *Annual Report* of the BHI also contained the *raison d'être* of this new institution. There were at that time, the anonymous writer recorded, 270 Hospitals and other institutions in England and Wales 'for the cure of disease'; however in England alone 80,000 people (of whom 50,000 were 'absolutely destitute') were dying annually from only three forms of *incurable* disease – 5,500 of cancer, 9,800 of 'dropsy', and 64,000 of 'tubercular diseases'.*[12] To meet this 'great and crying want' only one hospital (the RHI) existed in England and that was 'of recent date (i.e. 1854]'. But the BHI was not set up for 'fit objects for parochial relief' for which provision was made by Parish Rates and a recently formed Society to 'provide ... further aid for *Workhouse Incurables*'.

The designation of *incurable*, it stressed, is fraught with difficulty. A case of aphonia at the BHI believed by at least two medical practitioners to be incurable, subsequently recovered; the writer of the article concluded: 'What a triumph this case would have been for the "Faith Healers" *et hoc genus omne!*'[13]

Reed refuses to give up the encounter
In April of the following year, it was resolved 'That the next [crucial] meeting of the Board be held on the [Coulsdon] Estate, subject to the weather proving favorable.' A month later, Reed reported that several members of the Board (including himself) had met at the Estate and 'were of one opinion that the spot was perfectly healthy, and in every respect adopted for the erection of a dwelling for the afflicted inmates of the hospital'. Reed furthermore reported that the estate would be cleared up, the water supply investigated and plans for a building (to house 300 patients) obtained. There would be three classes of patient: '1: The decidedly bed-ridden, 2: Those less disabled for self-assistance, 3: Persons from whom it would be desirable to provide accommodation of the nature supplied by an almshouse, observing a degree of privacy and separation not required by other inmates.' This matter was referred to the Building Committee, which immediately invited the submission of designs; it was later agreed 'that the opinion of Miss Nightingale [Chapter 6] should again be sought, and that the dimensions of the Sanatorium of Bournemouth & the Victoria Park Hospital ascertained'.[14] Nightingale was clearly supportive of the proposed building in this vicinity which was free (or relatively free), in her opinion, from miasmas.

Death of Reed and a final solution at last
At a meeting on 27 February 1862 (a mere two days after the founder's death –

---

*These statistics were apparently derived from: Elliot and Cobbe. *Glasgow: social science meeting,* September 1860.

Chapter 2), Andrew (the RHI Secretary) reported to the Board that '4$\frac{1}{2}$ acres [of the Estate] had been let by the late Dr Reed from 25th March 1859 to Mr White of Croydon, at 30/- per acre, the agreement being verbal & the rent paid in advance.'[15]

It appears that Dr Reed took a somewhat dictatorial attitude as far as the RHI was concerned: it was his idea, and he would act if needs be *without* reference to the Board! It was more than a year after Reed's death that all ideas of utilising the land at Coulsdon as the definitive site for the RHI were formally brought to an end, and in August 1864, it was resolved unanimously (by the Board): 'That application be made to the Board of the Asylum for Fatherless Children for their consent to the sale of the land at Coulsdon.'

Some three months later, the necessary assurance was obtained at a further joint interview: '... the Fatherless Board will raise no unnecessary objection to the sale of the property', and at a 'Special Meeting' later that month, the Secretary opened the proceedings with this statement: 'To consider the desirability of offering the Coulsdon Property, subject to the consent of the [AGM] to the Board of the Asylum for Fatherless Children, at a price to be agreed on.' Both this and a following amendment: 'That the land at Coulsdon be offered to the Fatherless Asylum for the sum paid for it, adding thereto the amount since expended on the Estate, and interest of 5% on the purchase money and other outlay' were carried.[16]

The matter was not yet finalised, however, for the following reply was received from 'The Fatherless Board': 'That under present circumstances it is *not* [my italics] desirable to purchase the land offered by the Board of the Royal Hospital.' It was abundantly clear that the Board of the RHI was now anxious to sell the land back to the Asylum for Fatherless Children as soon as possible, for this 'would obviate any legal difficulty'. The matter was duly discussed by the Board of the Fatherless Asylum, who while fully supportive of the sale, laid down certain stringent conditions, e.g. '... that the right of way possessed by the Royal Hospital over the roadway be surrendered, – that an oak fence 7 feet high, with tenterhooks on the top, be fixed at the expense of the Royal Hospital at the foot of the embankment on the North Side of the said roadway ...'.[17]

In February 1865, the Board of the RHI resolved: 'That the whole question of the Coulsdon Property be referred to a Sub C^{ee} consisting of Messrs. Huth, Woodhouse & Woolley and that they be requested to bring up a report on the subject'. Further developments came before a Board meeting of the RHI held in August of that year when it was resolved (in the light of a letter from the Brighton Railway Co refusing to allow a roadway from the station at Caterham Junction): 'That the Coulsdon Property be put up for sale by auction ...'. And one month later, the Board resolved 'That a large board be fixed upon the property offering it for sale, or for Building purposes.'

However, at a subsequent meeting this latter strategy was totally negated and instead a motion was put 'That the Coulsdon Property be offered to the Board of the Fatherless Asylum for £2000'; this was put to the board in October and was lost 5 to 4! The whole matter was therefore put in the hands of Messrs Debenham and Tewson.[18] A notice from the South Euston Railway Co. was presented to a meeting in December 1865; this mentioned '... a cutting of 16ft. required for the enlargement of the line near the railway station'. The magnitude of this development on the sale is impossible to discern! Meanwhile, interest in the Coulsdon Estate was shown by 'the Managers of the Consumption Hospital, Brompton' (Chapter 6). At the same meeting, the Secretary was instructed to inform Debenham and Tewson that 'the price of the property was three thousand pounds'.[19]

Later, a letter which virtually clinched the issue was received from the Secretary of the Asylum for Fatherless Children and was read to the Board:

> Offices, 10 Poultry, EC.
> 3rd July 1867.

Dear Sir.

I am desired by the Board of Managers of this Institution to send you a Copy of a Resolution passed at their last meeting. 'That an offer of Two Thousand Pounds, payable in two years, be made to the Board of the Royal Hospital for the purchase of their land at Reedham [Coulsdon]'

> I am, dear Sir,
> Yours very faithfully.
> Geo. Stancliff
> Secretary.

Mr F. Andrew.

It was immediately unanimously resolved by the Board of the RHI that this offer be accepted on condition that 'payment ... be made in four half-yearly sums of £500, without interest; should any amount be left unpaid at the expiration of two years from the date of agreement to purchase, the same to bear interest at 5 per cent, the expenses of Conveyance to be shared equally by the two Charities.' The next entry regarding Coulsdon was in July 1867; the first payment (of £500) was made in March of the following year.[20]

In February 1870 'The Secy. informed the Board that the Fatherless Asylum had intimated, through their Secy. their approval of the draft conveyance ...'. And at a meeting held in March it was resolved that 'in reference to the land situated at Coulsdon, resold to the Board of the Asylum for Fatherless Children for the sum of £2000, in accordance with a minute of the 11th July, 1867, 1: The Marquis Townshend [together with 19 other gentlemen] be requested, and are hereby authorized, to convey the said piece of land to the

Trustees of the Asylum for Fatherless Children, as they shall direct or require [and] 2: That Henry Huth Esquire, The Treasurer, be requested, and is hereby directed to receive the said purchase money at sum of £2000 for and on behalf of the Royal Hospital for Incurables.'[21]

The whole saga had therefore taken over a decade to resolve. Had Dr Reed acted less peremptorily (against the wishes of several influential members of his Board), the RHI would *not* have lost over £500, the Board would have been saved a vast amount of unnecessary discussion, several major figures would have remained on the side of the RHI, and the BHI might never have been founded!

References and Notes

1. Board minutes. Book 2: 4, 81, 111.
2. Ibid: 141, 148-9, 258, 280.
3. Ibid: 386-7, 410-1.
4. Ibid. Book 3: 1-3, 7-15.
5. Ibid: 209-14.
6. Ibid. Book 3: 105-7, 125-7.
7. Ibid: 195, 225, 238, 242.
8. Ibid. Book 3: 208-9.
9. *Constitution: minutes of General meetings* 54-73. (Royal Hospital for Neuro-disability archive). *See also:* Board minutes. Book 3: 204-7.
10. Ibid: Book 11: 331-2.
11. Board minutes of the British Home for Incurables: Book 1 (21 March 1861-18 September 1863): 1-4, 59-77; *See also:* British Home for Incurables. First Annual Report of the Board of Management. 1861: 1-6, 227; J.W. Brown, 'The opening of the British Home and Hospital for Incurables, Crown Lane, Streatham Common' (Streatham: Local History Reprints): 1 and 8-22. *See also:* E. Carpenter, *Cantuar: the archbishops in their office* (London: Cassell, 1971) 300-11.
12. Op.cit. See note 11 above (British Home for Incurables Annual Report): 3.
13. G.P. Rugg. British Home for Incurables: aphonia: recovery of a supposed 'incurable'. *BMJ* 1887; **ii:** 70.
14. Op.cit. See note 1 above: Book 3: 92-3, 347-8, 359-61, 388, 415, 435.
15. Ibid. Book 4: 144.
16. Ibid. Book 5: 286, 331, 346-7.
17. Ibid: 350, 371, 397-8.
18. Ibid: 404, Book 6: 16, 16, 34-35, 44, 52-3, 53,63.
19. Ibid: 106-7, Book 7: 3.
20. Ibid: 84-5, 94-5, 283.
21. Ibid. Book 8: 235, 245 6.

CHAPTER 8

The definitive 'home' (from 1863): Melrose Hall, Putney West Hill

THE 1898-99 ANNUAL REPORT of the RHI eloquently summarises early days at Melrose Hall: '... in 1863, Melrose Hall ... rose to view, surrounded by twenty-five acres of wooded grounds, and became the property of the Institution and the future home of its inmates.' 'In that year a [north] wing was added, and in 1867 a second [south wing].' In 1879 the first stone of a 'handsome addition' was laid and this new building was opened in 1881. Accounts of Melrose Hall in the early days of the twentieth century, i.e. when the Charity was about 50 years old, and its history, have been preserved.

History of Melrose Hall
The first building on the site of the future Melrose Hall (formerly West-hill Park) is depicted in a publication of 1784; this *estate* had been carved out of John Spencer (1708-46)'s extensive park; he was Lord of the Manor of Wimbledon. G.A. Walpole included in his *The New British Traveller* a 'view of Lord Stormont's House, *near* Wandsworth *in* Surrey' (Fig 8.1). The seventh Viscount Stormont, K.T. (later the 2nd Earl of Mansfield) lived from 1727 until 1796.

The history of the *estate* can be traced back to 15 May 1759, when John Russell (1710-71) fourth Duke of Bedford, sold 41 acres of agricultural land on West Hill to Mrs Penelope Pitt – wife of George Pitt (1722[?]-1803), the Whig MP for Shaftesbury and later Dorset, who in 1776 became the first Baron Rivers, for £1,200. The *estate* was converted into parkland and Mrs Pitt had the first house (named 'West Hill') (a casino or retreat) built there out of her own personal fortune. The grounds were 'converted' by 'Capability' Brown (1716-83), and later Humphrey Repton (1752-1818), the leading Landscape Gardeners of the time, and were contiguous to the Spencer estate at Wimbledon Park. By 1784, this house had become the home of Stormont.

In 1786, however, Stormont sold the house and estate to Sir Samuel Hannay, Bt.; he, in turn disposed of it to a naturalised German, J.A. Rücker (1719-1804) on 27 June 1789. Rücker soon had the house razed to the ground, and employed Jesse Gibson of Hackney to design a *new* house on the site; this house still stands today as the *original* building (which includes the main entrance hall) of the RHI (fig 8.2). The land and property were inherited on Rücker's death, by his nephew Daniel (D.H. Rücker). Daniel married the following year, and he and his wife spent their honeymoon in Scotland –

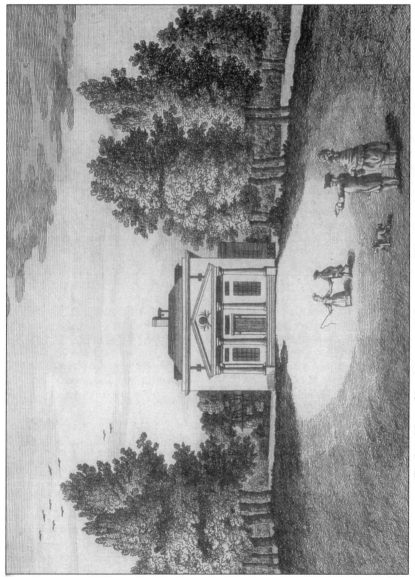

Fig 8.1: View of Lord Stormont's house near Wandsworth in Surrey in 1784.

111

where they met Sir Walter Scott (1771-1833); he apparently presented a copy of *Lay of the last Minstrel* – which had recently been published – to them. When Scott returned the visit, it is possible, but by no means certain, that Rücker decided to change the name of 'West Hill' to 'Melrose Hall' in his honour.[1] The following is a description (by an anonymous writer) of the house and grounds of West Hill whilst under the ownership of D.H. Rücker, i.e. about half a century before it was bought by the RHI:

AT the extremity of WANDSWORTH, and on the very highest part of WEST-HILL, the present mansion was erected, by the late John Anthony Rucker, Esq. From every part where it can be seen, the extensive park of Lord Spencer has a beautiful and dignified effect. The grounds of Mr. Rucker reach only to the bottom of the first valley, where a sunk fence divides it from that Nobleman's property. Though not to be compared with the park for extent, it is very spacious and picturesquely laid out: a gravel walk leads entirely round the grounds, which are near a mile in circumference, well wooded and diversified. At the South extremity, and at that part adjoining WIMBLEDON COMMON, there is an excellent supply of water, which is formed into an irregular serpentine, intersected with a small island; hence the plantation continues up to the house, in the way to which is a hermitage.

The gardens lay on the declivity of the brow, towards WANDSWORTH, below which is the farm and its appendages.

The house, from its elevated situation, may be seen for miles round, and is conspicuous from its white appearance. The fitting up, inside, is as elegant as it is possible: the walls are decorated in the modern style, with a running foliage, and subjects descriptive of the arts and sciences.

From the dining-room a very extensive view of LONDON presents itself; St. Paul's, Westminster Abbey, and the easternmost parts of the Metropolis are conspicuous. The scene on this side is closed by NUNHEAD-HILL. More to the left, and immediately below the sight, WANDSWORTH, bounded by the THAMES, on which may be seen vessels passing up and down, pleasingly terminates the prospect.

The view from the drawing-room, which is in the centre of the house, differs altogether from the former, presenting the most picturesque appearance, in which the turnings of the river, by intersecting the country, have a pleasant effect. The scene is altogether richer than the preceding one, from the woods and different objects traversing each other, without formality. The distance is closed with the hills of HAMPSTEAD and HIGHGATE. From the small drawing-room, the downs and country towards EPSOM are seen. On the ground floor, beside the above rooms, are a breakfast-parlour and correspondent room. The entrance to the house from the back-front is by a spacious hall. On the first floor are the library, billiard-room, and bed-rooms, one of which is fitted up from the manufactory of the late Mr. Rucker, when he carried on the printing business. The pattern, which is chintz, on an Indian dimity, is far superior to the shewy gewgaws of the present fashion.

The offices, stabling, &c. are in the form of a court-yard, and detached from

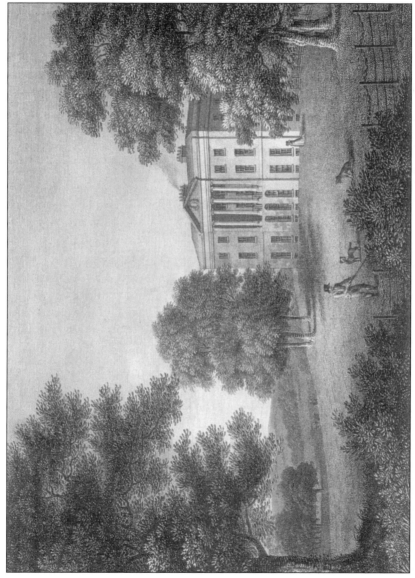

Fig 8.2: View of West Hill – the original building of the RHI – which was built in 1796.

the great house: a subterraneous passage of some length connects these buildings with the underground part of it.

WEST-HILL is six miles from HYDE-PARK CORNER, on the road to PORTSMOUTH, through KINGSTON.[2]

In 1824, falling on 'hard times financially', Rücker (junior) sold Melrose Hall (now nearly 50 years old), as well as part of the surrounding estate, to the wealthy (he had made a fortune during the Industrial Revolution), 2nd Marquess of Stafford to become the first Duke of Sutherland (1758-1833) on 28 January 1833. The deaths of two descendents of Rücker, Alderman J.M. (in 1908) and Miss Harriet (in 1932) Rücker were subsequently recorded in the local press.[3] On the day Sutherland died (19 July 1833), the 4th Earl Spencer (1798-1857), now the owner of Wimbledon Park, duly signed the conveyance documents for Melrose Hall. On Sutherland's death, the property was inherited by his son George Granville (1786-1861) who became the second Duke of Sutherland. At the relatively ripe age of 37 years Sutherland married Harriet-Elizabeth Georgiana, the daughter of the 6th Earl of Carlisle. The Duchess apparently 'increased [the fame of Melrose Hall by her] delightful receptions of the nobility and of distinguished foreigners, among whom were many of the crowned heads of Europe.'[4] In 1838, Sutherland purchased a further 38 acres from Spencer. West Hill Farm (see below) was then run to provide dairy produce for the family, and hay for the horses.

On 10 August 1842, John Augustus Beaumont (1806-86) an insurance company director and property developer, bought the Duke of Sutherland's estate (which included Melrose Hall) and in 1861, Wimbledon Park also; his intention was to develop the entire area for building; simultaneously Wandsworth as a home for the high ranking nobility came rapidly to a close! An anonymous writer during Beaumont's 'reign' recorded: 'The palatial character of the building [Melrose Hall], its commanding position, and the beauty of the surrounding scenery, covered with noble oaks of the richest foliage, have long rendered it one of the most charming of our country houses.' King George IV had himself been entertained at Melrose Hall.[5] When the Beaumonts left, the house was occupied for a short time by Lord Carysfoot.

Melrose Hall subsequently had a chequered history; in 1862, it was let briefly to the Viceroy of Egypt – Muhammed Sa'id Pasha, the founder of modern Egypt (who had visited London for the Great International Exhibition, held at South Kensington), as a palace. The Viceroy and his party (numbering 'a dozen officials and eighty slaves') were transported to Melrose Hall in cold, wet weather; the house was soon considered unfit for its envisaged purpose, and the Viceroy – but apparently not the rest of his entourage – moved out after a stay of one night only.[6]

Melrose Hall eventually becomes the home of the RHI

In June 1863, Melrose Hall became the definitive 'home' of the RHI. Amongst the 'appendages' of the house and estate were 'the Farm, the Dairy, the Baths and the Boat-house'. The precise location of Melrose Hall is given in fig 8.3.

The first mention of Melrose Hall in the RHI minutes was on 22 May 1862: 'The Secy. called attention to a mansion near Wimbledon being announced for sale in August, Melrose Hall.' On 20 August of that year, a *Special* Board Meeting was convened 'to view an Estate known as Melrose Hall, West Hill, Wandsworth'. After viewing the premises, the Board met (under the chairmanship of Huth, the Treasurer) at Putney House where a motion was put by William Woodhouse, seconded by Wickham, and carried: 'That Mr Debenham [the solicitor] be instructed to inquire the price by private contract of 1st the lots 1, 2 &3; 2nd the entire estate as advertised to be sold; the kitchen garden being, if practicable included in either case.'[7] It was then decided: 'That this meeting adjourn to 25th at the Office at three, 1st to receive a report on the inquiry as to the price of the Estate, 2nd To decide whether it be advisable to purchase the whole or any part of the Estate [and] 3rd To take measures in accordance with any Resolution that may there be passed.' At the continuation of the adjourned meeting, it was reported that 'The Agents had informed [Mr Debenham] 1st. That the price of Lots 1, 2 & 3 was 700 pounds per acre, and the mansion £7000, [and] the remaining lots were £500 per acre; the kitchen garden would probably be included at about the same rate. The timber & fixtures to be taken at a valuation. 2nd That they were willing to submit an offer of £700 per acre for Lots 1, 2 & 3 & £500 for the remainder, the mansion at the price of material, say £2000, and the timber at a valuation.' An alternative recommendation was that 'an offer be made at so much per acre for the land according to the price fixed, to include the mansion, timber, &c.'. In the event, the Board resolved: 'That no action at present be taken respecting the purchase of the Melrose Hall Estate.'[8]

Some five months later, at a meeting on 11 September, it was decided 'That the Estate at Wimbledon not having been sold by auction, a special meeting be summoned for Thursday next the 18th inst. at 12 o'clock to reconsider the propriety of purchase.' It was resolved unanimously, 'That Messrs Debenham and Tewson be authorised to offer for lots 1, 2 & 3 of the Melrose Hall Estate at the rate of £500 per acre, and £1500 for the House, Fixtures & Timber.' Towards the end of that meeting: 'It was agreed to adjourn [until] Thursday at the hour of the usual meeting, to be made special to receive the report of Messrs. Debenham & Tewson.'[9] A Board meeting a month later was told 'that the lowest offer Messrs. Chinnock & Galsworthy were willing to submit was, 1 For lots 1, 2 & 3, £1250, the timber by valuation. 2 for the whole property including the road & kitchen garden £20,000.' These were considered

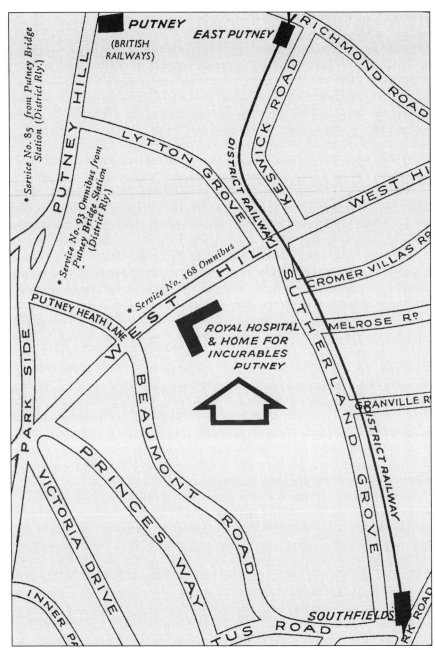

Fig 8.3: Map in the Annual Report of the RHI for 1937 – showing the location of Melrose Hall.

excessive, and the Board resolved '[that the amounts were] much higher than [they] would be justified in giving.'

But clearly the Board still had hankerings after Melrose Hall and in November, a sub-committee was set up to 'inquire further into the matter ...'. This sub-committee reported to the Board on 11 December: 'That seeing the entire Estate may be obtained on more reasonable terms ..., an offer of £500 per acre [which amounted to £15,000] be made for the whole, including the kitchen garden, buildings and timber.' Later that month the subcommittee's resolution was adopted by the Board, and it was agreed that an offer of this amount be made to Messrs Chinnock and Galsworthy. However, they replied 'that the offer was one they could not advise their client to accept.'

Still interested in this property, the Board again met at another *Special* Meeting in early January 1863, but a reply from the solicitors had not yet been received! Yet another *Special* Meeting was called a few days later when a communication had been received from Messrs. Chinnock & Galsworthy: '... the price of the whole Estate without the kitchen garden, and deducting one acre for a parsonage house, viz 26^1/$_2$ acres, was £20,000, the timber at a valuation, or a fixed price, say £500.' The proprietor, they said, was not unwilling to sell to the Hospital, provided the Board were disposed to purchase the whole property. 'The kitchen garden would be disposed of with farm buildings and adjoining lane, and if wanted would be sold at Building ground price.' In reply to this, the meeting resolved to make an offer 'not exceeding £15,000 for the 26^1/$_2$ acres ... inclusive of buildings and timber'. The assembled company later resolved 'That before making [this offer] Mr Debenham be instructed to negotiate for lots 1, 2 & 3 at a price not to exceed £10,000, the timber and buildings included.' At a Board meeting on 22 January, a letter from Chinnock & Galsworthy was read, indicating that 'they would recommend an offer of £20,000 for the estate [together with] 1 acre in Beaumont Road, value £500, the timber to be valued or taken at a specified sum. They believed that not a farthing less than this sum would be accepted.'[10]

In response, the Board resolved 'That an offer of £18,000 be made for the whole estate ... excepting one acre reserved for site of parsonage.' At another *Special* Board meeting the following month, a letter from Messrs Debenham and Tewson was read 'giving particulars of an interview with Messrs Chinnock & Galsworthy ...'. A meeting later that month resolved that '... the Board are not prepared to make the increased offer suggested in [Chinnock & Galsworthy's] letter.'[11]

By March 1863, alternative premises were *urgently* required and another sub-committee was set up with instructions to 'spend not more than £10 in advertisements'. They duly advertised for a *new* property in *The Times* and the *Builder*. In April it was minuted that: '... the efforts of the Commee to find suitable premises had been unsuccessful ...'. They had apparently viewed two other estates: one at Charlton and (the other) at Belvedere, but the Board recommended that '… the only alternative … appeared to lie in renewal of the negotiations for Melrose Hall …'.[12]

At a crucial meeting on 7 May, at which Debenham himself was present, a report indicated that a deputation had seen the Chancellor of the Exchequer on 2 May (ostensibly on the subject of the proposed taxing of Charities), but during that meeting, the Secretary 'presented a letter from Mr Debenham [it was in fact from Beaumont, but addressed to Chinnock & Galsworthy] in reference to the Melrose Hall Estate, and asked advice …'. It transpired that the letter indicated that Beaumont (the present owner of Melrose Hall) had been offered £20,000 for the house and site, to become a private residence, but that the Hospital could have the property on similar terms without any building restrictions, save 'the lot where [Holy Trinity] church stood' (which Debenham predicted would increase the value of the land by £1000).

Purchase of Melrose Hall

On 7 May the Board resolved unanimously: 'That Messrs Debenham & Tewson be instructed, … to purchase the Melrose Hall Estate on the following terms: for the Estate as advertised for sale on 27th August last, including site of proposed road, also fixtures and timber, and exclusive of one acre reserved for parsonage, the sum of Twenty Thousand pounds. The purchase to be free of conditions excepting as regards lots 2 and 4, and that in respect of these the restrictions not to exceed those mentioned in Messrs Debenham and Tewsons' letter of 17th Feby last, viz. that not more than one house be built upon each acre, the minimum value of each house to be £1500, exclusive of outbuildings. The proprietor to covenant to open a road into the Princes Road, and to give right of way therein … as the board shall have completed a road [to] access their Estate.'[13]

The completion of legal proceedings regarding the purchase of Melrose Hall (which was made on 12 June 1863) was fully documented at a Board meeting held later that month. The Board unanimously resolved that 'For the Estate … the sum of £20,000, deducting at the rate of £600 per acre for the plantation, allowing one acre, if necessary, in favour of the proprietor in making such deduction.' They also undertook to be responsible for the fencing of the Estate. The 'required sum' for the deposit was £18,000. To complete the transaction, a sum of £6000 had to be borrowed to make a total of £20,000. This left the newly appointed trustees with the task of inspecting the property and recommending repairs and alterations (see below), which was left to the Building Committee. The cost of alterations in fact amounted to £8,765.

Although it was agreed in October 1863 that the following resolution be submitted to the Annual Meeting held on 27 November 1863: 'That Melrose Hall, West Hill, Putney Heath, be the permanent Building for the purposes of the Charity – that the land at Coulsdon (subject to the concurrence of the Vendors) be sold, and the proceeds of the sale, with the amount of the Building Fund, be appropriated to the purposes of the new building, the option being given to those who subscribed to that Fund specially for a Building at Coulsdon of having their subscriptions returned and the votes arising from them forfeited'; at a meeting later that month, this motion was however withdrawn![14] Instead, in February 1864, the following resolution was passed unanimously: 'That this Commee recommend to the Board that in order to mark the fortunate circumstances of the acquisition of Melrose Hall, and in anticipation of the benefits arising to the Hospital and its Inmates upon the completion of the New [north] Wing [already under construction] the laying of the First Stone be attended with a fitting ceremonial, to be of a private character, and that Mrs Henry Huth [wife of the Treasurer] be invited to perform the ceremony.' This, she agreed to do.[15]

This wing adjoined the 'original' building. In May 1864, disquiet was registered by the Building Committee concerning the use of brick of a very inferior quality' for the building of the 'New Wing to Melrose Hall'. However, they were later deemed satisfactory by the Building Committee.[16]

After these lengthy negotiations, the Melrose Estate and the first extension to the house thus became the property of the RHI, and in June 1864, the female patients were moved from Putney House into Melrose Hall; in the summer of the following year the men followed.[17] In 1871, the Parsonage site (1½ acres) was also acquired by the RHI. Sadly, Reed did not live to see the definitive site of his fifth 'brainchild' as he had died in 1862.

A *Special* Board meeting was convened in June to consider 'an offer for a piece of land adjoining the Church at West Hill, and adjacent to the Hospital grounds.' It was agreed to purchase this for £1460 'to include the fencing next the road, and new trees planted all along & trenching two borders 6 ft wide and 2 ft 6 in. deep.' The condition(s) of the purchase included a proviso: 'That the Hospital [was] not to allow the land to be built upon anywhere for a period of 10 years under a penalty of £1200; and after that time to allow only one Villa Residence of the value of £2300, without stabling, which if built be of the value of £300. The said Villa not to be used for the purpose of any trade or profession, under a penalty of £1200.' The Board agreed to this purchase with certain modifications, and the transaction was completed the following month. In September: 'In accordance with a recommendation of the House C^{ee} an expenditure of £45 for clearing and trenching the piece of land ... and for removing and repairing the oak fence, was agreed to' by the Board.[18]

Alterations and a second extension

On 25 July 1867 'The First Stone of [another] New Wing [to the south of the 'original' building] was reported to have been laid on the 10th inst. by Lady

Elcho, according to arrangements'. This wing adjoined the Rücker building to the south. A minute in November of that year states (in an article for the subscribers): 'The building is now far advanced towards completion, and will shortly be finished, then there will be prepared for the benefits of the helpless sufferers for all time a house worthy of the philantrophy [sic] of the age.' The architect of both extensions was W.P. Griffith. It was agreed in October 1868 'to summon a *Special* Meeting of the Board on the 14th to receive [this] New Wing from the Contractors'.[19] Owing to the fact that Queen Victoria was unwilling to become Patron (see Chapter 9), the Board considered 'that it would not be fitting … to put up the Royal Arms on the pediment of the New Wing, as originally designed.[20]

With the Coulsdon property now duly sold, it was possible to pay the builders (Simms and Martin) £800, followed by £3700 'upon production of Architects certificate'. Subsequently a cheque for £1000 was also produced.[21]

On 28 January 1869 the following disturbing minute revealed: '… the Stone Work of the Roof of the New (south) Wing had been inspected, and found in a very defective Condition; it was considered that a competent person should be engaged to examine it.'[22]

Other contemporary developments
In December 1864, the Board was: 'read a letter from Mr Lee of Golden Square, informing the Board that a projected railway (North Surrey No. 2) proposed to pass immediately at the foot of grounds of Melrose Hall on an embankment 15ft. high.'[23]

The great extension of 1879-81
The matter of a 'permanent addition to the present Building' was considered by the Board in February 1878; plans were already under way to invite the Prince of Wales to 'lay the First Stone'. The architects for this enormous undertaking were Messrs Searle, Son & Hayes (of 66 Ludgate-hill, EC), and the builder, Mr Goodman (of Barnsbury). The cost of the enterprise was originally estimated at £19,988. The new building (260 feet in length) had been planned with a view to further extension in order to accommodate yet more patients at a future date. The underlying plan was to make the 'new' wing [or great extension] the eventual centre block, with its frontage on West Hill, and to build a future extension at the north-east end.

Fig 8.4 shows the *ground floor* plan of the new building. The *Basement* was to house the menservants' and porters' living rooms and dormitories; there was also to be extensive storage space, and rooms to contain 'warming apparatus', etc. The *upper floors* (which were to be approached by hydraulic lift* in addition

---

*The original lifts were worked by hand, but in 1909, electric ones were installed.

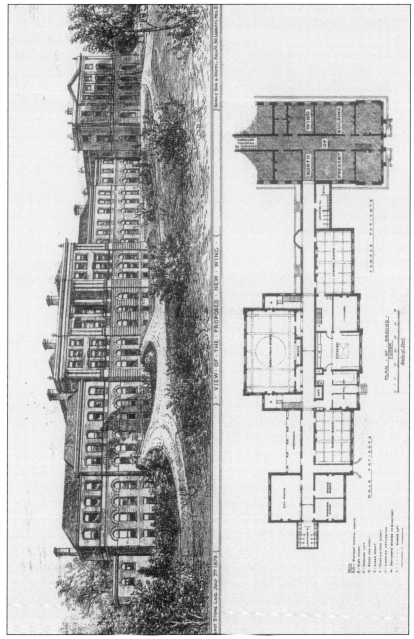

Fig 8.4: Plan of the ground floor of the great extension [Building News 1879, 37 (4 July): 8].

to 'spacious staircases') were designed to provide accommodation for about 100 *more* 'inmates'; the 'allowance [of air space] being about 100 superficial feet [per bed], and not less than 1,200 cubic feet of air space'. Warming of the new building was obviously a matter of great importance, and the Building Committee consulted with Charles Hood FRS who in turn conferred with the architects 'upon a plan of Warming the Building by Hot Water'. They also requested estimates for the cost of the work.[24]

A great deal of consideration seems to have been given to 'fire-risk' for which ample provision was given in the upper floors; in addition, all corridors were constructed of iron and concrete (with a 'finish on the surface with patent Victoria stone and red-tile borders').

Architectural options
Management affairs from early 1879 had been dominated by the urgent need for enlargement of the RHI. The hospital already had 185 'inmates', and it could have introduced a 'ceiling' at this level; however, the Board felt that an extension was the only real solution; they had rejected the idea of leasing a 'commodious house' in the vicinity. The new extension would ultimately accommodate 100 additional 'inmates', a new assembly room, dining room, kitchen and offices. It was later recommended that the Bakery be placed in the basement of the New Wing, and that the needful modifications be made in the plans. The Board were initially offered three options by the architects:

Scheme F: Capacity 285 beds: cost £12,783.
  "   H: "   312   " : cost £13,917.
  "   I: "   322   " : cost £19,061.

The first of these options was immediately rejected in the light of discussion (which objected to quadrangular spaces). Scheme J: Capacity 399 beds (men 92; women 307): cost £35,000 was also considered.

In view of the increased cost of J, the Board reverted to Scheme I; it is clear that they were opposed to going above the £20,000 limitation. In the light of this decision, the architects submitted a modified plan of Scheme J; this gave a total of 309 (71 for men and 238 for women) beds, at a cost of £20,000. They then produced an entirely new scheme (M) with a total accommodation of 350 beds, as well as a new assembly room, kitchen, offices etc., the cost of which was estimated to be £26,000. Although this was the favoured option of the Building Committee, the Board turned it down as too expensive. Yet another plan (Scheme O) was submitted by the architects in January 1879; the kitchen and assembly room were reduced in size (compared with Scheme H); the ultimate capacity would be 295 beds, and the estimated cost £18,300. The Board accepted this 'as a basis for the proposed New Wing'. Various minor modifications raised this amount by £350-£400. The architects' fees for the plans amounted to £100. The lowest tender, from the builder Mr William Goodman, (£19,988) was accepted, but the overall cost including lighting, warming, cooking, baking apparatus, hot water service, and a hydraulic lift (and, of course, the 'cost of the First Stone ceremonial') was estimated at 'not less than £25,000'. The Annual Report for 1877-8 recorded:

> The Board have under consideration ... a wing extending northward from the end of the present building next the Kingston Road, facing and running parallel to the highway. The rear will be open to the south, commanding the extensive landscape familiar to visitors of the Hospital.

In order to raise funds for the project, it was suggested that donors of £500 and £1000 to the Special Building Fund were to be given the privilege of naming a Ward in perpetuity.[25]

Having decided upon clear-cut plans for the proposed New Wing, the next step was when the first (foundation) stone should be laid.

The First Stone

The Prince of Wales KG (1841-1910) was requested to 'lay the First Stone of the New Wing' during the 'ensuing spring or summer'. In reply to the letter of invitation, Lt. Gen. Sir Dighton Probyn wrote that His Royal Highness would not undertake this role until after Easter 'in consequence of the recent bereavement'. In May, Probyn informed the Building Committee that 'HRH the Prince of Wales had consented to lay the First Stone of the New Wing on Monday 7th July next' and that it was 'highly probable' that he would be accompanied by the Princess of Wales.[26]

This set in motion the setting up of a 'Ceremonial Committee' to organise this important event. However, on Friday 20 June (only a fortnight before the proposed ceremony) the Private Secretary to the Archbishop of Canterbury (President of the RHI) called at the RHI office and informed Mr Andrew that HRH 'had received several Communications [they seem to have related to the Davis and Stringer cases – Chapter 14] in relation to the Management of the Hospital' suggesting that he should *not* carry out this engagement. His Royal Highness had therefore written to the Archbishop for advice! The overall conclusion was that 'the charges were [considered] groundless and the 'ceremonial' duly took place – not on 7th (which is inscribed on the plaque in the Assembly Room – Fig. 8.5) but 8th July.[27]

Incidentally, before the Assembly Room was available, the lady inmates had the use of what is today the library, whilst the male inmates had use of the north wing.

Their Royal Highnesses were received by the Archbishop of Canterbury, deputising for the Bishop of Rochester – who would have been present had the ceremony taken place on 7th July – who said prayers. A statement was read

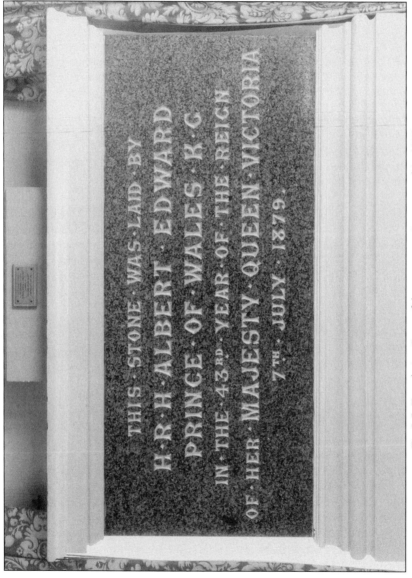

Fig 8.5: Foundation Stone of the great extension – started in 1879.

by the Chairman of the Building Committee (George Frederick White), and after a reply, HRH laid the First Stone. The Prince used a mallet (handed to him by Sir Charles Reed, MP) which had been 'used by the late Prince Consort on a similar occasion at Earlswood at Reedham in 1856 and also at the Infant Orphan Asylum in 1869'. Their Royal Highnesses then toured the Hospital, spoke to several 'inmates', and 'expressed themselves much pleased with the Institution'. It was announced that 'upwards of £9,600 [this amount was raised to £10,884 in the minutes of the Ceremonial and Building Committee], had been given as promised to the Building Fund.' 'The Morning Papers [the Board minutes record] gave excellent accounts of the Ceremonial, with the exception of the *Standard*.' The Hospital was described in *The Times* to be '... on the side of a hill half-way between Putney Church and Wimbledon Camp.' Their Royal Highnesses consented to their names being given 'to two Wards in the New Wing' and the Prince 'had much pleasure in becoming a Patron of the Institution'.

The ceremony was followed about a week later by a leading article in *The Times*. The tone of this was overall adulatory: 'The Prince and Princess of Wales [the writer stated], had extended to the hospital the powerful support of their patronage.' But this was followed by some comments regarding the 'method of selecting the objects of the Charity'; the writer was opposed to the voting system (Chapters 14 and 16), for 'it is by these [votes which are given in proportion to the subscriptions] that the admission of the beneficiaries is determined'. This had 'led to the establishment of agencies for canvassing and for the exchange of votes.' The 'worst result of these practices [he continued] is the difficulty which they place in the way of the really deserving poor ...'. And the leader-writer concluded with some words about the Council of the Metropolitan Hospital Sunday Fund – which, quite rightly, [he felt] did not support any 'voting charity'. This leader was followed by two letters, one drawing attention to the 'Free Ward', and the other commenting on the mode of voting, but the Council of the RHI decided to turn a 'blind eye' to this media criticism.[28]

Official opening of the great extension
The new wing was officially opened *not* by the Prince of Wales, but by his younger brother – HRH the Duke of Connaught and Strathearn KG (1850-1942) on Saturday 16 July 1881. The Prince of Wales and the Earl of Beaconsfield (Benjamin Disraeli KG (1804-81) had previously been invited to carry out the ceremony, but for various reasons both had declined.

The original day appointed for the opening ceremony was 9 July but this was later changed and arrangements for the occasion were spelled out in detail. However, this was not such a glittering occasion as the ceremony for placing the First Stone two years earlier. For that ceremony, the Heir to the Throne (to become King Edward VII on the death of Queen Victoria on 22 January 1901) had officiated.

The opening ceremony ultimately took place in the 'New Assembly Room' (used as a sitting room by the female patients), and HRH the Duke of Connaught was accompanied by the Duchess. The weather was described as beautiful. The occasion was reported in *The Times* for 18 July, when a detailed account of the Duke's speech was recorded. A 'subscription list of £5,093.10.0 headed by the Royal Visitors was announced.' For carrying out these duties, the Prince of Wales was given 20 Life Votes in the charity, and the Duke of Connaught a mere 10 Life Votes.[29] (Fig 8.6 shows the 'original' house, its first two wings, and on the left the great extension of 1879. Fig 8.7 shows the great extension about 1905.)

Some early problems

There seems to have been a great deal of discussion about the quality of the soil pipes in the new building. Instead of lead (which had been specified in the contract) iron pipes had been used.[30]

In 1881 a proposal (which was declined) was made 'to construct a path and gate from the grounds of the Hospital into those of Holy Trinity Church, so as to make a shorter and less public route for inmates in the habit of attending that church'. In 1893, the Board was keen to purchase 12 acres, known as Melrose Gardens; Messrs Debenham, Tewson & Co were requested to offer £8000 for the property, although they felt that £10,000 was a more realistic sum.

In June 1883, the Board were asked permission for a house to be built 'on the Beaumont Road frontage of a property called Ravenwood, opposite a part of the premises of Melrose Hall.' This matter, like so many contentious ones, was referred to the solicitor, William Freshfield, who wrote that his firm 'did not [possess] any power either to grant or refuse permission' for this exercise.

Drainage of Melrose Hall proved a major headache in 1905; this was a very costly problem. The Board asked the London Sanitary Protection association (LSPA) to draw up a scheme for drainage; the opinion of their engineer was given to the Board in July 1905 – the whole drainage, except that of the Restell Wing (which had only recently been completed) (see below) was 'out of repair' and £1000 needed to be spent on it. Although this report was accepted, the lowest tender was £1372, which was also accepted.

Later, the Board agreed to the 'inauguration of a building fund ... for the erection of a Paying Patients Home [Chapter 17], accommodation for the male staff, and any other building scheme proposed by the Board'.[31] A proposal that 'a Ward or Wing ... to accommodate forty men and women of the Hebrew faith [a 'Jewish wing'], in connection with this Institution' was declined by the Board.[32]

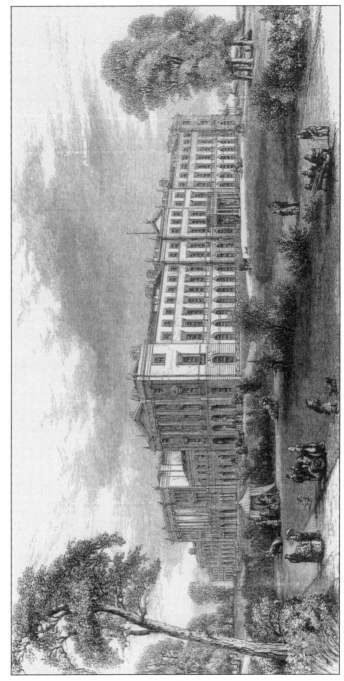

Fig 8.6: The 'original' house, its first two Wings, and (on the left) the great extension of 1879.

The Farm

The purchase of Melrose Hall in 1863 brought with it a farm situated to the south-east of the 'original' building on ground near that now occupied by Goodman House, which was kept up for some years by the RHI. It was useful in providing sustenance for the 'inmates'. There are, in the early days, several minutes referring to livestock; for example: in September 1869 '... the cows had been attacked by the foot and mouth disease, [but] were recovering', and in August 1871, the House-Committee minutes reveal 'that a Cow had been purchased for £28'. In March 1875 'it was now necessary to purchase the entire supply of food for the Cows'. Presumably the Melrose estate hay was by this time insufficient. But cows were not the only livestock; in May 1874 the Board ruled 'that the 12 sheep [which had been] purchased were approved, and that it was agreed to purchase 15 more'. In April 1876, the Board decided that 'it did not appear ... desirable to keep a Donkey [any longer]', this matter was referred to the House Committee.[33] In 1878 a 'new cow had been purchased for £30'. An interesting minute in January 1879 records: '... several Pigs had died from inflammation, and one from *typhoid fever* [my italics]. The rest, except one sow, had been killed, and the sties had been cleaned and disinfected.' And two months later, it was minuted: 'that two more pigs had died of typhoid fever.'[34]

Poultry were also kept, and they too provided a source of nutrition for the 'inmates'. In November 1879: '... an enquiry had been made into the yield of Eggs and Chickens from the Farm, which [at that time] was not regarded as satisfactory.' At the same meeting, the intention of the committee to purchase two [more] cows from Suffolk was also recorded. These were subsequently bought at £27 each, as well as 8 pigs for £10. The farm balance sheet for 1879-80 'shewed [an overall] profit of £142.17.7'. At the same meeting it was 'agreed to sell and to buy a cow'.[35]

Plans for *new* farm buildings were presented to a meeting of the Board in March 1876. These included a 'Cow-house, Piggeries, Stable, Cart-shed, Loft &c. and Gardeners' Rooms'. The estimated cost was £650 (which was accepted), or if the Gardeners' Rooms were not included, £500. Alterations were also required to the farmyard and there was a great deal of discussion on the siting of the farm buildings. The building and alterations were completed by January 1877.[36] In April 1881, the Building Committee ordered 'a plan for the New Fowl house', but the Board rejected a bid from Mr Gibbs to complete the project; his estimate was £142-00.[37]

A year later, 'the [House] C^ee recommended to the Board, on account of the nuisance arising from the cesspools, that it conduct the [farm] sewage into the main drain'. However, this strategy was not considered possible, and the assistance of the architects and also the 'professional services of Mr Dobson in dealing with the Farm Sewage' was sought.[38]

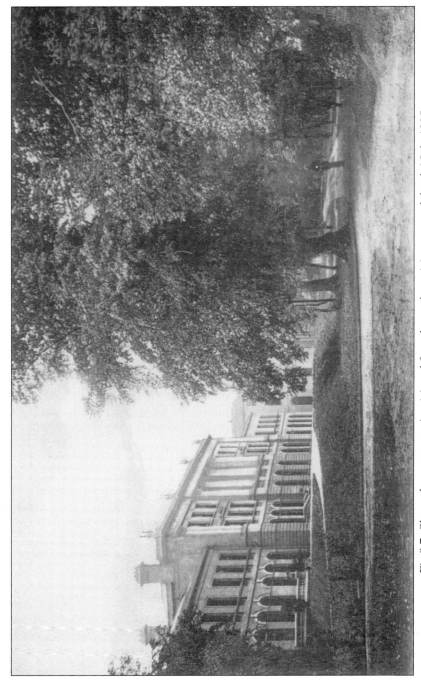

Fig 8.7: Shows the great extension (viewed from the north-east) in a postcard dated 6 July 1905.

Disease however continued to be a problem, and in October 1884: 'great mortality amongst the fowls was recorded, 82 having died.' Some five years later, a 'plan for affording shelter to the Pigsties [was] under consideration; [the] cost [was] estimated at £28.15.0.'[39]

But economics were central to the enterprise, and the Balance Sheet for the year ending 30 September 1889, for example, showed a profit of £80-2-3. In May 1890 a Board minute reads: 'Swine fever spreading amongst the Pigs; one had died; 3 more to be killed by order of the Veterinary Surgeon. Order to kill the rest except 2 sows.' Some six years later this disease again raised its 'ugly head': 'Outbreak of Swine Fever. Report of first case. Slaughter of Pigs by order of the Inspector to the Board. 49 pigs killed. The compensation would be £51.19.0 besides £3.5.2 proceeds of 3 carcases sold by the Hospital.'[40] In June of that year (1890) the following is recorded: 'A Cow removed [sic] by order of the London County Council, suffering from pleuro-pneumonia. Complaint by the Clerk to the Council of negligence in not reporting the case. Inquiry into the facts, and letter to be written to the Clerk of LCC Order for the removal of nine remaining cows.' In October 1896: 'Falling off in supply of milk from the farm [was recorded]. Agreed to reduce the number of cows kept. – Four sold. Agreement with the Dairy Supply Co. to supply not less than 20 gallons daily from 1st Novr. For one year at 9½d.'[41]

By the turn of the century, the livestock aspect of the farm was on the decline. For example, the death of yet another cow was minuted in May 1901, and it was agreed to dispose of the 'remaining two cows and letting of the field for grazing purposes'. The pig and poultry farm was ultimately given up in 1931 (see below). But at the same time, the orchard seems to have been thriving. In November 1900, for example, Mr Fowler '... kindly [made] a present of 100 fruit trees. And the Board gave an order 'for planting 150 more trees in the lower garden ground'.[42]

A 1916 update

A delightful (and well illustrated) fund-raising brochure entitled *A hospital farm in London* gives a somewhat romantic description of the RHI farm immediately after the Great War. The farmer, John Thatcher, who lived in a small cottage on the Melrose estate, had by then worked there for almost half a century! He had a staff of five or six men. His dogs guarded against poultry-thieves (and one was a rat-catcher); the farm at that time possessed 'about two hundred head of poultry'. There was also a ten-year-old 'big speckled' farm-horse whose major duty seems to have been 'drawing a heavy mowing machine across and across and again across the lawns'; the animal was also used for 'Sunday carting jobs'. In addition, there was a donkey – which went out daily 'with an invalid chair trailing behind him'.

The railed-off orchard, adjacent to the meadow contained at that time more than 1,200 young fruit trees. In addition, there were 'a few pear and plum trees, one fig-tree and a walnut tree'. A vinery produced 'about 150 lbs. of grapes a year'. The market garden yielded: rhubarb, celery, potatoes, cabbages, beans, pears, leeks, onions, turnips, vegetable-marrows, parsnips, carrots, radishes, lettuces, tomatoes and asparagus.

Some years before (the report continued), cows were kept on the farm (see above) – but milk was now supplied by a contractor, and the cow-shed was then used as an apple-store. There were about sixty pigs, including a pedigree hog, fed on 'waste food from the tables'. In addition there was a 'flock of pigeons'.

'The lawns [the anonymous writer recorded] are beautifully situated, and during the Summer months they are the scenes of garden parties and other entertainments'. The nurses used them for playing lawn-tennis, while the 'male attendants' were 'allowed a small space for a game of quoits'; there was a small bowling-green for the officers.

By the sale of pigs and hay, and the sale to the RHI of all vegetables, etc (at the current market price) the farm balance for the previous year (1915) 'showed a profit of £84.1s.4d'!

Thatcher duly retired in 1923 after 58 years service; the Board granted him a pension of £150 a year together with a 'bonus of six months' wages at his present rate'. He was replaced by John Wright.

In 1931 the Chairman (Turton Wright) informed a Board meeting that the House Committee wished to report to the Board their decision (which was accepted) to discontinue the keeping of pigs and poultry on the Hospital premises.

The vegetable farm continued, and in September 1939 (the month of the outbreak of war) the Board 'agreed to sanction an expenditure of £26 or £27 for ploughing, harrowing and dragging about five acres of the Hospital ground [for the cultivation of vegetables]'.

In 1935, grey squirrels became something of a problem on Hospital grounds, and advice was sought from the Ministry of Agriculture on the best means of exterminating them.[43]

Melrose estate: an expanding 'empire'

Although by 1881, three extensions had already been made to the 'original' house (see above), there were more to come. By then a laundry had been constructed and a dairy built in the old stables.

Another extension (Restell) – 1901-2

Under the terms of his Will, T.M. Restell, Esq. gave a legacy for another new wing at the RHI. This was at the east end of the great extension of 1879-81. The Board decided, in May 1900, 'that the architects be instructed to draw up plans' to meet the requirements. But there was obviously doubt concerning the precise nature of the proposed building, and legal advice was therefore sought. A case of 7 March 1901 was 'adjourned as it was considered necessary that the Attorney General should be present to represent the Crown'. The ultimate judgement confirmed that 'the Board could build a wing and utilize the new building for any purpose that might be useful to the Hospital ...'. And in April 1901, they were told that 'the contract should be read as £6,000 instead of £5,000'.

In June 1901, a letter from Freshfield (the Solicitor) suggested that the foundation stone for this new building (which Mrs Restell would be pleased to lay) should not be laid until the 'Contract had been signed & passed by the attorney general'. Ultimately, the date for the laying of the stone was arranged for 16 October 1901 at 3 p.m.[44] Also, in October: 'The Secretary was instructed to take ... necessary steps to secure if possible a member of the Royal Family to open [the Restell Wing] in July.' Neither the King (Edward VII) nor the Prince of Wales was able to perform the ceremony. It was then 'resolved to ask the President ... if it was possible to obtain the Prince of Wales if the opening was deferred to September or October'. Failing that, the Duchess of Fife might be invited to perform the function. It was later suggested that HRH Princess Christian might undertake this, and in May 1902 it was announced that she would indeed be pleased to perform the ceremony 'towards the end of October'. The date was subsequently fixed for 30 October 1902, when the Bishop of Southwark would also be present.[45]

The Times recorded (on 31 October): '[HRH] Princess Christian ... visited the [RHI], Putney-heath [where she was received by Lord Northampton, president of the hospital], yesterday afternoon, for the purpose of formally declaring open a new wing of the hospital ... This entirely new wing, which has cost about £8,300 ... will accommodate about 20 patients [and] is to be known as the "W. & T. Restell Wing".' The party was '... conducted to the assembly room, where prayer was offered by the Bishop of Southwark.'[46]

The De Lancey Lowe bequest

The De Lancey Lowe room which is a multi-purpose room, situated to the south of the great extension of 1879, and which forms a dominant feature of the present building, was added in 1909, i.e. 29 years after Lowe's death. This, and the Andrew Day room (named after the first secretary of the RHI), are spacious rooms used daily by the patients. The De Lancey Lowe room was built originally as a ladies' sitting room, through the Will of Mrs Lowe (at the time of her death, Mrs Waldo-Sibthorpe) in memory of her first husband, Edward De Lancey Lowe, who had died in 1880. It was first suggested in 1908 that 'the new Day Room which it is proposed to build at the Hospital should be called "The De Lancey Lowe Room"; the architect was therefore instructed to ensure that these words were suitably inscribed on a stone, the position of which should be agreed upon at the next Board Meeting.'

Edward William Howe De Lancey Lowe (1820-80) had had a very distinguished military career in India. He was the youngest son of Lieutenant General Sir Hudson Lowe (see below) and his wife Susan, the daughter of Stephen de Lancey, sister of Sir William Howe de Lancey, and widow of Colonel William Johnson. Born at St Helena, he was educated at the Royal Military College Sandhurst. In May 1837, he was appointed ensign in the 32nd foot (later, the Cornwall Light Infantry); he was subsequently promoted, respectively, to lieutenant (1841), captain (1845), major (1857) and lieutenant-colonel (1858). Lowe served with this regiment in the Second Sikh war (1848-9) and also at the outbreak of the Indian mutiny at Lucknow, in 1857; in May 1857, he and his company were dispatched to Cawnpore. When Inglis assumed the chief command (on Sir Henry Lawrence's death), Lowe took command (which he held throughout the defence of the Lucknow residency) of the 32nd. Later that year, after the second relief by Colin Campbell, Lowe commanded the 32nd both at the defeat of the Gwalior rebels at Cawnpore, and also during the campaign at Oude the following year. He later commanded the 2nd battalion 21st Royal North British Fusiliers, and the 86th Royal County Down regiment. Lowe retired on half-pay in 1872. In 1877, he was promoted to the rank of major-general. His wife was Anne Louisa Russell, the daughter of Maurice Peter Moore FSA (1809-66) a solicitor. There are portraits of both Lowe and his wife in the De Lancey Lowe room at the Hospital today (Figs 8.8 and 8.9).[47]

Edward Lowe was the son of an even more distinguished father – Sir Hudson Lowe KCB, GCMG (1769-1844), who had served, following an impressive army career, as governor of St Helena (which was at that time a possession of the East India Company) from 1815 until 1821, i.e. during Napoleon's captivity there. His father had been an army surgeon, who ultimately became assistant inspector of hospitals and subsequently head of the medical department at Gibraltar. He was the first officer to bring to England (on 9 April 1814) news of Napoleon Bonaparte's abdication, having apparently ridden a perilous journey from Paris to Calais. He was governor of St Helena when Napoleon died there on 5 May 1821; one theory is that Napoleon's death was due to arsenic poisoning, in which Lowe was involved; taking available historical evidence into consideration, this theory however seems unlikely. Although appointed governor of Antigua in 1823, he soon resigned on 'domestic grounds'; following this he was appointed (until 1828) to the staff in Ceylon [now Sri Lanka] and in 1831, he returned finally to England.[48]

Later extensions

In 1892, a new laundry was added, and in 1930 the dining rooms were

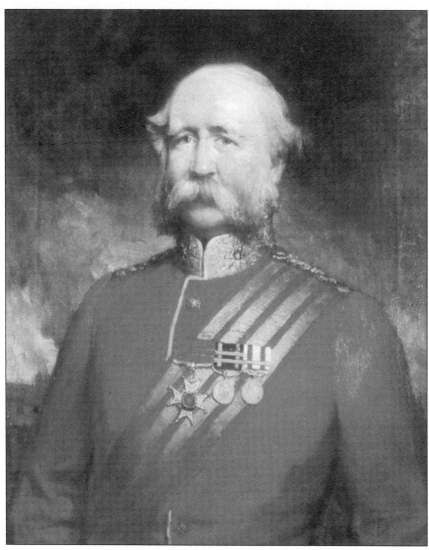

Fig 8.8: Portrait of Major-General E.W. de Lancey Lowe, CB (1820-80) – in the de Lancey Lowe Room at the RHN. He was the younger son of Sir Hudson Lowe (1769-1844).

extended outwards, towards the road; at the same time the men's dining room was enlarged and merged into that of the ladies'. During the twentieth century several other extensions have been added. These will be referred to in Chapter 18.

Insurance and rates at Melrose Hall and the Wimbledon Common Tax

Insurance of the hospital premises was obviously important. In 1870, insurance cover was as follows: '... on the Centre £8,000, and upon each Wing £6,000'; the 'Dairy [was also insured] for £150 and the Fowl House for £50.'

There was a move afoot also in 1870 to preserve the common land used by the public – principally for grazing, and as a source of firewood – of Wimbledon and Putney Commons. This belonged to Earl Spencer, the Lord of the Manor of Wimbledon. In January 1871 therefore: '... a Bill (which eventually received the Royal assent) was in preparation to be submitted to Parliament for the purpose of [conserving] Wimbledon Common'; this was of course in the neighbourhood of the Hospital. The interest of the Lord of the Manor, estimated at £1250 a year, had to be purchased. This meant that Spencer was to receive an annuity of this amount in perpetuity, and that was done by a rate levied upon the adjacent proprietors, of which the hospital was one. Du Cane (a member of the Board) asked for their support, and 'to sign a petition in its favour'. This, according to 'the agent of the solicitor for the Bill' would amount to 'an annual rate of 6^D in the pound'. A subsequent minute from the House Committee (endorsed by the Board) stated: '... it was considered advisable that the Board should refrain from taking part in any measure to aid or oppose the Bill.' However, it was later agreed by the Board 'that a request be addressed to [Sir] Charles Reed Esq. M.P., asking the favour of his proposing, in Committee, that the Hospital be exempted from the tax to be levied under the provisions of the Bill.' The Board subsequently appealed against this tax, and it was later agreed to 'engage Counsel to represent the Hospital'.[49]

Possibility of selling Melrose Hall

In March 1951 the question of the 'sale of part or all of the [Hospital] premises' was discussed by the Board. Alderman (later Sir Cyril) Black considered, however, in a letter, that to sell the entire property and move elsewhere would be neither practicable nor desirable; further, 'he did not consider it would be easy to dispose of a part of the land at a reasonable figure.' Whilst agreeing with these views, Sir Gerald Lenanton (another Board member) 'agreed that the legal position of the Home, in the light of the Town & Country Planning Act and the zoning schemes now being prepared, should be clarified.' In May, the Board 'decided to ask the Solicitors to object to the proposal to zone the Homes' property for hospital purposes only, [because] at

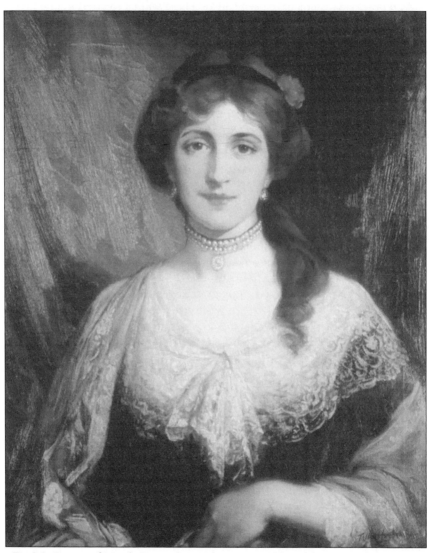

Fig 8.9: Portrait of Mrs de Lancey Lowe (later Mrs Waldo-Sibthorpe) – whose bequest allowed the de Lancey Lowe Room to be erected – in memory of her first husband. (RHN archive)

some future date the Board might wish to sell or develop part or whole of the estate.'

In response to a letter received from the London County Council (LCC) the Board agreed 'to take the advice of Weatherall, Green & Smith as to the value of the property and the LCC's powers and intentions'. A further letter from Black advised 'against the sale of any portion of the property'. That seems to have been the end of the matter![50]

References and Notes

1. Anonymous, 1898-99 Annual Report: 11; Anonymous, 'An abode of peace: the Royal Hospital for Incurables', *London Argus* 16 May 1902, 94-5; 'Incurable!: The Royal Hospital at Putney', *Daily Graphic* 16 February 1906; Anonymous, 'Royal Hospital for Incurables', *Wandsworth Borough News*, 1908; A.E. Stokes-Roberts, 'The original house', in: *A short history of the Royal Hospital and home for Incurables, Putney* (London: Royal Hospital and Home for Incurables 1972) 4-6; R.J. Ensing, 'West Hill: the making of a noble retreat', *Wandsworth Historian* summer 1990: 6-19. **Sir Walter Scott** (1771-1832) was a notable Scottish novelist and poet. Born and educated in Edinburgh, he is probably best known for the Waverley Novels, published in 1829-33. He latterly suffered from 'apoplexy and paralysis' and died at Abbotsford.

2. Anonymous, 'West-hill, the seat of D.H. Rücker, Esq.' *Wandsworth Borough News* (Battersea Library, London SW11 1JB).

3. Anonymous, 'Death of Alderman Rücker', *Wandsworth Borough News* 16 October 1908; Anonymous, 'Death of Miss Harriet Rücker: link with Old Wandsworth', *Wandsworth Borough News* 8 January 1932.

4. Op.cit. See note 1 above: Ensing.

5. Op.cit. See note 1 above (Stokes-Roberts).

6. D. Cumming, *Melrose Hall and the visit of the Viceroy of Egypt.* (Battersea Library, London SW11 1JB.)

7. Op.cit. See note 1 above (Stokes-Roberts); Board minutes. Book 4:210.

8. Ibid: 267-70.

9. Ibid: 278, 280-1.

10. Ibid: 290-1, 319-20, 330, 341-2, 351-2, 361-2.

11. Ibid: 390-1.

12. Ibid: 402-3, 425.

13. Ibid: 433-7.

14. Op.cit. See note 1 above (Stokes-Roberts); Op.cit. See note 7 above (Board minutes). Book 5: 13-18, 28-9, 57, 100, 107, 164.

15. Ibid: 172, 183.

16. Ibid: 13-18, 214, 226.

17. Op.cit. See note 1 above (Stokes-Roberts).

18. Op.cit. See note 1 above (Stokes-Roberts). Op.cit. See note 7 above (Board minutes), 3.
19. Op.cit. See note 7 above (Board minutes), Book 7: 417.
20. Ibid.
21. Ibid. Book 7: 86, 104, 211, 283.
22. Ibid: 491-2.
23. Ibid. Book 5: 364.
24. Ibid. Book 11: 482-3, 502-3; Book 12: 28-9, 39.
25. Ibid. Book 12: 2, 5-6, 7-8, 28-9, 30, 39, 48, 60, 70-1, 138-41, 181-2, 212, 219 220-1, 230, 241, 304, 410, 411, 481; Book 13: 133, 453.
26. Ibid. Book 12: 161, 172, 175-6, 181, 184, 240.
27. Ibid: 278-81, 304, 308-11; Book 13: 453; Anonymous, 'Royal Hospital for Incurables', *Times, Lond.* 7 July 1879: 11; Anonymous, Leading article, *Times, Lond.* 12 July 1879: 11.
28. Op.cit. See note 7 above (Board minutes), Book 12: 319-22, 354, 410-1; Anonymous, 'Visit of the Prince and Princess of Wales to Putney', *Times, Lond.* 9 July 1879: 10.
29. Op.cit. See note 7 above (Board minutes), Book 13: 108, 154, 188, 198, 267, 280-1, 293-4, 306-7, 307, 320, 372-3. *See also:* Anonymous, 'Royal Hospital for Incurables', *Times, Lond.* 1 June 1881: 12; Anonymous, 'Royal Hospital for Incurables', *Times, Lond.* 18 July 1881: 11.
30. Op.cit. See note 1 above (Board minutes): Book 14: 341-2, 350, 359-62, 369, 370.
31. Ibid. Book 13: 258-9, 272, Book 14: 194; Book 18: 323, 329, 421-2, 425-6; 436, 449; Book 23: 197, 199, 208-9, 211; Book 27: 243.
32. Ibid. Book 14: 227.
33. Ibid. Book 8: 133; Book 9: 21; Book 10: 107, 317; Book 11: 61; Book 12: 12.
34. Book 12: 229.
35. Ibid: 421, 452; Book 13: 146.
36. Ibid. Book 11: 49, 79, 92, 245.
37. Ibid. Book 13: 240.
38. Ibid: 460, 466, 467, 471.
39. Ibid. Book 14: 458; Book 16: 344.
40. Ibid. Book 17: 34; 143; Book 20: 34-5.
41. Ibid. Book 17: 153; Book 20: 188.
42. Ibid. Book 22: 220, 358.
43. Anonymous, 'Hospital Farming in London', *Hospital* 1915; 9 October. Anonymous, *A hospital farm in London* (London: Royal Hospital for Incurables, Putney Heath, 1916) 18; Anonymous, 'The Hospital Garden', *Agricultural Economist* March 1916; Anonymous, 'Fifty years a London farmer: John Thatcher's 25 acres at Putney: planted 1,040 trees', *Evening*

News 17 July 1923; Op.cit. See note 7 above (Board minutes), Book 25: 120-1, 188, 332; Book 26: 76, 84, 276, 279; Book 27: 28-9.

44. Ibid. Book 22: 91-2, 325, 332, 357, 368, 377, 405, 412.

45. Ibid: 413, 430, 463, 465, 485, 491; **HRH Princess Christian of Schleswig-Holstein** (1846-1923) was the fifth child and third daughter of Queen Victoria (1918-1901)'s nine children; *See also:* Anonymous, 'Princess Christian: funeral at Windsor: a touching incident', *Daily Telegraph* June 1923; Anonymous, 'The passing of HRH Princess Christian: The empire mourns a very gracious lady', *The African World* 16 June 1923: 276.

46. Anonymous, 'The Royal Hospital for Incurables', *Times, Lond.* 31 October 1902: 3.

47. Op.cit. See note 7 above (Board minutes). Book 23: 412; H.M. Chichester, 'Lowe, Edward William Howe De Lancey (1820-80)', in: S. Lee (ed), *Dictionary of National Biography* (London: Smith, Elder & Co. 1909); 12: 189; Anonymous, *Quarterly Review* vol 103; Anonymous, *Colburn's United Services Magazine* (1880).

48. H.M. Chichester, 'Lowe, Sir Hudson (1769-1844)' in: S. Lee (ed.) *Dictionary of National Biography*: 12, 189-193. *See also: Colburn's United Services Magazine*, April-June 1844; R.C. Seaton. *Sir Hudson Lowe and Napoleon* (London: 1893); S. Furshufvud, B. Weider, *Assassination at St Helena: the poisoning of Napoleon Bonaparte* (Vancouver: Mitchell Press 1978): 543; B. Weider, D. Hapgood, *The murder of Napoleon* (New York: Methuen 1982); M. Keynes, 'The medical health of Napoleon Bonaparte', *J med Biog* 1996, 4: 108-117; A.K. Kubba, M. Young, 'The Napoleonic cancer gene?' *J med Biog* 1999, 7: 175-181.

49. Op.cit. See note 7 above (Board minutes), Book 8: 132, 435, 440-1, 449; Book 11: 229, 238, 245, 313, 322, 343; Book 12: 47; *Wimbledon and Putney Commons conservation and Wandsworth Common conservation Bills (expense)* (London: House of Commons 15 April 1872).

50. Op.cit. See note 7 above (Board minutes), Book 27: 387-8, 395, 407.

CHAPTER 9

Difficulty in obtaining Royal Patronage, and the title of the institution

TODAY, THE HOSPITAL is fortunate in the great interest shown by several members of the Royal Family, including the Queen herself. Although the Institution had been founded as the *Royal* Hospital for Incurables, patronage from Queen Victoria (fig 9.1) was not immediately forthcoming. This was the fifth charitable foundation founded by Reed (Chapter 2), and he had seemingly had no difficulty in obtaining Royal recognition of previous ones! Reed had a highly influential contact in Prince Albert, the Prince Consort, and his untimely death (probably from typhoid) in 1861 – a mere seven years after the foundation of this Charity – must have come as a severe blow. The difficulty in obtaining Royal patronage in the early days of the Institution is well outlined in the following correspondence, some ten years *after* the foundation of the RHI. This both emphasises widespread feelings about a hospital for *Incurables* in the mid-nineteenth century, and also the enormous difficulty in establishing a *new* (unorthodox) discipline at that time, and probably today as well:

Hackney
2nd May 1864

Charles Reed, Esq.
to
Sir Charles Phipps, Esq.

Sir,

Among the private papers of my father the late Dr. Andrew Reed, is a letter from you bearing date, Osborne, July 27th 1854. and it has upon it this pencil note, 'renew the application in 10 years'.

The application was that you would be pleased to lay before Her Majesty, the Queen, the claims of the Hospital for Incurables, the last of five Charities founded by my father, and to four of which the Royal Patronage has graciously been extended.

In your reply to this application you are pleased to say that 'before her Majesty gave her name and countenance to an undertaking, a very large amount of public support should have testified to two things: first, that the Institution will meet a great public want, and secondly that it meets the public want in the right way; points upon which the general voice of society should have expressed its opinion before it would be desirable that the name of the Queen should affix the seal of her "sanction to the proposal".'

140

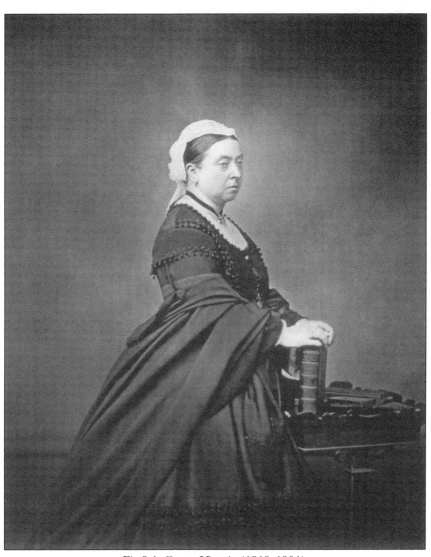

Fig 9.1: Queen Victoria (1819-1901).
Reproduced with permission from The Wellcome Library, London.

Dr. Reed's evident intention in placing this appeal in abeyance for ten years was to give ample time for the supply of this required evidence, if it could be produced and it is not too much to say that the growth and usefulness of the Charity well warrants the renewal of the application.

Dr. Reed indeed is removed from the midst of his philanthropic work [he had died in February 1862], but as his son and as one of the governing body of the Hospital, I am asked by my colleagues to discharge thus far a filial duty.

The Hospital has now been in full operation for ten years. It has received in contributions from the public upwards of £58,000. During the year 1863 it had an accession of Twelve Hundred New Subscribers.

It is held by the Physicians & Surgeons of the great Metropolitan Hospitals, to be of the greatest value.

It has at present *Ninety poor persons* (who are in receipt of small pensions for life) living in their own homes, but receiving medical advice of the best kind.

It has a Home for the Hopelessly Incurable at Putney, (Melrose Hall, a freehold lately purchased for the sum of £18,000) and here Eighty Two persons find a permanent abode, with the best care in nursing, medical skill, and food, which can be provided for them.

Prior to the year 1854 no Institution had been formed to meet the want so greatly felt and the result of the experience of ten years leads to the conclusion that within the range of the great Charities of England none within so short a period have taken so strong a hold of the best sympathies of the benevolent and good.

May I be allowed to hope that you will afford to us the help which we require to obtain the patronage of Her Majesty the Queen, so earnestly desired by the Founder and by those who succeed him.

I have the honor to be,
Sir,
Your most obedt. & Humble Servt.
Chas. Reed[1]

The reply to that plea (written two days later) is as follows:

Sir Chas. Phipps
to
Chas. Reed, Esq.
Osborne

May 4th 1864

Sir,

I have the honor to acknowledge the receipt of your letter of the 2nd May in which you remind me of a letter which I wrote in answer to an application from your respected father in 1854 – a part of which you quote.

You are perhaps not aware that about three years subsequently, in August 1857, a second application upon the same subject was made through Lord Alfred Paget to whom I stated in a private letter, the reason why I thought that that application, to which a favourable answer would not be returned had better not be made.

I enclose you a copy of the letter then sent, and for the reasons therein stated I would still recommend that no formal application should be sent for submission to the Queen.

I have the honor to be,
Sir,
Your most obedt. & humble Servt.
C.B. Phipps.

Chas. Reed, Esq.

The copy of this private letter reads as follows:

Osborne
8th Augt. 1857

My dear Alfred Paget,

I feel it difficult to answer the application of Dr. Reed to you, because I never like to have to discourage any person in a benevolent, and what they consider a good act, but the principle of an Hospital for Incurables is not considered to be a sound or advisable one.

The Establishment has none of the uses of an Hospital, it is neither curative, that is it does not take people in with a view of restoring them to Society in a sound and useful state, nor is it of any use to Medical Science by affording instruction to the Medical Men who attend in the train of the Officers of the Hospital.

In fact it is a false term to call it an Hospital, in the usual acceptance of the word, it is an Asylum. It seems also a cruel sentence upon a person to make it necessary for their admission into the Asylum that they should be certified as Incurable.

The good also that such an Institution can possibly do must be very limited. In an Hospital thousands of persons pass through the hands of the Doctors in the course of the year, they are cured, their diseases are modified, and others take their place in the Wards, or as Out Patients. In Asylums for orphans they grow to a certain age & quit the Establishment, but in this Institution when you have once filled the building with Incurables, there would remain for the rest of their lives, and all the rest of the Incurables in England would know that there is such an Establishment into which some two or three hundred may gain admission but the doors of which must then be closed unless they die off.

You can take your own means of letting Dr. Reed know that an application would not be successful, and therefore it had better not be made, as a refusal is always a discouragement.

It is necessary to be careful in making a selection from the very numerous list of those Establishments, to which the Queen should grant her Patronage, but it is never desirable that any good intentions should be discouraged.

Sincerely yours
C.B. Phipps.

Lord Alfred Paget.[2]

In April 1867 a Board minute records that: 'Colonel Herbert had presented a letter [to the House Committee] which he had received from Col. Biddulph … in answer to one which Herbert had written to him [at the 'request of the Secy. in accordance with the wish of several members of the Board'], in the hope of securing for the Charity, the patronage of the Queen'. However, the result was yet another declination![3]

Gift from the Queen
As evidence that the Queen was not fundamentally opposed to the RHI *per se*, is the following minute written in February 1868: '… the Queen [has] sent, through Dr [William] Jenner for the use of the patients, a copy of Her Majesty's Book – *Leaves from the Journal of our life in the Highlands*, and the Secy. had been desired to send a suitable acknowledgement.'[4] (See also Chapter 16.)

A Royal Title at last
In 1903, i.e. almost fifty years after the Charity had been founded and now in the reign of King Edward VII, a letter was received at the RHI from the Under Secretary of State requesting the 'date of permission for using the word "Royal" in the title'. Of course, no record could be found, and it was decided 'to see Mr Akers-Douglas [to] try and obtain the necessary permission'. In October of that year, the president was asked to 'secure H.R.H. the Prince of Wales [for the Chairmanship of the Annual Dinner, and] at the same time to express the hope that the question regarding the Title Royal might be soon settled.' The Prince however, declined the invitation because he only presided at 'the festivals of those hospitals of which he was President'.

Towards the end of that year, the following letter was received from the Under Secretary of State at the Home Office:

Whitehall
November 2nd 1903

No 108,329/11

Sir,

With reference to your letter of the 12th August last … I am directed by the Secretary of State to acquaint you, for the information of the Board, that he has had the honour to bring this matter to the notice of the King [Edward VII – 1841-1910] who has graciously been pleased to command that the Institution shall be styled 'The Royal Hospital for Incurables'.

I am Sir
Your obed^t. Ser^t.
M.D. Chalmer

The Secretary,
Royal Hospital for Incurables
West Hill. Putney Heath. S.W.

This patronage continued into the next reign; in July 1910, King George V signified his pleasure at becoming patron.[5]

A Royal Charter of Incorporation?

In December 1899, 'The attention of the Committee was drawn to a paragraph in the newspapers stating that the British Home for Incurables had obtained a Royal Charter of Incorporation under the name of the [BHHI]. Freshfield [the RHI solicitor] considered that had the Board known [that they i.e. the BHHI] intended to apply for a Charter, an objection would have been made of the appropriation by them of the name of "hospital". ... He advised that "at Putney" should be added to the style of the RHI, and that it might be advisable to obtain a Charter of Incorporation for this Hospital.' In January 1904, the Board received another letter from Messrs Freshfields stating that the cost of a draft Charter would be £500-600. On being told that 'the cost of [such a draft for] several other Institutions' was £220 or less, Freshfields 'verbally stated cost to be [only] about £300'. Col. Holland, a member of the Board, advised that at the next meeting (in February) he would therefore propose a change of solicitor. This proposal was carried by 7 votes to 1, and Messrs Farrer & Co. of 66 Lincolns Inn Fields were duly appointed 'official solicitors to the Institution' forthwith.[6]

In April 1904, Mr Rücker proposed, and Mr Carver seconded a motion, which was passed, to formally apply for a Royal Charter; Messrs Farrer 'had [by then] intimated the cost to be about £150.' Incidentally, at the same meeting, the Board decided (4 to 2) to retain the present title of the Institution, and *not* to include the word 'Home'. By September 1904, the Secretary had seen the draft charter – prepared by Farrers, and it was agreed to 'hold it over' until the Annual Meeting of 1905. In October 1905, 'the draft petition ... and Charter [were read by the Board] and subject to one or two slight alterations agreed to.' It was then proposed (by Rücker), seconded (by Dix), and resolved (5 to 3) that the word 'Home' be incorporated in the title so that it would read: Royal Hospital & Home for Incurables, Putney. 'An amendment to retain the old title was lost by 5 to 3.' Messrs Farrer were initially apparently opposed to 'the word "Home" being inserted', the reason being unclear. In retrospect, the decision to insert the word "Home" probably saved the RHHI from being taken over by the Minister of Health in 1948 (Chapter 15). In June the following year, the Board resolved that 'consideration [of the Royal Charter] be deferred until March 1907 for the Annual Meeting of that year.'[7]

There was evidently a great deal of indecision and procrastination surrounding this matter, and a letter, together with a report, regarding the 'proposed Charter of Incorporation' from Messrs. Farrer & Co, was read to the Board in February 1908; they required clarification on 'the liabilities of the Trustees of the Hospital'. In view of their comments the Board decided 'that the question of a Charter of Incorporation be not proceeded with'. Farrer & Co pointed out however, that there were certain advantages to be gained by the possession of a Charter of Incorporation; lists of London Hospitals with and without a Charter were submitted. The matter was therefore fully discussed at the June 1917 meeting of the Board, and following discussion, a motion was carried which instructed Messrs. Farrer & Co to 'put in hand an application for a Charter of Incorporation'. The details were to be thrashed out by the Solicitors, Chairman and Secretary, reviewed (and approved) by the Board, and submitted to an Annual Meeting. Also, the Board decided that special attention should be 'drawn to any alteration or amendment of the present Rules as set forth in the Constitution'.[8]

The matter was in the light of a 'rough *proof* of the Charter and Bye-laws' again discussed at a Special Board meeting in November 1917. The President (Lord Wolverton) was apparently in favour of a Charter! At this meeting 'A large number of suggested alterations were made' and a further draft was requested as soon as possible, and presented to the December meeting, when the amended draft was 'approved with one or two slight alterations'. Various minor alterations were subsequently made, and 'the Secretary was instructed to have copies printed in accordance with Farrer & Co's requirements.' At a meeting in September 1918, the Board reaffirmed its enthusiasm for a Royal Charter of Incorporation, inserting the word 'Home' in the official title of the insitution.[9]

Intervention of the British Home and Hospitals, Streatham

At this point, a temporary obstacle arose. In November 1917, a letter (dated 9 November) was read which was addressed to the Board, from the Secretary of the British Home and Hospital for Incurables (BHHI), Streatham. His Committee objected, he claimed, to the inclusion of the word 'Home' in the title, because it was felt that this was likely to cause confusion (between the two Charities), and that if the RHI went ahead 'they will feel bound ... to enter a protest against [the RHI] under the extended title'. A heated discussion took place, and the Board agreed a reply (dated 22 November) as recommended by Farrer & Co. In this the Secretary on behalf of the Board expressed the intention to proceed, and to 'apply to the Privy Council for a grant of a Charter'. A minute in June 1918 states: 'Mr North [of Farrer & Co.] informed the Board that the Home Office had intimated to his firm that the King had graciously sanctioned the change of name from "The Royal Hospital for Incurables, Putney Heath" to "The Royal Hospital and Home for Incurables, Putney Heath".' At a Special Meeting of the Board in September of that year, a Petition by the [BHHI] to the Privy Council, was read, and Arthur Farrer (of Farrer & Co.) 'expressed the opinion that he would be able to answer the arguments set forth'; he also recommended 'the best Counsel to employ in such matters'.[10]

The Royal Charter is at last granted
Despite a suggestion that a formal application for a Royal Charter of
Incorporation be further delayed, on account of the protest from the BHHI
(together with the 'inexpediency of any public dispute with another Charity')
the Board decided to proceed, and that 'Farrer & Co [be] requested to go
forward with the application for a Charter ...'. In November 1918, the Board
considered (but rejected) a suggestion from the Clerk to the Privy Council
that, in connection with the application 'this Institution shall be named "The
Royal Hospital & Putney Home for Incurables".' A further letter (dated 24
December) received by Farrer & Co. from the Clerk to the Privy Council was
read to the Board: 'I am directed by the Lords of the Council ... that the title
for the Charity now proposed by the Board, namely, "The Royal Hospital and
Home for Incurables, Putney", appears to meet the requirements of the case.'[11]
    At a Board meeting on 24 July 1919 it was announced that the Royal
Charter of Incorporation had been received from Farrer & Co. There was now
some uncertainty about 'designs for the Common Seal'. However, this was
finally selected in November when one prepared by Thomas & Sons was
chosen. Now that the Hospital had obtained a Charter, Farrer & Co.
recommended that the Hospital and *all* of its property should be transferred by
the Trustees to the Hospital as a Corporation.[12]

Royal Patrons and other regal matters

The matter of patronage has been, since the foundation of the Charity, of
immense importance to the Board (see appendix 1). Fortunately, to this day the
Hospital has always had one or more Royal patrons. The death of Queen
Victoria (who had reigned for sixty-four years) was announced at a Board
meeting on 24 January 1901; it was agreed to ask King Edward VII (who as
Prince of Wales had already been a patron for twenty-one years) to continue
his patrony – which he agreed to do. In February 1908, 'A letter was read from
the Hon. Mrs Pelham [indicating] that the Princess of Wales [1867-1953] had
kindly intimated her willingness to become a Patron of the Hospital'; she had
also presented a 'signed photograph' of herself.
    On the death of Edward VII, the president (Lord Northampton) sent
condolences via Lord Knollys, GCB on 'behalf of the Board of Management,
and the Patients of the Royal Hospital for Incurables, Putney Heath' to Queen
Alexandra and King George V (1865-1936) who was 'graciously pleased' to
become patron together with his Queen.
    The Board was subsequently informed of correspondence 'between Lady
Eva Dugdale and the [RHHI] respecting a Case in which Her Majesty the
Queen [Alexandra] is interested'. However, we do not seem to have further
information on this matter.[13]
    A later letter from the then President (Wolverton) to Princess Mary (dated

25 November 1921) congratulated her on her forthcoming marriage to the 6th Earl of Harewood, KG. And, at a meeting on 22 April 1926, the Chairman (Sir William Clerke) signed a letter of congratulations to the future Duchess of York presumably on her forthcoming marriage on 26th of that month to HRH the Duke of York (later King George VI – 1895-1952). A letter was also sent to Princess Mary inviting her to become a Patron 'in place of the late Princess Christian (1846-1923)'. She presumably declined however, because in October 1923, HRH the Duchess of York (1900-2002) was sent, and accepted, an invitation to succeed Princess Christian as a Patron.[14]

Queen Alexandra (by then the Queen Mother) who had always taken a very keen interest in the Charity died in 1925; a letter of condolence (dated 24 November 1925) was duly sent by the President, Lord Cave on behalf of the Board to Lord Stamfordham at Buckingham Palace.

On the death of King George V, the Board decided on 27 February 1936 to invite King Edward VIII (1894-1972) to become a Patron. He duly accepted and as a result received 25 honorary votes!

As recently as June 1952, the Board was informed 'that Her Majesty [Elizabeth II] had been pleased to grant Her patronage to the Hospital.[15]

Royal events
When the Charity had City offices, these provided an ideal venue for witnessing Royal events. For example, in 1911: 'The Secretary was authorised to use the Board Room for the office staff and their friends on 22 [June] inst. should no offer be received from an outside source to hire the windows [to view the Coronation procession of King George V in Ludgate Hill].'[16]

Title of the Institution
As early as 1879, some members of the Board had considered that 'the name of the Hospital was inappropriate, and that it should be changed to "Home".' (See above.) In November 1953, '… the Board approved the draft of a circular letter … to all Governors with the Annual Report, asking their views as to the desirability of changing the title of the Hospital & Home'.

Controversy at this time centred on the word 'Incurables'. The voting was:

In favour of change:	Governors:	352
	Patients:	24
		376
Against a change:	Governors:	548
	Patients:	126
		674

The Board decided in March of the following year that in view of the large majority against a change, no alteration could be made to the title of the Institution at the present time but that publicity should be given whenever possible to the controversy ... which was of public interest.

In 1964, the Finance Committee had recommended that 'Putney' be omitted from the official title of the Charity, because, it was said, this implied that 'the Hospital and Home is not a *national* [my italics] charity but [is] confined to Putney and district'. The Board however, after discussion, again felt that the title should remain unchanged.

A year later (in 1965), there was a move to drop the word *'incurables'* from the title. The general feeling of the Board was however 'to leave the title as it is unless the Board can think of a better one'; the Board hoped at that time that the *Hospital and Home* would become better known as the RHHI in the same way that BOAC (British Overseas Airways Corporation) and MCC (Marylebone Cricket Club) mean something! The Board also felt that by the retention of the word 'incurables' on application forms, there was a tendency to diminish the shock following admission, and that this would demonstrate what sort of institution was being applied to![17] In 1987, it was decided to omit the now out-dated term 'incurables', and the name was altered to *The Royal Hospital and Home, Putney*. It was not until 1995 that the name of the institution was ultimately changed to its present one – *The Royal Hospital for Neurodisability*. Thus, the term *incurables* which had formed an integral part of the title since 1854 was in latter years excluded.[18]

References and Notes

1. Board Minutes. Book 5: 219-224; C. Reed to C. Phipps 2 May 1864, [RHN archive]; **Sir Charles Beaumont Phipps** KCB (1801-66) was appointed Equerry to Queen Victoria in 1846, and Private Secretary to Prince Albert the following year. In 1849 he became Keeper of the Queen's Purse, and Treasurer to the Prince of Wales. In 1862, he became Receiver-General of the Duchy of Cornwall. Phipps had previously served in the army in which he had reached the rank of lieutenant-colonel and from 1835 to 1839, he had been steward to the vice regal household in Ireland.

2. C.B. Phipps to C. Reed 4 May 1864, [RHN archive]. **Lord Alfred Henry Paget** (1816-88) was Chief Equerry, 1846-74, and Clerk Marshal of the Royal Household, 1846-88. He was the son of the first Marquis of Anglesey, and between 1837-65 had been the liberal MP for Lichfield; C.B. Phipps to A. Paget 8 August 1857: [RHN archive].

3. Op.cit. See note 1 above (Board minutes). Book 7: 12-13. **General Sir Thomas Myddleton Biddulph** KCB, PC (1809-78) was the Keeper of Queen Victoria's privy purse from 1867. From 1851, he had been Master of the Queen's Household.

4. Op.cit. See note 1 above (Board minutes). Book 7: 265; **Sir William Jenner,** GCB, FRCP, FRS (1815-98) was physician extraordinary to Queen Victoria (from 1861), and in 1862 was appointed physician in ordinary. In 1863, he was also appointed physician to the Prince of Wales. Jenner was an authority on typhoid fever and was one of the first physicians to distinguish it from typhus fever.

5. Op.cit. See note 1 above (Board minutes), Book 23: 46, 65, 69-70, 75; M.D. Chalmer to F. Andrew 1903, 2 November, (RHN archive); Anonymous, 'The Royal Patronage', *Morning Post* 20 July 1910; Anonymous, *Hospital* 6 August 1910.

6. Op.cit. See note 1 above (Board minutes), Book 21: 460-1; Book 23: 85-6, 92.

7. Ibid: 102, 103, 131; Anonymous, *Medical Times* 15 December 1917.

8. Op.cit. See note 1 above (Board minutes): 214, 216, 265, 355, 359.

9. Ibid. Book 24: 251, 256-7, 270, 276, 285, 329, 340.

10. Ibid: 277-9, 329, 340.

11. Ibid: 345-6, 352-3, 355, 359.

12. Ibid: 383, 389, 395, 400, 453.

13. Ibid. Book 22: 280-1, 289, 333, 349; Book 23: 354-5, 461-2, 475, Book 24: 25-6

14. **HRH Princess (Victoria Alexandra Alice) Mary** (1897-1965) GCVO, CBE, Princess Royal, was the only daughter amongst the six children of King George V (1865-1936) and Queen Mary of Teck (1867-1953); Op.cit. See note 1 above (Board minutes), Book 25: 30-2, 132, 139, 142, 218, 312.

15. Ibid: 279-80, Book 26: 334-5, 346, 348; Book 27: 438.

16. Ibid. Book 23: 501-2.

17. Ibid. Book 12: 438; Book 27: 483, 495-6; Book 28: 349-50, 371-2, 375-6.

18. Cowan, architects, *Conservation study for the Royal Hospital for Neuro-Disability, West Hill, Putney, London* (London: the Board of Management of the Royal Hospital for Neuro-Disability, 2000).

CHAPTER 10

Seaside House at St Leonard's-on-Sea: a great success during the latter years of the nineteenth century

THE FIRST MENTION, in the RHI minute books, of a *home by the sea* (a forerunner of John Howard House which was opened in Brighton in 1974 and sold some 25 years later) was in November 1884 (i.e. thirty years after the charity had been founded). In January 1885, a resolution was passed by the Board:

That the desirability or otherwise of providing a temporary Seaside House for the reception, from time to time, of such Inmates as may, in the opinion of the Board and medical officer, be likely to derive benefit therefrom.

The matter was subsequently discussed under three heads: I Necessity on medical grounds; II Locality (a preference was given to Brighton); III Capacity ('provision should be made for 6 Inmates and staff of 3 or 4 persons'); and IV Cost (an estimate was '£700 a year'). It was soon decided to set up a small Seaside House and to give it a twelve-month trial.[1]

A temporary house
A subcommittee appointed by the Board (which was empowered to find suitable premises and to 'appoint the staff') then visited St. Leonard's and inspected several houses. They agreed in recommending: 1st 135 London Road – Rent £85; and 2nd 137 Marina – Rent £90. Ultimately 2 (or 3) Whiterock Gardens, Hastings, was also considered at '£100 a year for three years, or £120 for one year only'. A substantial delay in negotiations resulted from tardiness on the part of the solicitors, but all these premises were ultimately rejected and 'a house [at no 18] St. Margaret's Road, St. Leonard's was then considered, and accepted at a rent of £70 for one year. Miss Hodges was duly appointed by the Seaside House Committee as housekeeper at £40 a year. In June of that year '.. the Secy. [was] instructed to purchase a Piano suitable for Seaside House at a cost of say £21.' In July 1885, it was reported '... that the furnishing of the House at St. Leonards was complete, and that four Inmates would be received on Monday the 20th.' These patients stayed for four weeks, and returned

151

'much benefited', and were immediately replaced by six others. From then onwards, six Inmates stayed at the Seaside House for a period of six weeks. It should be noted that the parties were either all male or all female; mixed sex parties were not acceptable!

In February 1886 (i.e. after one year) an update of the *progress* of Seaside House was presented to the Board, who decided to keep the project going; it was minuted: '... that an application be made to Mr Francis H. Fowler [the landlord], to renew the tenancy of the House at St. Leonard's on Sea (which will expire next June) for [the following year, beginning in Midsummer].'[2]

The cost of the first year was defrayed in entirety by the generosity of the treasurer, John Darby Allcroft.[3] Frequent Seaside House Reports in the Board minutes contain, amongst other things, details of the prevailing weather on the South Coast of England.

Permanent premises

The question of permanence (and a definitive building) for a Seaside House was first aired in October 1886. The following month, the Secretary wrote (on behalf of the RHI) to Miss Briscoe, presumably an estate agent, asking her if she possessed a site – preferably in 'unoccupied ground, north of St. Margaret's Road, and [or alternatively at] a spot contiguous to the Corporation Improvement at [a location which went by the name of] Bopeep' – which the RHI could purchase. However, she declined the first option on the grounds that the site must be developed as a whole. As to the Bopeep site, she felt that this was 'too bleak and exposed for Invalids'. It was subsequently agreed to seek a medical opinion on the suitability, or otherwise, of the Bopeep site.[4]

In the event, both sites were eventually deemed unsuitable for building, but the Board had by this time gone ahead and obtained 'a plan and elevation [for a] proposed Seaside House'. Negotiations began for Sussex House, but these were soon dropped on account of expense. A 40$\frac{1}{2}$ year lease on a house – 29 Marina – for £1500, or alternatively 55 Marina, which was on a 29-year lease at a yearly rental of £140, were also suggested. The Board requested Mr Longsdon (a member of the Board who incidentally died the following year) to pursue the former option. However, a deputation from the RHI to St Leonard's recommended that the latter was 'best adapted for the purposes of the Home', and that 'the offer of 29, Marina ... be declined'. The lease was, however, considered too short, and the Board resolved in February 1887 'that an offer of £2750 be made [for] No. 55 [which was situated on the sea-front] Marina, St Leonard's on Sea – which was on a 95-year lease.' Later that month, they agreed to raise this sum to £2800, and trustees were named. Agreements were subsequently signed and repairs to this property duly carried out.[5] The *temporary* Seaside House had been closed 'prior to Midsummer [1887].'[6]

When the *new* Seaside House was opened, the Board decided to 'receive ten persons for a period of six weeks, five to be changed every three weeks'. Also, it was minuted: 'arrangements must be made for night-nursing'. In late 1887, the matron, Miss Hodges, resigned, somewhat precipitously, due apparently to the fact that 'the Board appeared not to have confidence in the truthfulness of her statements'. It was agreed at a Special Meeting in early January 1888, to advertise for a *new* matron 'at a commencing salary of £40, in [the] Daily Telegraph & Christian World'. The new matron – Mrs Morfee (her salary was increased to '£50 a year' in June 1889) – was duly appointed to take up her duties on 2 February 1888; she had already been introduced to Mrs Linicke, matron at Melrose Hall (Chapter 10). However, not all was well, and in September 1891, on 'account of ... frequent disturbances at the Seaside House, the Comm^ee [gave] the Matron a month's notice.'[7]

A report of a visit of a Deputation from the Committee on 20 February 1894 was minuted in detail; it transpired that the 'consumption of Beer, Milk and Soda Water [was] in each case in excess of the limit allowed at Putney ...'. But overall the conclusion was that the *Seaside House* was being run satisfactorily.[8]

The future of Seaside House always hung in the balance. The 1893-94 *Annual Report* recorded that in view of the 'accumulation of burdens upon their funds', there was 'only one alternative, viz., the abandonment of the Seaside House at St. Leonards'. But the Board shrank from such a dismemberment '[feeling that] its relinquishment would be warranted only by the clearest necessity'. Therefore, Seaside House was allowed to continue 'at any rate, at present'.

Final days of the St Leonards project

In January 1896, it was decided to admit 'pensioners' (out-patients) to Seaside House. In February 1900, the Board decided, in principle, to put 'Seaside House' at the disposal of the Government for the reception ... of soldiers returned in a sick or wounded condition from the War in South Africa.' However, the finance committee (supported by Freshfield) raised doubts 'as to whether the Board had power to apply the funds of the Hospital to such a purpose'. By January 1901, the question of continuing with Seaside House – owing to difficulties experienced in filling it – was debated by the Board and the House Committee, and later that year they agreed, reluctantly, to the closure. Before selling the property, the Board was advised by Freshfield that 'it would be necessary to obtain the sanction of the Charity Commissioners'.[9]

After a great deal of careful consideration, therefore, the Board decided in 1901 to close *Seaside House*. It had survived for a mere sixteen years. Seaside House was, while it lasted, hailed as one of the great successes of this charity, during the latter days of the nineteenth century.

Transport from Putney to Seaside House

Early on, the Board requested a saloon carriage to convey inmates to and from St Leonard's. However, the London, Brighton & South Coast Ry. Co. proposed that they would provide only a second class carriage. The offer was therefore declined. In March 1890, it was recorded that '… the assistant manager [of this Railway], had promised to inquire as to the possibility of constructing a double door in one of the carriages and also of issuing special second class return tickets available for two months.' 'The Saloon Carriage [which allowed admission of invalid chairs as well as patients in a recumbent position] provided by the London, Brighton & South Coast Ry Co. [had apparently proved a] great success', and the thanks of the Board were conveyed to the Directors of the railway.[10]

References and Notes

1. Board minutes, Book 14: 471, 496-7; Book 15: 15, 21, 188-9.
2. Ibid. Book 15: 55, 63, 70, 76, 84, 92, 107, 112, 125, 135-6, 242-3, 257.
3. Ibid: 188-90, 315-6.
4. Ibid: 369, 374-5, 384-5.
5. Ibid: 395-6, 418, 427-8, 435-6, 441-2, 449-50, 460, 468, 477-8, 494; Book 16: 7-8, 19-20, 24, 35, 77, 78, 82, 106.
6. Ibid: Book 16: 13.
7. Ibid: 92, 108, 131, 136, 157, 307; Book 17: 455-7.
8. Ibid. Book 19: 66-7, 172.
9. Ibid. Book 20: 33-4, 205; Book 22: 13, 15, 284, 349, 445-6.
10. Ibid. Book 16: 138, 144; Book 17: 90, 222, 257.

CHAPTER 11

Nursing at the RHI, and a
Nurses' Home at last

THERE IS ONLY sparse reference to nursing in the early Board minutes. Since the RHI was both a long-stay *Home* as well as a *Hospital,* this fact seems anomalous. Nursing was *not* of course at that time considered (in the mid to late nineteenth century) a 'respectable' profession, and many nurses were of the Sairey Gamp variety as portrayed in Dicken's *Martin Chuzzlewit*;[1] amongst other vices, alcoholism was rife!

In the very early days of the Charity, conditions not only for the nursing staff, but for the patients also seem to have been very inadequate by present day standards; in October 1861, for example, the Matron told the Board that at the Branch (the annexe to Putney House), patients 'partook of their meals in the bedroom, there being no room of assembly in the house'.

In March 1865 (more than a decade after the Charity had been founded) a Board minute states: '… steps were being taken to engage a Head Nurse …', and at the same meeting 'It was agreed to refer the whole question of nurses to the House Comm^ee with power to revise the staff of nurses at their discretion. It was considered that three trained nurses should be chosen'; the following month, the same Committee decided that 'Mrs Turner [who was later the subject of a complaint on account of alleged inefficiency and insolence] had been engaged as Head Nurse, at £35 a year, and that a situation as Under Nurse @ £25 a year had been offered to Mrs Aylin.' In June of that year: 'the Secy was desired to advertise for a Superintending Nurse @ £25 a year, to be appointed by the House Comm^ee, and to inform the matron that that [sic] Grace Sugg would fill her place pro-tem.' Many years later, nursing problems continued; Dr Woodhouse, the Medical Officer, considered that although in the day nursing was satisfactory, that at night was not; he therefore 'advised on the engagement of another permanent night nurse', and in a subsequent report he also wrote of the need for 'an additional Day Divisional Nurse'.[2]

A year later, the Board recommended that the Nurses should receive a 'minimum of £13 with an addition of £1 a year to a maximum of £10, and a rise at Lady Day of £1 to each nurse'. Later, in 1866, the Board agreed 'to supply to the nurses a uniform dress of dark blue, and … an order had been given accordingly.' And in May 1866 '… [it was] considered expedient to engage for the first time a female night nurse'.

In January of the following year: 'The Secy produced letters from the authorities of Addenbrookes' Hospital, Cambridge, and from the District Nursing Society at Ipswich in reply to inquiries respecting Lennora Biscoe, candidate for the situation of Head Nurse.' The Secy and the Governor also reported interviews separately held with Mrs Wardroper, Matron of St Thomas's Hospital, from which it appeared that the conduct and character of Miss Biscoe, when in that Hospital, had been good. She had however been dismissed from the Nightingale Fund on account of '... intemperance when at Cambridge, ... which [as] seemed likely, [was] attributable to the hostility of some of the Under Nurses in that Institution.' Despite this blemish on her character, it was resolved 'that [she] be engaged as Head Nurse on the terms arranged at the Meeting of the House C^{ee}.' We later read that she was soon 'dismissed for using bad language', and a new Head Nurse was appointed almost immediately.[3]

A few years later, in March 1879, in order to 'secure an improvement in the staff of ordinary nurses,' the salaries were raised to £18 for the first year, and afterwards £20 a year'.[4]

Discipline

In October 1866 a Board minute records that one of the nurses 'had been discharged for drunkenness', and in February 1871, a further one records: 'that a female nurse ... had been reported for intoxication and warned against a second offence.' Later that year, '... two Female Nurses ... had been reported for drunkenness, but as it was the first offence, they were warned that dismissal would follow a repetition.' In November 1871: '... the Head Nurse had been charged with making statements of a prejudicial character respecting the Governor and Matron, and two of the Inmates, and that the House C^{ee} were engaged in inquiring into the matter.' These charges and the inquiry were soon 'terminated in a pacification between the parties concerned'.

Fig 11.1 shows the rules for nurses in 1911.

The Matron

The first Matron (at Carshalton) was Mrs Crossthwaite (Chapter 1). The resignation of the second matron (Mrs Eliza Bellringer) was reported to the Board in February 1866. She had been Matron for 9½ years, had served the institution well at Putney House and the early days at Melrose Hall, and retired due to ill-health. The Board agreed to give her a testimonial, as well as a gift of £100, and this was subsequently altered to £25 per annum. She was later admitted 'as a paying care' and she died at the RHI on 27 December 1881.[5] Her successor, Mrs Haughton, did not stay long, and the following minute relates to the fourth matron. 'A New Governor and Matron, Mr & Mrs Darbyshire* [took up] their duties on 28th July [1869].' In September however, this matron

---

*A married couple often took on these responsibilities in the days of the workhouses.

Royal Hospital for Incurables,

PUTNEY HEATH.

RULES FOR NURSING STAFF.

1. Quiet and orderly behaviour must be maintained at all times. Conversation in the corridors and on the staircases is not allowed, either when on or off duty.

2. No one may absent herself from any meal without permission and no food is to be taken in the ward kitchens without permission.

3. Waste of water, gas, and electric light must be carefully avoided. Nurses may not go into each other's rooms after 10 p.m., and all lights must be extinguished by 10.30 p.m.

4. Beds must be made, slop-pails emptied, and rooms left perfectly tidy before going on duty in the morning.

5. Bedroom fires must not be lighted before 2 p.m. or made up after 7 p.m., unless in case of illness.

6. It is forbidden to put nails or pins in the walls or anything on the window sills. A few fresh flowers may be kept in the rooms, but plants in pots are not allowed.

7. Two cardboard hat-boxes only are allowed and they must be kept straight and tidy on the top of the cupboards and not under the beds.

8. The washing of small articles, such as stockings, handkerchiefs, &c., is forbidden. Soiled linen must be sent without fail to the Laundry every Monday not later than 7 a.m.

9. Bedroom furniture must not be rearranged without permission, and members of the Nursing Staff are cautioned against leaving money or valuables about.

Trunks are not allowed in bedrooms.

10. Any Nurse who is not feeling well must immediately report herself to her Ward Sister.

By order of the Board,

LUCY S. BEGG,

Matron.

April, 1911.

Fig 11.1: Rules for the nursing staff of the RHI in April 1911.

was reported pregnant and 'her confinement was expected in the latter part of November or early in December …'. A month later: '[The House Committee were] of opinion that the Matron's expected confinement in November or December next was improperly with-held from the Board [when she and her husband had been appointed], and that the intentions of the Board, as advertised will be frustrated by the birth of an infant at the Hospital.' However, the Committee decided not to take further steps 'in the hope that the interests of the Institution will suffer as little as possible by the anticipated event'. In November, it was minuted: 'that the accouchment of the Matron had taken place on 9th inst. and that leave had been given for the accommodation of the Nurse.' Mrs Darbyshire was able to resume her duties on 28 December.[6]

In September 1877: '… the attention of the House Committee [was] drawn, at the instance of the Matron [who had held that position 'for upwards of eight years'], to certain statements made by several nurses and servants … who alleged that they had witnessed acts of *undue familiarity* [my italics] between Mr Darbyshire [her husband] and Miss Mapleton, the Head Nurse.' The Matron subsequently suggested that he be suspended from his post for 'a few months'! But the House Committee did *not* accept this idea. Instead they resolved that: '… the House Committee be requested to engage a [new] Matron at a salary not exceeding £100 a year, and a Steward at a salary not exceeding £80 a year'. This whole episode was referred to in the *Annual Report* for 1876-7: '… lately, domestic troubles have cast a cloud over the household, and occasioned anxiety to the Board, yet the shadow has now passed away …'. Meanwhile, a new Head Nurse was also appointed in place of Miss Mapleton; the new one was a widow of 35 years and had been Head Nurse and Assistant Matron at the Poplar and Stepney Sick Asylum.[7]

The House Committee, therefore, proceeded to the election of a *new* Matron. They unanimously appointed Miss Emma Mason, 'some time Head Nurse [of the RHI], and lately Matron of the Sussex County Hospital at Brighton', who would take up her duties 'about the 1st Dec'. The new Matron soon made a positive impact! In March of the following year, for example, she made recommendations for 'Improvement of the Nursing of the Hospital'; the Nurses were to be relieved of 'the duty of cleaning the Wards, and … a class of servants, to be called Ward-maids [would be engaged at £14 a year]'. She also introduced Divisional Nurses who were directly answerable to the Head Nurse. In April 1881 (i.e. after about three years), '… Miss Mason … verbally tendered her resignation'. Her reason was that 'the Cee had not given her the help she required' and also the 'larger responsibilities involved in the New Building [i.e. the great extension]'. Her resignation was formally accepted and she left 'the service of the Board on the 23rd [July 1881]'. Miss Mason was paid her salary (of £25) to Michaelmas, and a 'further sum of £25, making together £50'.[8]

At a meeting on 26 April 1881, the Board addressed the question of the superintendence of the Hospital; should they have: I a Medical Man; II a man and his wife, as Governor or House Steward and Matron; or III a lady as Matron?[9] The last option was chosen and in 'accordance with the understanding arrived', Mr White recommended Mrs Linicke (Superintendent of Sir Patrick Dun's Hospital, and of the Nurses' Training Institute, in Dublin).

The *Annual Report* for 1880-1 had recorded 'The Board have the pleasure to report the accession to their number of Surgeon-General T. Graham Balfour, MD, FRS, whose experience of hospital work has already proved of great service to them'.[10] He clearly favoured Miss Macdonald 'whom he considered highly qualified for the position'. The Secretary said that a member of the Board, Mr Lobb, was also prepared to submit the name of a lady [who was] in his opinion entirely fitted for the office of Matron'. The Board resolved, however, that they would like the House Committee to interview Mrs Linicke.

Appointment of Mrs Linicke
Clearly, Balfour had his doubts regarding the suitability of Mrs Linicke for this important position. In April-May 1881, he sought advice from Florence Nightingale on a suitable recruit. In reply to a letter from him, she wrote (from 10 South Street, Park Lane, W) on 29 April 1881 (Fig 11.2):*

> I cannot tell you the pleasure with which I saw your handwriting again. How many recollections we have together.
>
> Your decision as to the Hospital for Incurables <u>establishment</u> is a most wise one. I will immediately <u>try</u> to find some lady suitable to recommend to you as Sup[t]. But we do not like to recommend any one but those of whom we have had experience. And there are those who have been not only trained but tried & employed by us. And for those there is such a demand to head & conduct Trained Staffs which we are asked to send out to Hosps that we are often at our wits end. Nothing can be more important than your Hospital for Incurables. I bid you "God speed" with all my might. To put it on a good footing is a noble work. I wish we may be able to help you in it.
>
> Yes: Sir John M[c]Neill sent me his reprint of the Chelsea Commission. And Mr Kinglake had sent me his book last autumn. I have never opened it. It was enough to hear what was in it. It was too painful. I rejoice, like you, that Sir John fought the battle 'o'er again'. I read all my old friends over again.
>
> in haste, & hoping to write to you again, & with kindest regards to Mrs Balfour, pray believe me ever sincerely yours

Florence Nightingale[11]

The following two letters – which were clearly also addressed to Balfour – begin in a more formal vein; she began 'My dear Sir', rather than 'My dear Dr Balfour'. The first of these (from the same address) is dated 14 May 1881:

---

*As with the letters transcribed in Chapter 6, this correspondence has not, as far as is known, been published before.

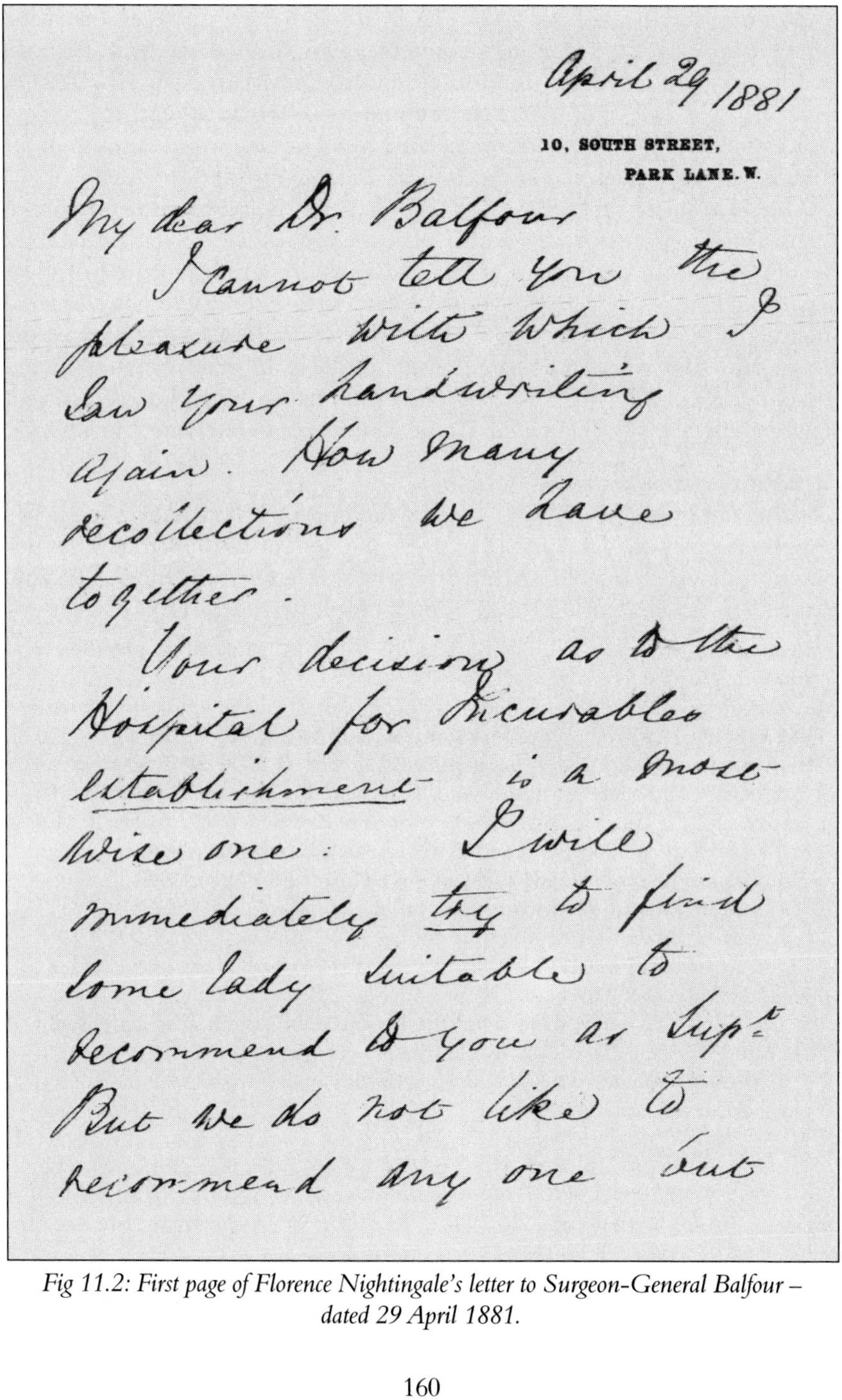

April 29 1881

10, SOUTH STREET,
PARK LANE. W.

My dear Dr. Balfour

I cannot tell you the
pleasure with which I
saw your handwriting
again. How many
recollections we have
together.

Your decision as to the
Hospital for Incurables
Establishment is a most
wise one: I will
immediately try to find
some lady suitable to
recommend to you as Supt.
But we do not like to
recommend any one but

*Fig 11.2: First page of Florence Nightingale's letter to Surgeon-General Balfour –
dated 29 April 1881.*

160

I am grieved to find that we cannot conscientiously spare one lady among those whom we have trained & proved, the only ones we could recommend for such a post as yours, the Lady Sup^ed. of the Putney Royal Hosp^l for Incurables. They are all serving in posts from which we could not suggest a removal, even for promotion. We have no reserve. And we never recommend from those who have had only a year's <u>training</u> for a position as Head. They must have passed thro' Ward Sisterships, (i.e. Head Nurse Ships) or Assistant Matronships or Matronships of Small Hospitals to the satisfaction of their employer first before we offer them such a responsible post as that you mention. Then there are others in important posts whom we cannot disturb.

We have never anything like the number ready for the posts that are offered us. The harvest truly is ready but the labourers (of the right sort) are still few.

There is nothing I should have liked so well as to have been able to help you with a Lady Sup^t., both for the sake of the poor Patients in your great Institution – which I rejoice to know is creating such a position as you describe – & for auld lang syne between yourselves and us.

That you may find some lady to carry out your wise intentions is my most earnest wish. I am so glad you are busied [sic] with the Putney Hospital.

I have consulted our Matron, Mrs Wardroper, & our Secretary Mr Bonham Carter, & gone thro' all our experienced "ladies" with the result I am sorry to report. May you be more fortunate!

I will write again about other things. May I give you joy, you & Mrs Balfour upon your boy? And may he realize all you would have him be!

You kindly ask after me – it is always severe pressure of overwork & illness – & I am not growing younger [Nightingale was 61 at this time, but lived until she was 90].

You are working at Statistics, I am sure. And I may perhaps be troubling you soon about some matters of Military Hospitals. formal references given ~~were~~ are always the Matron & Secretary of our Training School. <u>Not</u> myself. I have not time to make this tedious explanation shorter. But I am sure that you, – who are so well skilled on the great care required in these kinds of negotiations, & in the total want of conscience displayed by Testimonials in general, – will approve & think necessary the kind of carefulness we are obliged to ~~take~~ observe, in order not to make our recommendations as much a 'dead letter' as most are – keeping up, as we do, our interest in the careers of our trained women for a great number of years, during which they are not immediately under our own eye. Mr Bonham Carter told Mrs. Linicke that she must rely upon the testimonials of <u>her</u> <u>own</u> (Dublin) Comm^ee. as the best proof of her capacity for <u>supervision</u>.

Please forgive me, & set Mrs Linicke's position right with your Comm^ee. (& prevent me from being referred to officially.)

Most Private
I think there is some truth in what you fear about Mrs Linicke's "hardness" but I think it would shew more with her subordinate staff than with <u>the</u> <u>Patients</u>. And I cannot say that it appeared at St. Thomas'. I earnestly hope that she will be a success with you, as you deserve.

Pardon this hasty scribble & believe me ever yrs sincerely

Florence Nightingale[12]

The second (much shorter) letter (marked <u>Private</u>) written from the same address, later on the same day, is obviously written to Balfour – although again, she begins 'My dear Sir'.

> About Madame Linicke, as a candidate for the appointment at the R. Hospital for Incurables, – <u>hers</u> was one of the names I brought before my "colleagues" for the office.
>
> Mr Bonham Carter's objection was: "I should be very averse to disturbing Mad. Linicke. She had her salary raised to £100 last July, & is only in her third year of service."
>
> [She was trained by us & we obtained for her the post at Dublin. She cannot accept another post without our consent; but if you offer it to her, I don't suppose <u>we</u> should refuse it.]
>
> To tell you all this is to tell you that we think her a competent woman, & that you might "go farther" "& fare" a great deal "worse". But as I am writing <u>confidentially</u> to you, will you allow me to write more ~~by n~~ tomorrow. As I have not a moment to day?
>
> In answer to your question she is much too clever a woman to do the "C.O. [Commanding Officer]" "over every body – & every thing" –
>
> … Ever yours sincerely.
>
> F. Nightingale.[13]

The two remaining letters from Nightingale were both headed 'Private' and both of them concerned the possible appointment of Mrs Linicke; both were clearly addressed to 'My dear Dr Balfour'. The first (dated 15 May 1881) is as follows:

> Now about <u>Mrs Linicke</u> – she has had a very difficult position in Dublin where she has now been for 2½ years – difficult because of the elements which <u>might</u> be jarring that she has to work under & with – viz. <u>two</u> Boards and a Ladies' Committee, a Medical Staff, House Surgeon, Probationers & servants & &. Neither (private & Hospital) properly speaking she is the head of the <u>Training School for Nurses</u>, attached to Sir Patrick Dun's Hospital but independent of it. Nursing it & two other small Hospitals. In answer to your questions, I believe I may say that she has "administrative ability" & "powers of organisation". She has very remarkable powers of observation & of expression, which are most useful in her position. It will be for the authorities of the Training School, at Sir Patrick Dun's Hosp^l where she is in charge of the nursing, – to speak to her qualifications. I believe they will be very sorry to part with her. We understand that she is very successful in charge of the female servants (Irish) also. She has a Matron at the "Home". Sir Patrick Dun's Hosp^l has something more than 100 beds. To return to your questions. I think she has "<u>firmness</u>" & gentleness to "carry out her plans & the Committee's orders", and in "dealing with the subordinate staff". And she is very kind to Patients. I think she has both a "firm" and a <u>light</u> hand in <u>all</u> the above matters. I ask myself again your query, "would she be likely to work amicably with the Medical Officer or would she try to come

C.O. over every body & every thing"? I don't think it would have been possible
for her to work these somewhat conflicting elements of the Dublin concern, & to
make them so well, as we believe, – if she had had any such nonsense in her
head. Confidentially to you I will say, she has a very good opinion of herself. But
this is, I do believe, one secret of her success. She takes a pride in making things
go amicably. If they did not, it would be a slur upon herself in her own
estimation. Self-satisfaction, you know, prevents some women from being
imperious or irritable. It is not at all obnoxious or prominent in her. And I don't
know that your Committee would remark [sic] it. I mention it to you only,
because you have asked the pointed questions. And I am writing private
experience to you to enable you to judge. Success to all you do.

Let me be always for now & for auld lang syne. Yours most sincerely

Florence Nightingale

Do you sometimes see Lady Tulloch now? Please send her my love when you
write.[14]

The last (10 pages long) in this series of letters (also from 10 South Street) is
dated 23 May 1881:

…I write rather in haste to catch you before your Tuesday's Comm^ee & to say that
Mrs Linicke was not authorized to refer to me but to Mr. Hy Bonham Carter as
Secretary of the "Nightingale Fund", or to Mrs. Wardroper as Lady Sup^t of the
"Nightingale Training School" at St. Thomas Hospital.

I should wish any communication from me to be treated as unofficial & quasi
[sic] private, as you have so kindly already done.

Mrs Linicke, when here, had not yet mentioned the subject to her own Dublin
Committee, I think. [She had been telegraphed for, I understood, by a Member
of your "R. Incurables Hos^l" Committee]. And Mr Bonham Carter did mention
to her that her application must be made with the knowledge of her own
(Dublin) Committee &, this being done she might refer to him or to Mrs
Wardroper.

The proper course for her to pursue would have been to write & tell Mr.
Bonham Carter that she had applied for the Matronship of the Putney Hosp^l
with the knowledge of her own Comm^ee and to ours.

We do not like to run the risk of appearing to have assisted her in applying for
the post "unbeknown" to her Comm^ee – which is, as you know, so far from the
truth, that, tho' I had thought of her & placed her name before my "Colleagues",
I answered you that we had "no one to recommend" – until you asked me for my
private opinion, you has proposing Mrs Linicke.

Besides this, I am obliged to decline giving formal official recommendations
myself to our trained nurses, except they be those whom I have personally
watched & known in their work for years (which was could not be the case with
Mrs. L.) And even then the [sic] she is certainly a very clever woman. She came
to our Training School when she was, I think, nearly 40. And she had had much
experience in management, tho' not in Hospital life, before she came. We thought

she would not cotton to Hosp¹ life. But she <u>did</u> [I should say that when she first came to us, during an interval of about a month when our admirable "Home" Sister (Mistress of Probationers) was away for health, she managed the "Home" for us, & did not do it remarkably well. But this would not tell against her in my mind. It was a most difficult post – quite new to her – a large number of Probationers, with a ~~large number~~ great proportion of gentlewomen, many her Seniors in the work. I think it would have been a miracle if she had attached them all to her.

And I must say to her credit that, she being a person of "consideration", as you will say when you see her, "knocked under" as I heard it expressed, & was herself most obedient to our "Home" Sister & our rules; to be under authority was quite new to her & speaks well for her power of wielding authority properly herself in her turn.]

With <u>you</u>, <u>if</u> she goes to you, instead of her being new to her work as she was with us, she will have had the advantage of 2½ years of Hospital management, besides her year's training.

I have tried to put her before you, that is <u>confidentially</u> before you <u>personally</u>, as I think her, to enable you in a measure to judge for yourself.

I will ask you now to wait a day or two, if that is possible, till I again consult my "colleagues", Mr Bonham Carter, our Secretary who, you will see, is very anxious that she should not be "disturbed" at Dublin, & Mrs. Wardroper, our Matron, [these of course know more about her in some respects than I do] as to what character they would give her.

I had, as I think I mentioned, placed Mrs. Linicke's name before them when I consulted them about names for your "Incurables Hosp¹". But they came to the conclusion that we would not "disturb" <u>any</u> of <u>ours</u>.

Now you have found out Mrs. Linicke for yourselves. And I should not be at all surprised if you were delighted with her. But you will see it would not "do" for <u>us</u> to <u>offer</u> her.

I should say that she is pre-eminently good in domestic arrangements, working with a Matron or Housekeeper under her.

But, after all, her Dublin employers must have of course the last word about her.

If you cannot wait "to use" this till you hear again from us, please kindly use ~~say~~ only what I have told you <u>generally</u>, without mentioning such things as I have told you for your own judgement only – e.g. her good opinion of herself, & her not having been good at management among our "gentle" Probationers during her month's rule.

Can <u>you</u> not send us some Probationers, whether "gentle" or "simple", for our work from time to time? We have always more applications, ten times more, than we can admit. But not <u>always</u> of course, the right material, especially not among the "gentle".

Ever yours sincerely

Florence Nightingale

It strikes me that you may be fearful of Guy's Hospital disaster in choosing Mrs. Linicke. Thank God, we have been able to keep quite clear of such unseemly doings at St Thomas', & are always on the best terms with the Medical Officers who are our best friends. And as to our setting ~~them~~ ourselves up against them, it is a thing not even to be thought of among us: 'a question not to be asked': it is so far from us.

in haste F.N.[15]

In the light of Nightingale's comments, Mrs Linicke was duly interviewed. She outlined her plans, if appointed; she was also happy to 'bear the title of "Matron", the domestics being under the supervision of a "Housekeeper".' Mrs Linicke said that:

> ... if appointed, she should take control of the Nursing, dispensing with the office of Head Nurse, as now existing, and communicating personally with the Nurses through the divisional nurses; she should herself report to the House Committee of the nursing; this was a matter in which she had no alternative, being under pledge to Miss Nightingale. At the same time she would avoid sudden or rash changes, and did not contemplate the dismissal of the present head nurse. She would also report on the Housekeeper's department; but considered that the Steward should report direct to the Comm[ee].

Following the interview, the House Committee were unanimous in recommending that Mrs Linicke be appointed at a salary of £200 a year. She was later to meet the Board. A minute states: 'N.B. Mrs Linicke stated starkly that her age was 46, and that she was a Protestant (Lutheran).'[16]

Mrs Linicke's time as matron was not without its health problems; in October 1894 she 'was suffering from neuralgia and sleeplessness', and it was later reported that she had rheumatic fever (for which she was seen by Dr Munk). However, by November her health was 'greatly improved' and she had been sent to Bournemouth for convalescence. A further minute states that she had been 'ordered to take baths and waters ... on the Continent'; while she was away for at least six weeks, the Steward was directed to 'take the supervision of the establishment'.

In March 1902, her 70th birthday was approaching and she had by then held the office of matron for 21 years; she wrote to the Board asking that 'if [they] would grant her a pension she would be quite willing to retire'. The Board decided to grant a pension of £150 per annum and to ask her to stay until 1 January 1903.

Subsequent matrons

In July 1902, the rules for the matron's duties were altered (see below), and it was agreed to advertise for a new matron who must be between 35 and 45 years old.

The Board duly interviewed nine candidates for Mrs Linicke's position, and appointed Miss J. Harding at a 'salary of £110 per annum together with board lodging and laundry ...'. She presumably rejected the appointment.

The office of Matron to the RHI must have been a difficult (if not impossible) one, by any standard, during the first part of the twentieth century. Fig 11.3 shows the rules for the Matron in 1902. There were for example, calls in 1908 for the resignation of the then Matron (Miss J. Stirling Hamilton) whose 'attitude towards the House Committee was [said to be] unworthy of one holding her position'. After a lengthy discussion at a Board meeting a proposal for her resignation was withdrawn, and this, it was minuted, 'would end the matter'. However, shortly afterwards, in March 1909, she offered her resignation on the grounds that 'difficulties in connection with the Nursing and Management of Incurable Patients and the Staff do not lessen as time goes on'. Her resignation was accepted by the Board, who in turn blamed the Ladies Visiting Committee who had apparently made a 'specific charge against [her] with regard to her duties concerning nursing matters'. This in turn led to the resignation of the Hon. Secretary of the Ladies Visiting Committee and also the Vice-President (the Hon. Mrs Norman Grosvenor). There were 75 applications for Miss Stirling Hamilton's post, of whom the Board short-listed seven.[17]

Miss Lucy Sarah Begg was duly appointed, at a salary of £130. On 25 March 1915 (i.e. soon after the Great War had begun) Lucy Begg requested three months leave for 'Nursing duty in France' (see later). Her formal letter, addressed to 'The Board of Management', was dated 31 March 1915. The Board agreed in principle, albeit reluctantly, to her request but asked her 'not to make any final arrangements before she saw the House Committee on Wednesday, March 31st.' The House Committee agreed, and Miss Begg duly wrote a letter of thanks from an Eastbourne address, on 13 April. Soon after this, her health was reported (in January 1920) to be less than satisfactory, and she was undergoing a 'rest-cure'.

In 1921, the Board discussed at length evidence pointing to some friction between Miss Begg and the Assistant Matron; this led to a letter from the Secretary on behalf of the Board (as a result of a resolution – a copy of which he enclosed) to the Matron, in which he gave her three months to settle her differences! In a reply Miss Begg took this as a serious criticism of her 'personal character', and vehemently denied a rift between herself and the Assistant Matron. The Chairman, after further discussion, wrote to Miss Begg indicating that although there was no 'personal animosity [to yourself] as you appear to suspect', the resolution cannot be rescinded. In 1930, after much discussion, the Board decided to ask Lucy Begg to resign on a pension of £250 per year. (She died some fifteen years later, on 27 January 1945.) On this occasion, there were 90 applicants, of whom 11 were interviewed by a sub-committee; the number was then reduced to three.[18]

THE ROYAL HOSPITAL FOR INCURABLES.

RULES FOR MATRON.

1. The Matron must be a lady who has received three years' training in an ordinary Hospital. Preference will be given to a person who has also held a similar position of responsibility in a large Institution.

2. At the date of her appointment she shall be between the ages of thirty-five and forty-five years, and must retire at the age of sixty-five years.

3. The Matron is held responsible for the engagement, dismissal, and proper control of the assistant nurses and female servants, and for the efficient nursing and dietary of the Hospital, and is expected to see that the directions of the Medical Officer are faithfully carried out.

4. The Matron must visit each ward every day, and more frequently if necessary, and in the event of any inmate being in such a state of ill-health as to necessitate the presence of the Medical Officer, she shall at once summon him.

5. The Matron is held responsible for the cleanliness and order of the Hospital, and shall have charge of the Kitchen, Laundry, furniture, fittings and linen. A requisition must be presented to the House Committee for their sanction for all renewals and requirements.

6. The Matron is held responsible for the engagement of the divisional nurses. In the event of a divisional nurse being guilty of gross neglect of duty or insubordination, the Matron may suspend such nurse—reporting the same at the next meeting of the House Committee.

7. The Matron is not permitted to have friends to sleep at the Hospital, except in the case of being summoned by the Medical Officer through the serious illness of the Matron.

8. The Matron is allowed a holiday not exceeding five weeks a year, and it must be arranged that the Matron and the Steward are not both away from the Hospital at one and the same time.

9. The Matron is expected to receive visitors and show them over the Hospital if required to do so, and is expected to use every endeavour to further the interests of the Institution as occasion may arise.

ADVERTISEMENT.

The Royal Hospital for Incurables, Putney Heath. 250 beds.—Required a lady to act as Matron ; aged 35 to 45. Fully trained, good disciplinarian. One experienced in work of a large hospital preferred. Commencing salary, £110 per annum, and board, residence and laundry. Applications, with three copies of recent testimonials, to be forwarded to Secretary, 106, Queen Victoria Street, London, E.C., on or before September 15th, 1902. Rules sent on receipt of stamped addressed envelope.

Fig 11.3: Rules for the matron of the RHI in September 1902, i.e. following Mrs Linicke's resignation.

Miss Rose E.A. Potter of the Chester Royal Infirmary was ultimately elected at a salary of £300 a year. In late December 1935 (i.e. after five years service) she sent, somewhat reluctantly, a letter of resignation, and this was accepted by the Board. She had been asked by the Board to do so, she claimed without 'an adequate reason'. The Board did state however, that in their view she had not 'won the affection of the patients, or the confidence of the outside public, in the way which the Board consider necessary for the success of their Institution'; they also referred to 'defects of temperament and organisation'. It was decided to advertise on this occasion in *The Times, Daily Telegraph, Morning Post, Nursing Times,* and *Nursing Mirror.*

A sub-committee was set up to do the short-listing; four ladies were seen, and Miss D.W. Rosier was appointed. She intimated that she would begin duty on 16 May 1936, and was 'desirous of carrying on the Examination work in connection with the General Nursing Council'; the Board decided that she 'be allowed to attend the final examinations for 27th to 29th October [1936]. In 1942, Miss Rosier resigned, and she was succeeded by Miss K.M. Corbett, who held the position until 1954. Six applicants were short-listed in March 1955; Miss Alnutt and Miss Howard were considered outstanding and both were interviewed.[19]

Miss Clare Annie Howard was ultimately appointed in April at a 'salary of £775, less £195 for board & lodging charge'; she retired at the end of June 1966. A sub-committee to select a successor to Miss Howard was duly set up; 12 enquiries had already been received, and the closing date for applications was 31 October 1965.[20]

Mrs Margaret Clara Bodington was duly elected.[21]

Other nursing matters

Mrs Linicke's pension

Madame Linicke (see above), who had held the office of Matron from 1881-1903, died in Dresden during the second year of the Great War (1914-18); a claim for £112 was made on a pension due to her, by her Estate. As the claim was in German, the matter was referred to Farrer & Co., but the Board later refused the claim. Another request, from Berlin, for the £112, being a pension claim for June 1914-March 1915 was received, but the Board again declined to grant this, and 'stuck to their guns'. However, a letter from Farrer & Co. indicated that the matter was shortly to come up before the 'Mixed Arbitral Tribunal' based in London. At a meeting on 25 October 1923 the Board ultimately resolved that the £112 be granted to the heirs of Mme Linicke 'on proof of the claimant's title'. In fact, £151.9s.7d. was paid.[22]

Difficulties with recruitment

The Times carried an article in 1941, indicating the difficulty with recruitment at all levels at the RHHI; much was associated with the massive demands on manpower resulting from the war efforts.[23]

A training School for Assistant Nurses
In 1956, the Board decided to endorse a recommendation from the House Committee that the General Nursing Council be approached for authority to set up a training school for assistant nurses. This had been a 'topical' issue since a report of a committee of the Royal College of Nursing, chaired by Lord Horder (1871-1955), recorded its views in 1942 – that a two-year, rather than a four-year teaching programme was adequate. It was later reported (1960) that there had been a 100 per cent success rate in the first group.[24]

An infestation with rats
In October 1873, i.e. long before the nurses' home was built, it was agreed to 'replace the floor in the nurses' kitchen by one of concrete ... in order to exclude the rats which infested this room ...'.[25]

A new Nurses' Home?

Since 1864, the nursing staff had resided in the main building. Sir Merton Russell-Cotes of Bournemouth 'intimated [in 1918] that he might be disposed to make a gift of £5,000 towards a new Nurses' Home' provided the Board undertook to 'raise a similar amount by public subscription'. This, the Board agreed to do! And, in April 1919, the members asked whether some of them could visit the Nurse Cavell Nurses' Home at the London Hospital in order to find out exactly what a *new* nurses' home was like.[26]

To build this Nurses' Home, which was therefore badly needed, was approved in principle on 24 July of that year. The urgent need for a *new* Nurses' Home was summarised in the following letter to an architect:

January 23rd, 1920.

Dear Mr Ellis,

In the hope and belief that you will easily be able to put our case before the Local Council successfully the Board of Management of this National Charity direct me to send you the following facts:

Before the War started in the year 1914 it had been fully decided to erect a Nurses' Home in our own grounds at Putney for the accommodation of our nursing staff. The nurses were then, as they are now, occupying sleeping quarters in the basement of our Hospital. The nurses sleep four and six in a room, which is divided into 'cubicles' by means of curtains. Complaint has been made from time to time that the basement rooms are damp.

We have at present about seventy nurses, but this staff is really inadequate, if the eight-hour day is to be worked regularly and smoothly. The new Nurses' Home (for which plans have been prepared) is to provide ninety to one hundred separate bedrooms.

At the majority of other London Hospitals the nurses are provided with separate bedrooms and are made as comfortable as possible, this being necessary in view of the great difficulty there has been for a long time in securing the right type of young woman for nursing.

It will occur to anyone with practical knowledge of the subject that it is even more difficult to obtain nurses for Incurables than it is to get them for ordinary medical or surgical cases. For this very reason the Board of the [RHHI] are persuaded that good and comfortable quarters must be provided for the nursing staff, if the great work of this Institution is to go on.

When the Board have only basement rooms to offer to its nursing staff (as is at present the case) it follows that young women cannot be induced to enter our service or to stay.

The extreme urgency of the position may be imagined when it is explained that we have now 232 suffering and incurable patients to look after. We have also a long waiting-list of incurable men and women who are eager for admission. Many of the patients are unable to feed themselves. They have to be washed and waited upon as if they were helpless infants.

The beneficiaries of the Hospital are mainly those who before being overtaken by illness led industrious lives. They could, in very many instances, be described as the members of the upper working classes, for whom the Government is now anxious to build dwellings.

It is a point of general agreement with all public authorities and by the recognised heads of the nursing profession that nurses should each have a separate bedroom, as well as suitable recreative quarters.

A Nurses' Home has for years been a stern necessity and the Board trust there will be no obstacle whatever to the erection of a sensible and not extravagant building without delay.

Yours truly,

CHARLES CUTTING,
Secretary.

HERBERT O. ELLIS, ESQ.,
46 Fenchurch Street,
E.C.3[27]

This letter also provides a great deal of information about nurses' conditions in 1920 as well as conditions at the RHHI.

Plans were to be obtained from Ellis & Clarke, architects (for which they charged £1,087), but a site had not yet been 'definitely fixed upon'. The House Committee later recommended that the 'Meadow Site' should be used. The names of contractors and quantity surveyors (a fee of £848.7s.6d. was charged) were sought at a meeting of the Board in January 1920.[28]

However, not all were in agreement that a *new* building costing some £60,000 (sic) was justified; Glegg (a member of the Board) for example, felt that they should rent a house in the neighbourhood as a 'temporary Nurses'

Home'. At this point, the Board resolved unanimously to put the matter 'on hold'. This, however, left them in an awkward situation, because HRH Princess Mary (1897-1965) had already consented to lay the Foundation stone on 12 May 1920; however, they wrote a letter to her, and also to 'the newspapers' explaining that the stone-laying ceremony was being postponed, but she would be most welcome as part of a fund-raising campaign; £3,478.13s.9d. was in fact collected from 80 purses; the overall amount raised being £4,171.13s.7d.[29]

Temporary facilities
Negotiations were therefore begun to purchase two empty houses – nos. 170 and 172 (which would accommodate 'about fifty nurses') opposite the Hospital, on West Hill, as a *temporary* Nurses' Home; these were considered by the RHHI architects to be worth about £3,700 after necessary alterations and decorations. A formal offer for this amount was made, but the vendor insisted on £4,200 and this was soon agreed. A minute for June 1920 states that letters relating to the purchase of these houses, as well as 7 Keswick Road (for the Secretary) and the contract for the former properties, was sealed. These premises were therefore adapted as a Nurses' Home.[30]

Final approval for a new home
The urgent need for a Nurses' Home was clearly still a highly topical matter. However, at a Board meeting in May 1932, the Chairman (Turton-Wright) 'reported that he had had letters from two or three members of the Board, who were *not* [my italics] in favour of the building of a Nurses' Home at present.' Despite this, at a meeting in May the following year, after a great deal of discussion, a sub-committee under the chairmanship of Dr Belfrage was set up to look into the requirements and cost of a Nurses' Home on Hospital grounds. And in November the Board resolved that the report of this sub-committee be referred to the House Committee; the main point at issue was whether the necessary accommodation could be provided by extensions or additions to the existing hostel, or whether it would 'be preferable to build a new hostel within our own grounds'. In reply to the Board, the House Committee pointed out that it was necessary to have accommodation for 75 (64 nurses and 11 'other employees') persons, and that this was *not* possible by extending or adding to the existing hostel. It was necessary therefore to erect a *new* building in 'Hospital grounds adjoining [Holy Trinity] Church'. The overall cost would be £20,000. Also, they had asked the hospital architect (Pigott) to 'prepare ... a scheme for utilizing the rooms in the existing Hospital which will be vacated on the completion of the Nurses' Home.' This outline was approved by the Board at their meeting in December.[31]

Objections were however raised by residents on the Beaumont Estate, and this led inevitably to legal interventions. The Official Arbitrator gave his decision to proceed on 20 June 1934. Details of the new Nurses' Home were given by Pigott and approved by the Board on 26 July 1934, and it was agreed that 'as soon as the Secretary is informed by Farrer & Co that the legal obstructions are removed, he shall notify Mr Pigott to proceed with the quantities and tenders.' The tender of James Carmichael Ltd – £20,477 – was subsequently accepted, and the Board decided that 'there should not [after all] be a Foundation Stone Ceremony'.[32]

Opening of the Nurses' Home
The Duchess of York (later Queen Elizabeth the Queen Mother) opened the new Nurses' Home which had cost £25,000 on Wednesday 24 July 1935.[33]

This left the Board with the difficult problem of what to do with the two houses on West Hill, currently in use as a Nurses' Home. In September (1935), it was decided to auction them, and that 'the sum of £1,600 for the two, or £800 each house, should be the minimum' reserve price. At auction, the reserve price was *not* reached; therefore the Board agreed to a sale 'for £1,500, or failing this, £1,450'. But, the sale was, 'for the time being … withdrawn' because the two houses might provide better accommodation for the male servants. On 22 July 1937, it was reported that £1,350 had been offered for 170/172 West Hill, and had been accepted! So the saga ended.[34]

7 Keswick Road
This left the other property then owned by the RHHI unsold – namely 7 Keswick Road. The 'freehold' of this house (then the official residence of the Secretary) was offered in 1924 for £250. (It had been built in 1889, and the lease was due to expire in 1958.) The Secretary reported in late 1937 that three offers had been received for this property; the highest of these (£1,050) was accepted.[35]

Nursing Homes Registration Act, 1927
This Act was passed by Parliament in 1927. There was great uncertainty at the time as to whether it was relevant to the RHHI. However, Farrer & Co concluded that the RHHI was *not* 'a Nursing Home, within the meaning of the Act, and therefore registration under the Act [was] unnecessary'. However, the minute continued, 'the Royal Midland Counties Home for Incurables, Leamington, is not controlled by a party of persons constituted by special Act of Parliament or incorporated by Royal Charter'; therefore that Institution 'is a Nursing Home within the meaning of the Act …'.[36]

There seems, in retrospect, little doubt that the future of the two institutions in the light of the National Health Service Act and the subsequent result of arbitration (in 1950) were influenced by these events (Chapter 15).

References and Notes

1. G.C. Cook, A.J. Webb, 'Reactions from the medical and nursing professions to Nightingale's "reform(s)" of nurse training in the late 19th century', *Postgrad med J* 2002, 78: 118-123.

2. Board minutes. Book 4: 130-1; Book 5: 416-7, 424, 448, 464; Book 22: 24, 44, 45-6.

3. Ibid: 166-7; Book 6: 50, 210, 212, 447; Book 8: 69, 104.

4. Ibid: Book 12: 219.

5. Ibid: Book 6: 143, 184; Book 11: 55-6, 70-1, 82; Book 12: 229, 385.

6. Ibid: Book 8: 115, 140-1, 146-7, 177, 186.

7. Ibid: Book 11: 384, 397, 399-400.

8. Ibid: Book 11: 403-4; Book 13: 239-40, 298, 305.

9. Ibid: 248.

10. Ibid: 367. **Thomas Graham Balfour** FRCP, FRS (1813-91) had studied medicine at Edinburgh University, and took his doctorate in 1834. His uncle was a grandfather of Robert Louis Stephenson, the novelist. Two years later he joined the Army and was employed by the statistical branch. He was one of the earliest (with Southwood Smith) of sanitary reformers. At Nightingale's suggestion, he was appointed Secretary to the Sanitary Commission. Balfour subsequently became principal medical officer at Netley (with the rank of Surgeon-General) and later Gibraltar. Later in life he became a member of the Metropolitan Asylums Board. *See also*: Anonymous, *Lancet* 1891, **i**: 228-9; Anonymous, *BMJ* 1891, **i**: 204-5; *Munk's Roll* 4: 123-4; C. Woodham-Smith, *Florence Nightingale 1820-1910* (London: Constable, 1950): 271, 273, 281, 313; *Roll of the Army Medical Service* 4449.

11. F. Nightingale to T.G. Balfour 29 April 1881: 3 (Royal Hospital for Neuro-disability archive). **Sir John McNeill** (1795-1883) had obtained an MD (Edinburgh) in 1814. He served as surgeon at the East India Company's Bombay establishment from 1816-36, and later became a distinguished diplomat. McNeill also served on the Commission of Inquiry into the Commissariat Department and General Organisation of the troops in the Crimea (1855). *See also*: Z. Cope, *Florence Nightingale and the doctors* (London: Museum Press Ltd. 1958): 65-74; Woodham-Smith (note 10 above): 204, 218, 264, 271, 274, 280, 344, 381, 385, 393, 408, 454, 471, 560, 588. **Alexander William Kinglake** (1809-91) had written a *History of the Crimean War*. He was educated at Eton and Trinity College, Cambridge, and was present during the Crimean War. Kinglake later became the major historian of that campaign; Lady Raglan had apparently invited him to undertake this 8-volume historical account.

12. F. Nightingale to T. G. Balfour 14 May 1881: 7 (Royal Hospital for Neuro-disability archive). **Sarah Wardroper** (1813-92) was matron of St

Thomas's Hospital, London for 33 years (1854-87). *See also*: F. Nightingale, 'The reform of sick nursing and the late Mrs. Wardroper', *BMJ* 1892; **ii**: 1448; Woodham-Smith (note 10 above): pp 336, 338, 344, 345, 347, 348, 569. **Henry Bonham Carter** (1827-1921) was a cousin of Florence Nightingale; he served as Secretary of the Nightingale Fund for 38 years and was a devoted servant who helped run the nurse training-school at St Thomas's Hospital. *See also*: Woodham-Smith (note 10 above): 504, 506; B.M. Dossey, *Florence Nightingale: mystic, visionary, healer*, (Springhouse, Pennsylvania: Springhouse Corporation 1999): 261, 294, 298, 300, 348, 378, 380, 398-9, 400, 412, 413.

13. F. Nightingale to T.G. Balfour 14 May 1881: 3 (Royal Hospital for Neuro-disability archive).

14. F. Nightingale to T.G. Balfour 15 May 1881: 5 (Royal Hospital for Neuro-disability archive). Sir Patrick Dun's Hospital, Dublin had been founded in 1808, and had 100 beds. The medical staff in 1881 consisted of: four physicians and four surgeons; there was also a consulting surgeon. *See also*: *The Medical Directory for 1881; 37th Annual issue* (London: J & A Churchill, 1156). **Lady Tulloch** was the widow of Major-General Sir Alexander Tulloch KCB (1803-64). Educated for the law in Edinburgh, he had joined the 45th regiment in Burmah in 1826, and subsequently served in the Crimean War (1854-6). With McNeill, he investigated the condition of the British Army in the Crimea. In 1857, Tulloch published *The Crimean Commission and the Chelsea Board. See also*: Note 11 above (Cope).

15. F. Nightingale to T.G. Balfour 23 May 1881: 10. (Royal Hospital for Neuro-disability archive). In 1880, there was a colossal dispute centred on Guy's Hospital involving nursing. The senior consultant staff were 'up in arms' at the introduction of the Nightingale system of nursing which was replacing the old (well established) system of old fashioned ('Sairey Gamp') figures whom they seem to have favoured. *See also*: Note 1 above.

16. Op.cit. See note 2 above. Book 13: 261-2, 265-7; Book 19: 223, 251, 357; Book 22: 456, 461, 476-7, 481, 490.

17. Ibid. Book 23: 371-3, 402-4, 412-3.

18. Ibid. Book 24: 158, 165, 408, 410-1; 492-4, 497-8, 499-500; Book 26: 48-50, 55. 'Death of Miss Lucy Begg, former matron of Incurables' Hospital'. *Wandsworth Borough News* 9 February 1945.

19. Op.cit. See note 2 above: Book 26: 63-4, 321-2, 325-332, 334, 343, 354-5.

20. Ibid. Book 28: 23-4, 369.

21. Ibid: 380, 384.

22. Ibid. Book 23: 488, 501-2; Book 25: 123, 129-30, 135, 140, 152-3, 156.

23. Anonymous, 'Scarcity of hospital staffs: high wages in industry, *Times, Lond.* 1941.

24. Op.cit. See note 2 above. Book 28: 59, 189; Anonymous, 'The assistant

nurse: proper control suggested: a closed profession', *Times, Lond.* 1942, 11 October.

25. Op.cit. See note 2 above. Ibid. Book 9: 458.

26. Ibid. Book 24: 359-60, 377.

27. C. Cutting to H.O. Ellis. 1920: 23 January: 2 (Royal Hospital for Neuro-disability archive).

28. Op.cit. See note 2 above. Book 24: 384, 394, 396, 400, 404, 412, 413-14, 421, 423-4, 426-8, 452, 460.

29. Ibid. 404-5, 414, 426-9, 430, 438, 440, 443-4, 445-6; *See also:* Anonymous, *Daily Telegraph* 30 March 1920; Anonymous, *Surrey Comet* 7 February 1920; Anonymous, 'Princess Mary and Hospital for Incurables', *Daily Chronicle* 31 March 1920; *Times, Lond.* 13 May 1920; Anonymous, 'A busy afternoon for Princess Mary: visiting the young and old', *Nursing Mirror & Midwives Journal* 22 May 1920.

30. Op.cit. See note 2 above. Book 24: 430-1, 434-8.

31. Anonymous, 'Royal Hospital for Incurables: need of Nurses' Home', *City Press* 6 December 1929; Op.cit. See note 2 above, Book 2: 453-4, 467, 482; Book 26: 142, 180-1, 206-7, 213-4, 218, 233, 238.

32. Ibid. Book 26: 236, 240-1, 242-3, 245-7, 255-6.

33. Ibid: 272, 276-7, 288-9, 291-2; Anonymous, 'New Nurses' Home: Duchess of York to receive purses', *Daily Telegraph* 5 July 1935.

34. Op.cit. See note 2 above, Book 26: 272, 277, 289, 297, 301, 336, 400.

35. Ibid. Book 25: 166-7; Book 26: 413.

36. Ibid. Book 25: 494-7.

CHAPTER 12

The tragic case of Joseph Merrick (the 'Elephant man') in 1886

A N ISSUE IN WHICH the RHI seems to have come out somewhat discreditably involved Joseph Merrick (the 'Elephant man'). In a letter published in *The Times* for 4 December 1886, and written on 30 November, the Chairman of the (Royal) London Hospital (Mr F.C. Carr Gomm) outlined the sad story of this, by then, legendary figure. He wrote:

> The [RHI] and the British Home for Incurables both decline to take him in, even if sufficient funds were forthcoming to pay for him' [and Gomm went on to ask for help:] Can any of your readers suggest … some fitting place where he can be received?

In this letter, Gomm both outlined the case-history of this pathetic individual, and also outlined his justification for bringing the matter before the public:

> I am authorized to ask your powerful assistance in bringing to the notice of the public the following most exceptional case. There is now in a little room off one of our attic wards [at the London Hospital] a man named Joseph Merrick, aged about 27, a native of Leicester, so dreadful a sight (fig 12.1) that he is unable even to come out by daylight to the garden. He has been called 'the elephant man' on account of his terrible deformity. I will not shock your readers with any detailed description of his infirmities, but only one arm is available for work.

> Some 18 month ago, Mr. Treves, one of the surgeons of the London Hospital, saw him as he was exhibited [by Tom Norman] in a room off the Whitechapel-road. The poor fellow was then covered by an old curtain, endeavouring to warm himself over a brick which was heated by a lamp. As soon as a sufficient number of pennies had been collected by the manager at the door, poor Merrick threw off his curtain and exhibited himself in all his deformity. He and the manager went halves in the net proceeds of this exhibition, until at last the police stopped the exhibition of his deformities as against public decency.

Treves (with assistance from [Sir] John Bland-Sutton) gave a full account of Merrick's deformity at a meeting of the Pathological Society on 2 December.

> Unable to earn his livelihood by exhibiting himself any longer in England, he was persuaded to go over to Belgium, where he was taken in hand by an Austrian, who acted as his manager. Merrick managed in this way to save a sum of nearly £50, but the police there too kept him moving on, so that his life was a miserable

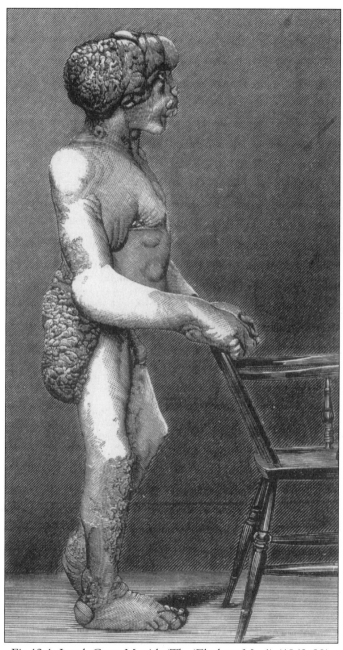

Fig 12.1: Joseph Carey Merrick (The 'Elephant Man') (1862 90).
Engraving of his right profile. British Medical Journal *1886, ii: 1188.*

and hunted one. One day, however, when the Austrian saw that the exhibition was pretty well played out, he decamped with poor Merrick's hardly-saved capital of £50, and left him alone and absolutely destitute in a foreign country. Fortunately however, he had something to pawn, by which he raised sufficient money to pay his passage back to England, for he felt that the only friend he had in the world was Mr. Treves, of the London Hospital. He therefore, though with much difficulty, made his way there, for at every station and landing-place the curious crowd so thronged and dogged his steps that it was not an easy matter for him to get about. When he reached the London Hospital he had only the clothes in which he stood. He has been taken in by our hospital, though there is, unfortunately, no hope of his cure, and the question now arises what is to be done with him in the future.

He has the greatest horror of the workhouse, nor is it possible, indeed, to send him into any place where he would not insure privacy, since his appearance is such that all shrink from him ... The police rightly prevent his being personally exhibited again; he cannot go out into the streets, as he is every-where so mobbed that existence is impossible; he cannot, in justice to others, be put in the general ward of a work-house, and from such, even if possible, he shrinks with the greatest horror; he ought not to be detained in our hospital (where he is occupying a private ward, and being treated with the greatest kindness – he says he has never before known in his life what quiet and rest were), since his case is *incurable* [my italics] and not suited, therefore, to our overcrowded general hospital; the incurable hospitals [i.e. the RHI and the British Home for Incurables] refuse to take him in even if we paid for him in full, and the difficult question therefore remains what is to be done for him.

Terrible though his appearance is, so terrible indeed that women and nervous persons fly in terror from the sight of him, and that he is debarred from seeking to earn his livelihood in any ordinary way, yet he is superior in intelligence, and can read and write, is quiet, gentle, not to say even refined in his mind. He occupies his time in the hospital by making with his one available hand little cardboard models, which he sends to the matron, doctor, and those who have been kind to him. Through all the miserable vicissitudes of his life he has carried about a painting of his mother to show that she was a decent and presentable person, and as a memorial of the only one who was kind to him in life until he came under the kind care of the nursing staff of the London Hospital and the surgeon [Treves] who has befriended him.

It is a case of singular affliction brought about through no fault of himself; he can but hope for quiet and privacy during a life which Mr. Treves assures me is not likely to be long.

Gomm proceeded to ask what could be done with Merrick on a long-term basis:

[When suitable accommodation is found] charitable people will come forward and enable me to provide him with such accommodation. In the meantime, though it is not the proper place for such an incurable case, the little room under the roof of our hospital and out of Cotton Ward supplies him with all he wants.

The Master of the Temple on Advent Sunday preached an eloquent sermon on the subject of our Master's answer to the question, 'Who did sin, this man or his parents, that he was born blind?' showing how one of the Creator's objects in permitting men to be born to a life of hopeless and miserable disability was that the works of God should be manifested in evoking the sympathy and kindly aid of those on whom such a heavy cross is not laid.

Some 76,000 patients a year pass through the doors of our hospital, but I have never before been authorized to invite public attention to any particular case, so it may well be believed that this case is exceptional.

Any communication about this should be addressed either to myself or to the secretary at the London Hospital. ...[1]

This account was followed by an illustrated one in the *British Medical Journal* for 11 December of that year. Treves seems to have been one of the first members of the medical profession to be intrigued by the curious deformity afflicting Merrick, previously the subject of discussion by the *Pathological Society of London* in December 1884 and again in March 1885; details of the case were also recorded in the *Transactions* of that society for 1885. Further information on Merrick has been provided by Trombley, and by Howell and Ford.[2]

The London Hospital's charter apparently stated specifically that it was *not* a hospital for incurables; it could not therefore offer permanent shelter to such an individual.[3] Merrick became the subject of intense interest in the media of the day, and he apparently had many visitors, including the Princess of Wales (later Queen Alexandra) (1844-1925). He suddenly died in the London Hospital, on 11 April 1890, where he 'had been [resident for] four or five years', and where his health was clearly deteriorating. Following a post-mortem examination, *The Times* for 16 April carried a full report entitled '*Death of "the Elephant Man"*'; he had died suddenly of 'asphyxia', and the jury at an inquest recorded a verdict that 'death was due to suffocation from the weight of the head pressing on the windpipe'. Shortly after Merrick's death, Carr Gomm again wrote to *The Times*, repeating his assertion that 'no incurable hospital would take him in [but as] an exceptional case the committee [of the London Hospital had] agreed to allow him to remain in the hospital upon the annual payment of a sum equivalent to the average cost of an occupied bed.'[4]

Why did the RHI and the British Home for Incurables *not* accept this *incurable* individual for admission? A search of the Board minute books for the relevant period, as well as the case-books (which include reasons for rejection) has failed to reveal a documented reason for refusal of his admission. It seems most likely that he was either considered to belong to the 'pauper class', and hence a responsibility of the workhouse and *not* the RHI, or that his appearance was so revolting that he would have been unacceptable on those grounds.

Another case from the London Hospital

On 27 October 1887 (about a year after his first letter to *The Times*), a note from Gomm was read to the Board; in it, he requested that the Board 'receive, without election, a male patient upon whom an interesting and successful operation [has] been performed'. The minute continues: 'The Secy was desired to express the regret of the Board that they were unable to accede to Mr Gomm's request.'[5]

References and Notes

1. F.C.C. Gomm, 'The Elephant Man', *Times, Lond.* 4 December 1886: 6. **Sir Frederick Treves**, Bt, GCVO, FRCS (1853-1923) received his medical training at the London Hospital, where he spent most of his subsequent medical/surgical career; he was appointed full surgeon there in 1884. He advocated surgical treatment of appendicitis, which was revolutionary at that time. He was surgeon-extraordinary to Queen Victoria and later sergeant-surgeon to King Edward VII (on whom he performed a surgical operation for appendicitis – which delayed his Coronation) and King George V. *See also*: S. Trombley, *Sir Frederick Treves: the extra-ordinary Edwardian* (London: Routledge 1989) 36-51; Anonymous, 'The elephant-man', *BMJ* 1886, **ii**: 1188-9; M. Howell, P. Ford, *The true history of the elephant man* (Harmondsworth. Penguin Books, 1980): 223; Anonymous, 'Congenital deformity', *BMJ* 1884, **ii**: 1140; 'Congenital deformity', *BMJ* 1885, **i**: 595; *Trans Path Soc Lond.* 1885, 36: 494. **Sir John Bland-Sutton** Bt. FRCS (1855-1936) was first employed at Thomas Cooke's school of anatomy at Brunswick Square. He then joined the Middlesex Hospital (he was appointed assistant and full surgeon in 1886 and 1905, respectively), where he spent most of his distinguished surgical career. He became president of the Royal College of Surgeons (1923-6). J. Bland-Sutton, *The story of a surgeon* (London: Methven, 1930): 204; *See also:* Anonymous, *Times, Lond.* 21 December 1936.
2. Op.cit. See note 1 above: (Trombley), 37-40; (Howell, Ford): 33-44, 140-151. *See also:* V. Kierman, 'X-rays expose secrets of the elephant man', *New Scientist* 1996, 7 December: 2.
3. Op.cit. See note 1 above: (Trombley): 42.
4. Anonymous, 'Death of "the Elephant Man"', *Times, Lond.* 16 April 1890: 6; F.C.C. Gomm, 'Death of "the Elephant Man"'. *Times, Lond.* 16 April 1890: 6.
5. Board minutes. Book 16: 95.

CHAPTER 13

The changing face of illness
at the RHI – 1854-1901

IN SEPTEMBER 1904, the Board of the RHI were made aware of several newspaper cuttings referring to 'the difficulty of obtaining admission to the Hospital by the lower classes', but it decided 'to take no notice of them'.[1] Admission to a *Poor Law Infirmary* ruled an individual out as far as a pension was involved.

There was also a widespread feeling that this was no longer a Christian 'home'. Thus in 1924, Mrs Annie Casher wrote to the Board complaining about 'the blasphemous errors of Christian Science and those hardly less of Christadelphianism [which were] sadly spreading in the [once Christian] Home.' She asked for a far more rigid regime, in which only *bone fide* Christians should be admitted. In a letter to her, the Chairman (expressing the opinion(s) of the Board) agreed in principle about these 'heresies', but felt that her idea of a member of the Board giving a formal address in order to eliminate such tendencies would not solve the problem, and might even be counter-productive. He felt that the House Committee should deal with such matters as they occurred.[2]

During the late nineteenth century, in-patients were often entertained by well-known performers (fig 13.1). Amongst these were Jenny Lind (1821-87) and her husband Otto Goldschmidt (a German pianist) who lived locally – in Parkside; they were frequent visitors, and also regular worshippers at Holy Trinity Church. Lady Jenkinson also gave concerts, primarily to raise funds, and Sir Squire Bancroft, a highly talented actor, read Dickens' *A Christmas Carol*. Another entertainer was the celebrated magician, David Devant.

The diagnoses of individuals seeking either *admission* to the Royal Hospital for Incurables (RHI), or *out-patient* management, in 1854-5, i.e. shortly after the foundation of the institution have been summarised in chapter 4. The present chapter seeks to compare the patients in these two eras of the hospital's development – almost half a century later!

Table 13.1 gives details of the first 100 entries in Case Book 11 (nos. 8501 to 9500); these individuals presented to the Board of Directors in 1901-2.

A marked preponderance of women, i.e. 76 compared with only 24 men should be noted; the reason for this remains unclear. Many were severely incapacitated and a considerable proportion confined to wheelchairs (fig 13.1). Although all patients in this sample chose to enter by 'election' rather than

181

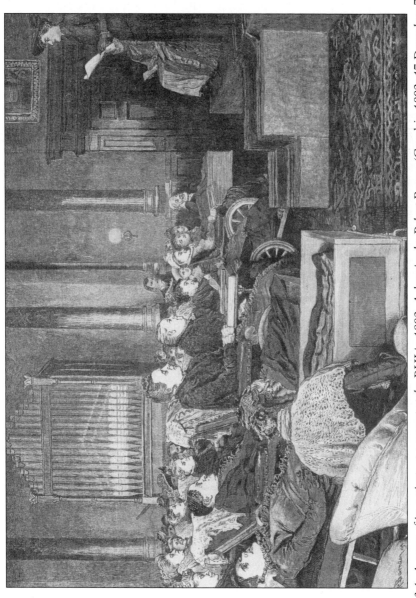

Fig 13.1: A group of in-patients at a concert at the RHI in 1892. A drawing by Robert Barnes (Graphic 1892; 17 December: 729).

'payment', only a minority (22 individuals) applied for in-patient ('inmate') care.

A huge predominance of neurological cases is noted, compared with the 'breakdown' of diagnoses shortly after the RHI's foundation (in 1854-5). Approximately half of the presentations involved some form of neurological disease. At this time there is good evidence of multiple (disseminated) sclerosis, the long-term effects of poliomyelitis, and Parkinson's disease (paralysis agitans). The second largest category (diagnosis-wise) is represented by disease of the locomotor system – 'rheumatism', rheumatoid arthritis, osteoarthritis and gout. Cardiac and respiratory disease account for a minority. *Mollities ossium* (case 9) is now known to be a malignant disease – myeloma involving plasma cells;[3] and 'paralysis agitans' (cases 19 and 92) is a disease of the basal ganglia. Some (perhaps all) of the cases of 'spinal curvature' were probably due to Pott's disease of the spine, resulting from tuberculosis. There were also cases of 'phthisis', 'lupus' and bone tuberculosis. As in the earlier sample (1854-5), malignant disease(s) accounted for only a very small minority (probably only two) of these cases.

Table 13.1: Details of 100 consecutive individuals 'presented' to the Board in 1901-2

No.*	Sex	Date of Birth (nineteenth century)	Diagnosis	Duration of illness (yr)	Date presented (twentieth century)	Category+
1	M	22 5 70	'Paralysis, from spinal injury'	4	15 5 01	I
2	F	4 9 39	Chronic rheumatism	'from girlhood'	"	I
3	M	28 10 55	'Spinal sclerosis'	8	"	P
4	F	30 11 51	Disease of right knee joint	Approx 34	"	P
5	F	20 2 52	Chronic rheumatic gout	Approx 18	"	I
6	M	10 2 69	'Paraplegia, caused by spinal injury'	3	"	P
7	F	8 6 58	'Spinal curvature'	'from infancy'	"	P
8	F	'1833'	Chronic diarrhoea	34	"	P
9	F	17 8 42	'Mollities ossium'	10	"	P
10	M	25 10 55	Disseminated sclerosis	15	"	P
11	F	1 3 53	Hemiplegia	Approx 1	"	P
12	F	5 11 26	Bronchitis. Ulceration of leg	Approx 0.5	"	P

No.*	Sex	Date of Birth (nineteenth century)	Diagnosis	Duration of illness (yr)	Date presented (twentieth century)	Category+
13	F	2 1 57	Spinal curvature	'from childhood'	15 5 01	P
14	F	29 11 41	'Cerebro-spinal neurasthenia'	26	"	P
15	F	17 8 55	'Rheumatoid arthritis deformans'	Approx 5	"	I
16	F	25 5 43	Wasting of muscles of hands	7	"	P
17	F	29 7 66	Spinal disease – deafness – partial blindness	Approx 2	"	I
18	M	24 4 69	'Tumour of medulla oblongata'	$4^1/_2$	"	I
19	M	16 11 48	'Paralysis agitans'	7	?	P
20	F	23 5 40	Cataract of both eyes	Approx 2	15 5 01	P
21	F	21 11 48	Cancer of breast	Approx 1.5	"	P
22	M	? 8 56	'Spinal sclerosis'	Approx 3	"	P
23	F	? 12 32	Bronchitis	Approx 1.1	"	P
24	F	13 6 60	Epilepsy	'from girlhood'	22 5 01	P
25	F	16 5 66	Rheumatism	12	"	I
26	F	27 5 41	Gout & bronchitis	9	"	P
27	F	10 8 58	Epilepsy	Approx 20	"	P
28	F	29 10 43	Hernia	>5	"	P
29	F	12 9 45	Hernia & spinal weakness	30	"	P
30	F	10 11 66	Myelitis or disseminated sclerosis	3	"	I
31	F	5 9 68	'Paralysis affecting one leg, hand, and hips'	29	"	P
32	F	27 1 44	Rheumatoid arthritis	6	"	P
33	M	3 8 59	'General paralysis'	Approx 2	"	P
34	F	18 5 67	Rheumatoid arthritis	14	"	P
35	F	19 10 63	Phthisis	Approx 8	"	P
36	F	17 7 55	Chronic rheumatoid arthritis	12	"	P
37	M	'1865'	Rheumatism affecting joints	12	"	P
38	M	7 6 61	Spastic paraplegia	Approx 5	"	P
39	F	10 6 70	Spinal paralysis	18	"	P

No.*	Sex	Date of Birth (nineteenth century)	Diagnosis	Duration of illness (yr)	Date presented (twentieth century)	Category+
40	F	1 7 65	Loss of both legs, scalp wound, neuralgia and prostration [resulting from railway accident]	22	12 6 01	P
41	F	17 9 67	Rheumatoid arthritis	10	"	I
42	M	21 4 68	Paralysis affecting both legs	'from early childhood'	"	I/P
43	F	30 11 62	Chronic rheumatism affecting joints and heart	7	"	P
44	M	29 6 36	Paralysis – Hemiplegia – Hydrocele	Approx 35	"	I
45	F	13 8 36	Rheumatoid arthritis	4	"	P
46	F	4 7 49	Defective sight; deformity of legs	'from birth'	"	P
47	F	24 6 27	Lameness & weakness caused by an accident	2½	"	P
48	F	18 9 58	Chronic rheumatism	Approx 4	"	I
49	F	27 2 52	Rheumatism	Approx 4	"	P
50	F	1 3 63	'Paralysis, complete of left leg, partial of right leg'	Approx 5	19 6 01	P
51	F	1 3 63	'Creeping paralysis'	2	"	P
52	M	19 12 37	Rheumatism	7	"	P
53	M	3 5 34	Chronic rheumatic arthritis	25	"	P
54	F	12 9 39	Deafness	17	"	I
55	M	17 10 49	Paralysis – complete of right leg – partial of left leg	Approx 3	"	P
56	F	27 5 71	Neuralgia; indigestion; constipation; membranous colitis	Since age of 10	26 6 01	P
57	F	28 10 70	Spinal curvature & deformity – hernia	'from infancy'	"	I
58	F	26 1 51	Lupus	'from childhood'	"	P
59	F	14 2 71	'Gradual loss of power in legs'	8	"	P

No.*	Sex	Date of Birth (nineteenth century)	Diagnosis	Duration of illness (yr)	Date presented (twentieth century)	Category+
60	F	22 1 39	Hemiplegia	Approx 1.5	10 7 01	P
61	F	6 3 44	Emphysema Bronchitis	'some years'	"	P
62	F	14 11 67	Paralysis of legs & weakness of arms	Approx 3	"	P
63	F	26 11 53	'Dilated heart & swollen legs traceable to scarlet fever'	31	"	P
64	F	17 2 43	Paralysis	1.5	"	P
65	F	17 7 65	Paraplegia – confined to bed	20	11 12 01	P
66	F	10 5 71	Disseminated sclerosis	Approx 7	"	P
67	F	25 5 56	Rheumatic gout	Approx 12	"	I
68	M	19 4 49	Caries of bones of face and foot – foot amputated	Approx 3	"	P
69	F	25 4 59	Rheumatoid arthritis	Approx 10	"	P
70	M	'1842'	'Complete paralysis of left side'	13	"	P/I
71	F	14 12 53	Uterine fibroid – neurotic	Approx 28	"	I
72	F	? 1 66	Paralysis & muscular atrophy of left leg	24	"	P
73	F	21 12 34	Paralysis affecting left arm & left leg	58	"	P
74	F	16 10 46	Abdominal hernia & spinal sclerosis	Approx 15	"	I
75	M	21 5 69	Disseminated sclerosis	1	"	P
76	M	28 5 63	General paralysis – loss of left leg ('fell off a mast')	19	"	P
77	F	1 4 47	Osteo arthritis with ankylosis of many joints	Approx 10	"	P
78	F	15 6 51	Paraplegia	38	"	P
79	F	'1828'	Fracture of thigh & paralysis	Approx 0.3	"	P
80	M	22 9 43	General paralysis	Approx 4	"	P
81	F	17 10 62	Asthma & bronchitis	10	"	P
82	F	13 5 69	Spinal curvature and club foot	'from infancy'	"	I

No.*	Sex	Date of Birth (nineteenth century)	Diagnosis	Duration of illness (yr)	Date presented (twentieth century)	Category+
83	M	30 9 54	Rheumatoid arthritis in all joints	Approx 3	8 1 02	P
84	M	22 8 33	Aortic regurgitation & bronchitis	Approx 15	"	P
85	F	20 1 56	Leg removed – inflammation of knee joint	18	"	P
86	F	6 3 31	Hemiplegia	4	"	I
87	F	'1844'	'Heart disease'	Approx 12	"	P
88	F	24 10 46	Rheumatoid arthritis	Approx 11	"	I
89	F	9 9 61	Displacement of kidney and dilatation of stomach	<4	"	P
90	M	18 7 58	Paralysis of lower limbs	15	"	P
91	F	1 5 65	Tubercular disease of bone – quiescent	'from childhood'	"	P
92	F	5 3 41	Paralysis agitans	6	"	I
93	F	6 9 68	Locomotor ataxy (sic)	4	"	P
94	F	16 4 41	Epilepsy	15	"	P
95	F	26 12 59	Muscular paralysis	Approx 3	"	P
96	F	26 10 57	Spinal weakness: incipient paraplegia – Rickets in childhood	'from infancy'	"	P
97	F	2 8 57	Epilepsy	Approx 28	"	P
98	F	4 10 36	'Tumour in lower jaw, diseased bones of left leg and right arm	30	"	P
99	F	14 8 69	Rheumatoid arthritis	Approx 8	"	P
100	M	'1849'	Paralysis (lateral sclerosis)	6	"	P

*The numbers of those accepted are in bold. +I = inmate; P = pensioner.

References and Notes

1. Board minutes, Book 23: 133.
2. Ibid. Book 25: 196-200.
3 M J Stone, 'Henry Bence Jones and his protein', *J med Biog* 1998, 6: 53-7.

CHAPTER 14

Serious criticism of the management of the RHI

As I will attempt to show in this chapter, the management of this Charity had been carefully monitored *externally* since its foundation. Not only were the mass media interested, but a Select Committee of the House of Lords was also concerned about the way the RHI was being run. Being a hospital governor must, in the mid-nineteenth century, have been a demanding and exacting job; management was always open to criticism. In 1862, for example, *The Times* published a letter condemning the fact that of the 200-250 governors of the Bridewell and Bethlehem hospitals, a mere eight had to be present at an Annual Court to make the business viable. Being a member of a hospital Board seems also to have been a stressful undertaking; Lt.Col. A.G. Holland (a member of the Board of Management for 17 years, and a brother of a celebrated preacher – Canon Scott Holland), for example, died during a meeting at the RHI in 1914.

Beginning of hostilities: an outburst from the *Athenaeum*

The RHI had been in existence for little more than a decade when an anonymous writer focusing on London's Charities published a hostile assessment of a recent Annual Report (apparently that for 1865) in the *Athenaeum* for August 1867. This was one of several 'intellectual' weekly journals of the day. The article considered that the present premises, i.e. Melrose Hall, were 'just as unfit a place for an hospital as any old family mansion of the last [eighteenth] century might be expected to be'. In fact, 'No building could be worse adapted for the purposes of an hospital ...'. To bring about the 'necessary alterations and improvements' (the article continued) had cost 'far in excess of the amount spent on the incurables themselves'. The balance sheet, he wrote, supported this assertion. The 'Receipts' for the year had been 22,823*l* (£), whereas the 'Expenditure' was:

On the Incurables.	
Housekeeping	£2,199
Medical expenses	123
Wines and spirits	123
Payments to pensioners	1,966
Medical expenses of ditto	62
	£4,473

General Expenses.

Salaries and wages at Hospital	579
Laundry wages	173
Estate wages	121
Furniture, fittings, &c	1,336
Rent of houses	535
Tithe and rates	84
Rent of London offices	150
Salaries, &c. at office	610
Office and election expenses	110
Printing and stationery	146
Advertisements	241
Postages	105
Travelling expenses	54
Festival expenses	143
Legal expenses, auditors, and small items	95
	£4,482

On Building and Estate Expenses, Balances, &c.

Estate expenses	922
Building expenses	5,036
Repayment of advance	2,000
Purchase of stock	2,000
Balance	4,003
	£13,961

The writer questioned whether the subscribers (who amounted to nearly 6,000) would be happy with the knowledge that their gifts were being used predominantly on overheads, including 'salaries, office expenses, and charges of the establishment' rather than on the patients! He continued by indicating to his readership that according to the Constitution, 'all the donations and subscriptions of five guineas and upwards … are not only carried to a permanent fund, but that that permanent fund is practically placed beyond the reach and control of the subscribers, and left to the control of the "board of management", to deal with as they please!' He was also sceptical as to the suitability of the institution to care for *seriously-ill* incurable cases – 'people suffering from paralysis, softening of the brain, spasmodic affection of the muscles, and so forth'. These patients should, in his opinion, be segregated from the milder incurables: 'A malformation is incurable; asthma is incurable; disease of the heart is incurable, affection of the nerves is, in many cases incurable.' Also, in the spring of 1867 there had been a number of coroner's inquests 'into deaths which had occurred with unusual rapidity at the [RHI]'.

The nursing staff too did not escape criticism; they were accused in the article of 'very rough treatment of some of the poor helpless creatures committed to their care'. Another 'bone of contention' was that there was no (well qualified) *resident* doctor! A 'medical attendant … residing in the neighbourhood' apparently visited daily, but this was not considered good enough. Doubt was also expressed about the necessity for a new wing – which would cost 10,000*l* of public money. There seemed sufficient space in the existent building for the 'present inmates', the writer asserted. Not surprisingly the article was heavily criticised by the Board of Management of the RHI – 'There were grave inaccuracies in the statement … and its conclusions were mostly unfavourable.'[1]

In a 'supportive' rejoinder, which aimed at negating all of this criticism, from the Secretary of the RHI (Andrew) written on behalf of the Board of Management, it was pointed out that the 'inmates' constituted a *family* and Melrose Hall was 'a *home* for life'. This article was written from the Hospital's City Office, 10 Poultry, on 27 August. Although he corrected a number of factual errors, his reply was by no means convincing, and the anonymous writer to the *Athenaeum* must be given credit for revealing to the public that this was not at this time an altogether first-class Charity. The writer of the original article clearly thought little of Andrew's reply, and ended a further short contribution with: 'We shall have more to say about the mismanagement of this great charity ere long.' A subsequent article by Dr W.T. Gardiner, MRCP indicated that he was in any case opposed to the concept of *incurables* (beyond hope of recovery); he preferred to distinguish *curare* ('to take care of, with a view to healing') from *cura* ('care').[2]

The writer of the original article launched into print again on 21 September; it was his (and the journal's) intention, he claimed, to *improve* the management of the Royal Hospital, not to destroy it! An 'informant', it was stated, knew (as did most members of the Board) the limitations of Melrose Hall as a hospital building; there was, for example, no inclined plane for the cripples, or a lift. It was the vision of the founder, Dr Reed, he maintained, to erect a series of self-contained almshouses ('as we see erected by our City companies, … for their decayed members'), and Melrose Hall was not at all what he had in mind. The method of appointment of 'a skilled head nurse' was also criticised, as was the absence of a 'committee of ladies' (since the majority of the patients were female); the offers of ladies 'of the highest position in the aristocratic neighbourhood of Wimbledon' to form themselves into a 'visiting committee' had been rejected by the Board (Chapter 3).

Although there was a sizeable Committee of Management, 'less than twelve [whom he named, together with their addresses and occupations] constitute the responsible management [the 'House Committee']' he claimed. And this body is 'virtually self-appointed!', and is 'composed for the most part, of an *inferior class* [my italics] of men.' This committee meets once a fortnight and there are 'frequently not above two or three members present, and sometimes not [even] a quorum'. The hospital had, in his view, 'grievously failed' the extreme and dying cases. What should be done, was to improve the present conditions (the hospital after all was 'not one-half occupied'), rather than appeal for funding for an 'additional wing'.

Charles Dickens, he maintained, had pleaded for a hospital to take in *urgent* cases (who were 'discharged uncured from ordinary hospitals, and those who had no home to go to') who 'should have admission, free, at the discretion of the Board'. Although it was the original intention to admit patients from the London hospitals (including 'Guy's, Middlesex, and the hospital at Victoria Park') this was *not* now the case. Finally he called for a 'committee of investigation' into the entire management of the RHI. So strongly did the Board of the RHI view these articles, that a *Special* Board Meeting was called on 3 October. At this meeting (which resolved to submit the articles to the Governors at the AGM), the Secretary also referred to an article in *The Lancet* of 28 September (*Lancet* 1867; **ii**:: 403-4) 'containing a re-publication, in substance, of the article of the *Athenaeum* of the 21st ult.'. At a subsequent meeting of the Board (on 24 October) it was decided to write to Thomas Tilson (Editor of the *Athenaeum*) 'intimating that [they] might feel it necessary to state that they had not received from him any [direct] communication upon the subject referred to.'[3]

In a subsequent issue of the *Athenaeum*, a correspondent (who was also a Governor), Robert Wilkinson, told the readership that he would 'be glad to receive the names of any "subscribers" to unite with [him] in making the necessary investigations'. This same correspondent followed up this offer with a further (joint) letter (with another Governor) to the same journal, in November: they recommended on the basis of a visit to the RHI (accompanied by two lady visitors) that: (i) there should be a Ladies' House Committee, (ii) additional nurses were required in the 'paralytic and epileptic wards', (iii) 'extreme care' was needed in the selection and supervision of 'subordinate nurses and attendants', (iv) a 'professionally-trained nurse' should be employed under the matron, (v) fewer patients should be put in some of the wards, (vi) there should be thicker partitions between the wards, but (vii) that the 'present governor, matron and medical officer [Dr Woodhouse] should be retained in their posts'. An investigation into the female wards also had been carried out by Mary Ann Westbrook; on the whole, she found the *status quo* (including ventilation) satisfactory, but felt the need for a 'Ladies' Committee, chosen from the wives and daughters of the managers'. She emphasised that more nurses were clearly required for 'the epileptic and paralytic wards'. Despite these reassurances, the Editor of the *Athenaeum* demanded 'a competent official inquiry' (see below) conducted by a 'committee appointed by the subscribers'.[4]

The correspondence in this volume of the *Athenaeum* was 'rounded off' by a letter from the (then) Archbishop of Canterbury, Charles Thomas Longley (who was also President of the RHI):

Addington Park, Croydon, Nov. 12, 1867.

Sir, – I have read all the articles in the *Athenaeum*, which you have forwarded to me, and I should think that after such statements the subscribers generally would wish for an impartial inquiry, and that the Committee themselves would hardly wish otherwise for their own sakes. I hardly think, however, that as President of the Institution I should move at the suggestion of one individual only; while if called upon by a requisition of several persons interested in the establishment, I would at once take steps to carry out your suggestion. – I am, Sir, your faithful and obedient Servant,

C.T. CANTUAR.

On the same day as this letter appeared in the *Athenaeum*, the Secretary had written to the President:

The Royal Hospital for Incurables
10 Poultry, 30th Novr. 1867

My Lord Archbishop,

Permit me to send your Grace a proof Copy of the statement submitted by the board to the Governors at the Annual General Meeting yesterday, in reference to the criticisms of the 'Athenaeum'. I may mention that it was adopted with but one dissentiant – the Revd. William Woodhouse, who did not deny his alleged connexion with the articles of that paper.

I take the liberty of sending also a copy of the 'Athenaeum of this day's date containing a copy of a letter from your Grace as a Member of the Board. The publication of your Grace's letter is entirely without the knowledge of the Board of Management –

I have the honour to be
My Lord Archbishop
Your Grace's Obedient Servant

Frederic Andrew
Secretary

His Grace
The Lord Archbishop of Canterbury.

As an 'after thought' the editor of the *Athenaeum* wrote: the 'Committee … have taken no steps whatever to secure an "impartial inquiry" … On the contrary, from all we gather, the Committee, as a body, are doing all they can to avert further investigation,' and he finished on a highly critical note:

As we write, the Autumnal Election of this institution is advertised to come off at the London Tavern, not under the Presidency of the Archbishop of Canterbury, but of that of 'Sir Benjamin Solomon Phillips, Knight.' 'The election will commence at twelve and close at two.' 'Thirty applicants will be elected,' – out of nearly 300 candidates! – every one of whom might receive the advantages of the institution if its funds were properly applied. It is lamentable to think that, where so much good might be done, so many poor and deserving candidates are destined to disappointment, entirely in consequence of the determination of the Committee not to expend the funds at their disposal.'[5]

It was now abundantly clear that there had been an 'inside' informant to the *Athenaeum* – none other than a member of the Board of Management itself. At a meeting held on 12 December 1867 it was resolved unanimously: 'That the Reverend William Woodhouse be requested to retire from the Board of Management.'![6]

The electoral (voting) system (Chapter 3) under attack
Five years after the *Athenaeum's* outburst, *The Times* published an account of the 36th election of the Charity, again held at the London Tavern. They had, according to the Chairman of the meeting, Henry Huth, to select '20 candidates from rather a long list'. 'Much [the anonymous writer continued] had been said of late against the system of canvassing for votes'. Fig 14.1 summarizes advice given to candidates seeking admission to the RHI in 1910 and fig 14.2 shows an example of an appeal for votes for a potential out-patient of the Charity in 1898. If the system were to be abandoned, however, it would result in 'a large falling off of the funds of the institution'. The alternative was 'that the selection … be made by the Committee of Management'.

The next mention of the election system was in *The Times* later that year; the article began by stressing to the readership that 'We have been requested to publish the following interesting [signed] document.' It is not totally clear as to who had made the request, but it is almost certain to have been the Charity Organization Society; the 'document' (dated November 1872) was signed by John Walter and George C.T. Barley, who were Chairman and Secretary, respectively, of that Society. The whole body of subscribers had apparently been sent circulars. The three alternatives given to them were:

1. That the outdoor and indoor patients should be elected by the whole body of the subscribers as at present, and that the existing system of canvassing and voting should be maintained.

2. That the indoor and outdoor patients should be chosen, after a careful investigation of comparative claims, by a managing committee, elected by the whole body of the subscribers, whether resident in London or the country, as suggested by the Council of the Charity Organization Society.

3. That some other plan (which would have to be described by the subscriber proposing it) should be adopted in preference to both the others.

ADVICE TO CANDIDATES.

When an incurable invalid has been accepted by the Board of Management of the ROYAL HOSPITAL FOR INCURABLES, PUTNEY HEATH, as a candidate for the benefits of the Institution, he, or she, should, of course, do all that is possible to secure election.

Election is only possible by the votes of subscribers. It should be borne in mind that whether a candidate is seeking admission to the Hospital, or the pension of £20 a year for life, very great benefit is sought and some effort is necessary on the part of the candidates and their friends.

The Board have ~~difficulty in securing~~ *t secure* year by year the £35,000 necessary to maintain this National Charity, and, since the successful candidates are those who alone benefit, it behoves them to leave no stone unturned to make known the good work of the Hospital, profiting their own candidature in the process.

A List of Subscribers to the Hospital is published and may be obtained, post free, for 1s. 3d. from the Secretary. In this List will be found the names and postal addresses of those who possess votes.

Candidates and their friends should send their cards to subscribers in the hope of receiving votes.

Candidates should also let their friends know that votes for one Election only are obtainable at the rate of four per guinea.

Fig 14.1: Summary of advice given to candidates seeking admission to the RHI in 1910.

194

Out of 6,454 circulars issued, answers were received from a mere 1,090! It was assumed that this sample represented 'the average' opinion of the subscribers. The *results* of the questionnaire were summarized; Option 1 was preferred by 165 subscribers, 2 by 847, and 3 by 78, i.e. 'more than five-sixths … express a decided wish [the article continued] for some complete change in the present mode of selecting the recipients of the charity':

1. Number of subscribers in favour of retaining the present system of election and canvass who vote for alternative No. 1	165
2. Number of subscribers in favour of abolishing the existing system, and adopting alternative No. 2 – that is, leaving the appointment of patients in the hands of a committee – or some other plan	925
Number of subscribers who replied	1,090
1. Votes in favour of retaining the present system –	
Life votes	441
Annual votes	172
Total votes in favour of the present system	613
2. Votes in favour of abolishing the existing system -	
a. In favour of alternative No. 2 – that is, leaving the appointment of patients in the hands of a committee:-	
Life votes	1,023
Annual votes	1,094
b. In favour of some other mode of selection of patients, which they describe:-	
Life votes	189
Annual votes	69
Total votes desiring to abolish voting, &c.	2,375
Number of votes held by the subscribers who replied	2,988

Of the 165 subscribers who were therefore *against* a change, 86 were life (with an overall 411 votes) and 79 annual (with 172 votes) subscribers, whereas of the 925 *in favour* of a change 426 were life (with 1,212 votes) and 499 annual (with 1,163 votes) subscribers. This result, although the number of replies was disappointingly low, '[suggested very strongly] that a change in the system of selection was favoured'.[7] However, nothing was done!

More criticism from the *Athenaeum*

In February 1873: 'The Secy presented [to the Board] copies of the "Athenaeum" Journal, for Jan 18th and Feby. 1st containing [more] strictures upon the management of the Institution, and the mode of election.' It was resolved 'That the copies of the "Athenaeum" now presented do lie upon the

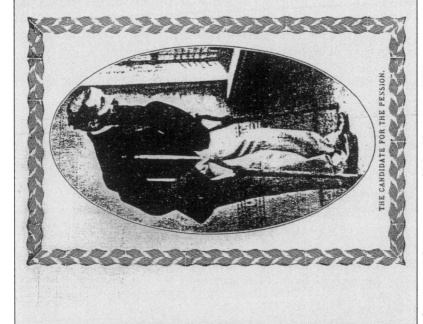

NOVEMBER ELECTION, 1898.

To the Governors of the

Royal Hospital for Incurables,

WEST HILL, PUTNEY.

Your VOTES and INTEREST are earnestly solicited
on behalf of

WILLIAM JAMES SHAVE

MARRIED. AGED 32.

CANDIDATE FOR THE PENSION,

Who for fourteen years has suffered from Rheumatism, and has been under treatment at St. George's Hospital, has been to Bath twice, and to the Local Hospital without benefit, and for four years has been quite disabled and is now entirely dependent upon his friends for support.

The case is personally known and strongly recommended by

Major-General Sir CHAS. D'OYLY. Bart., Newlands. Blandford
Major-General DENNE, The Down Wood, Blandford
Rev. C. H. FYNES-CLINTON. Rector of Blandford
C. B. HUMPHRYS. Esq., L R C P. & S ED. &c. Eagle House, Blandford

The Candidate is thankful to say that at this last May Election, his first attempt, he has secured 288 Votes, he again asks your kindly interest for November next, or for the following May, if November Votes are already promised

THE CANDIDATE FOR THE PENSION.

Fig 14.2: An example of an appeal for votes for a potential out-patient of The Charity, in 1898.

table.' The Board considered issuing a circular to attempt to squash this criticism, but this tactic was felt undesirable![8]

Both of these articles were printed under the following headings:

'LITERATURE

LONDON CHARITIES

Letter addressed to Subscribers to the Royal Hospital for Incurables. By Henry Carr. (Dryden Press.)

Proceedings of the Council of the Charity Organization Society. (Bell & Daldy.)

Report of the Committee for ascertaining the Wishes of the Subscribers to the Royal Hospital for Incurables. (Spottiswoode & Co.)'

The first (which pointed out that this was now a very wealthy Charity) addressed the theme of the 'overheads' of the Charity, the main 'message' being that the funds could, in the interest of the patients, be put to far better use. In the report of the RHI for 1870-1, there was mention of 132 'inmates' and 280 pensioners (each of whom received £20=00 annually), but the total income was no less than £25,449.13s.3d. This equated with an expenditure of £150 annually ('a great deal too large') on each inmate. The writer felt that £60 annually would be more acceptable. In place of this, the anonymous author suggested, the RHI could be supporting '990 more pensioners [out-patients]'. As a result the Hospital would be 'relieving 1,270 sufferers instead of [a mere] 412'. At present, the first article continued, 'one pound out of every three ... goes for general management'.

The second article was targeted at the 'paternalistic' system of election of which, it was claimed, 'a large majority of the subscribers' disapproved. He then provided details of the voting system. 'The inmates and pensioners are elected at half-yearly meetings, at which all the Governors ['close upon 10,000 in number'] vote, either in person or by proxy. Each subscriber possesses votes according to the value of his subscription. An annual subscriber has one vote for each half-guinea; a life subscriber one vote for each five guineas.' 'One gentleman [he continued] can give no less than 465 votes at each election'! In the autumn election of 1868, there were 40 vacancies and 307 competitors, and in November 1871, the corresponding figures were 20 and 298! 'It is almost impossible [he continued] that an election such as this should bring the most deserving candidates to the front ... those who are elected are ... those who have influential friends.' In addition, the writer repeated his previous assertion that 'Melrose House is as unsuited to its purpose as it well can be ...'. 'Melrose House is a noble mansion, fit only for the college of Mr Tennyson's Princess'![9] 'What is wanted ... is that the elections should be confined to a competent committee, upon which, as a matter of course, would sit one or two experienced medical men'. They would 'elect the worst cases'. He then referred to the founder's views on the *raison d'être* of the RHI:

> We quote the words [the article continued] of a gentleman who was originally associated with Dr. Reed in the management of the charity. The italics are his own:-

> In the early history of the charity, under the humane management of the founder, *destitute patients were admitted to all the benefits of the Home without payment or election.* In the founder's view this rule was the charitable feature of the charity. His often-repeated words were, 'We exist for the worst.' It was this which obtained for the institution in its infancy the invaluable 'Medical Testimonial' [Chapter 3]. Under the present management that rule has been altered, and the idea of charity obliterated. If Dr. Reed were living, he might say now, 'We exist for the wealthiest.' And, instead of his motto 'All the good for the good of all,' we must say, 'All the good for the good of all *who can best pay for it;*' or, 'All the good for the good of all *except the friendless*'.

The *greatest* blunder of all, in the eyes of the writer, had been the purchase of Melrose Hall in the first place; if it was sold it would yield a great deal of cash, and if spent on a building in a less salubrious locality 'would have held four times the number of patients at present resident at Putney'.

Yet more adverse publicity

In May 1874 a Board minute states: '… with regard to the Visits of the Hon. Mrs [Hamilton] Ward [a visitor to the RHI] evidence had been given by five of the Inmates shewing that that lady had spoken to the serious disparagement of the Committee, whom she had accused of mismanaging the funds. However, this view was immediately challenged by her husband William R. Ward of Oakfield, Wimbledon, SW, in a letter dated 4 May 1874. The Board resolved at a meeting later that month: 'That Mr. Ward be informed that the statement in question is grounded upon a letter written on the 6th March last by the Honble Mrs Ward to Miss Grant, an Inmate of the Hospital, in which the following passage occurs: "Enclosed is the paper I promised you, with Mrs Chapman's address – in the event of your leaving the Hospital you would I am sure find a comfortable home with Mrs Chapman, and she would take you for the same sum as you now pay".[10]

The allegation was that Miss Grant had told the Treasurer 'that the Hon. Mrs Ward had recommended her to leave the Hospital, and reside with Mrs. Chapman …'. There was also evidence that Mrs Ward had made 'charges of mismanagement … to the Matron, and in one instance, in the hearing of the Head Nurse.' The Board 'stuck to their guns' on this matter, and the following was subsequently minuted: '… in the opinion of the Board … the attempt of the Honble Mrs Ward to induce an Inmate to leave the Hospital was entirely uncalled for; it was also an undue use of the privilege of a visitor to the Hospital, and was calculated seriously to disturb the mind of a patient who needed repose, and who, with the advice of her friends, had recently entered the Hospital in the hope of securing it.' Mrs Ward was thus prohibited from visiting the Hospital! Both she and her husband seem not to have challenged the matter subsequently.[11]

The Stringer Case

A *Special* Board Meeting was called in April 1879 'on account of the reports, which had appeared in [several] Newspapers' about a controversy regarding the 'disposal' of one of the 'inmates'. The saga was to assume importance because the matter was reported to HRH the Prince of Wales, in an attempt to dissuade him from laying the foundation stone of the Great Extension to Melrose Hall (Chapter 8).

Mr Francis Stringer had been removed (from the RHI) to the Union Workhouse on 10 April (at the recommendation of Freshfield, the RHI Solicitor), but he was 'ejected from the precincts of the workhouse by the Relieving Officer', following which the Steward was told to take him 'back to the Hospital'. Stringer had been an inmate of the RHI for about four years, and a fixed annual payment of 100 guineas had been made by his friends; however, they had declined further payment, and on the advice of Freshfield, he was taken to the 'Poor House', and abandoned there. When the Steward returned to the workhouse (on the instruction of the RHI Secretary), Stringer 'had been received' despite the fact that he was not 'destitute' and the Steward was told by the Clerk that in consequence 'the Guardians had ordered a letter to be written to the "*Times*"'. Freshfield then advised that a letter also be sent which would be published simultaneously with the Guardian letter. These two letters appeared on Friday 11 April (other letters had apparently been sent to the *Telegraph* and the *Standard* – the latter paper had devoted a 'leading article' to the subject on 12 April).[12]

The RHI Board resolved that the 'real facts' of the case be sent to the Board of Guardians of the Wandsworth & Clapham Union (the Chairman was Canon Clarke), and also to 'the Press'. However, Freshfield's colleague, Mr Peter Williams, felt that this latter action was unwise as it could 'render the Board liable to an action for libel. The matter clearly engendered a great deal of hostility, and Mr Darbyshire, the late Governor of the RHI, wrote a letter (which the Board considered to be 'substantially untrue') which was published in the *Standard* on 19 April.[13]

A letter in reply to one from the Clerk to the 'Board of Guardians' was duly sent by the Secretary (Andrew):

To the Clerk to the Board of Guardians
Wandsworth & Clapham Union, S.W.

Sir,

I am directed by the Board of Management of the Royal Hospital for Incurables
to reply to your letter of the 12th inst; and to say, that they were not aware they
were acting with irregularity in seeking to obtain admission for an Inmate of the
Hospital into the Union.

In doing so, they acted under advice; and because they considered that the
Guardians alone could exert proper authority over Mr. Stringer's relatives, who
had left him in the hands of the Hospital, after full and proper notice given to
them to remove him.

The Board conceived that, as rate-payers in the Parish, they were entitled to
this amount of assistance from the Guardians.

They submit further that the removal of Mr. Stringer from the Hospital to the
Union, can not be said to have been effected against his will; because, when the
position of matters was explained to him, he acquiesced in the course which the
Board felt it right to adopt.

The Board had, doubtless, instructed their offices that Mr. Stringer must be left
at the Union; but it is a matter of regret to them, that in informing the Guardians
of this order on the part of the Hospital, he did not succeed in making heard
his intention to telegraph to [the office of the RHI in] London for further
instructions, when he found that Mr. Stringer would not be received.

The result of such enquiry on his part was that the decision to leave Mr
Stringer at the Union was reversed, and an order given to the Steward to take
him back to the Hospital, pending further communication with the Guardians.
This order would have been complied with, but for the fact of the Board, on his
return, having broken up, and Mr. Stringer having been received into the
Infirmary in the meantime.

Such are the facts of the case, and the Board instruct me to add that, as they
had no intention of burdening the Rates with the expense attending Mr.
Stringer's removal, they will, if required to do so, refund to the Guardians any
costs they may have incurred in the temporary maintenance of Mr. Stringer, or in
communicating with his friends.

I am
Sir,
Yours truly

(Signed) Frederic Andrew,
Secy.

P.S. I may add with regard to Mr. Stringer's designation as 'Captain', it cannot be
found, on reference to the Adjutant General at the Horse Guards, that any person
of that name served as an officer in the Army during the Crimean War, or in the
years 1853 to 1856.[14]

This letter apparently had the desired effect, for the Board of Guardians resolved 'that no further controversy on the subject take place'. The matter was followed by further correspondence in the *Times*; however, the Chairman of the Reigate Union Board of Guardians, for example, wrote that the RHI was not alone, 'for the Earlswood Idiot Asylum had in the past behaved in an exactly similar fashion'. *The Times* carried a brief 'post-mortem' on this case, and that seems to have been the end of the saga.[15]

The rumblings continue

There seems to have been continuous unease in the latter part of the nineteenth century, about the inadequacy of the management of the RHI; for example, a letter (sent on 17 January 1881) from a Mr Hill complained 'of the non-fulfilment of conditions proper to a Hospital for Incurables' but he declined 'to put the matters of complaint in writing' and alleged that the Board had attempted to 'suppress the report of his speech in the *Times*'. Despite denials by the Board, Hill again wrote (on 31 January) on the same lines and Freshfield recommended 'a simple acknowledgement of the letter, and request to the Manager of *The Times* seeking to 'trace the origin of the report quoted by Mr Hill'.

Some years later a letter was received by the Chairman of the Committee (in June 1890) from one of the Vice-Presidents – the Duke of Portland. He had heard a great deal of criticism concerning: the 'quality of food, want of supervision, management, ... religious needs of the Inmates, there being no Chaplain, and no facilities afforded for the patients attending early Communion.' The Secretary had replied on behalf of the Treasurer and the Board, and since no further letter had been received from the Duke, it was assumed by the management that the Secretary's replies had been satisfactory!

The following year the *City Press* apparently carried an article criticising the Matron and Nursing at the Seaside Home (Chapter 10); 26 female inmates, however, wrote to the Chairman of the Board indicating that these criticisms were 'most untruthful'.[16]

The House of Lords Report

A Report by the Select Committee of the *House of Lords* (which was reviewed in *The Times* in June 1892) succinctly outlined the hospital's structure at that time, i.e., nearly half a century after its foundation. There were currently 218 'inmates' (38 men and 180 women); in addition, 'Pensions of 20*l* [£] per annum are allowed to poor people [elected from the list of applicants] in any part of the country, totalling 11,000*l*.' The receipts for the previous year (1891) were 44,509*l* and the expenditure (including pensions of 11,129*l*) about 28,000*l*, leaving a balance of 16,509*l*. The Secretary (Andrew), who had filled that position since the RHI's foundation, received a salary of 500*l*. The matron, Mrs Linicke (Chapter 11 – who was German by birth, and it was said had a 'terrible temper') had a salary of 200*l* plus board and lodging; she yielded absolute power over the nursing staff, and was 'responsible for the ventilation of the wards'. She was directly answerable to the House Committee. Two grades of nurses existed: in grade 1 were five trained nurses (three on duty by day [each had charge of 'one corridor of 40 beds'] and one by night); grade 2 consisted of untrained nurses. In addition there were 'male attendants, mostly old soldiers, who [had] been employed in lunatic asylums; they [were] mostly employed in lifting patients': the steward (who had 'control of the male servants and also the drains') received 150*l* plus board and lodging. The medical officer who was *not* resident received 200*l* per annum; in addition, there was a consulting staff. There was 'no paid chaplain, but voluntary service [was] performed from outside'.

There was an annual meeting of governors (who paid half a guinea annually, or alternatively a lump sum of five guineas), as well as 6-monthly meetings for the election of in- and out-patient candidates. The Board of Management consisted of 20 governors (quorum 5) which sat every fortnight; from the Board, a House Committee was appointed – which met every week, when six or seven governors usually attended.

The food was 'contracted for', the contracts being made on the recommendation of the finance committee. The meat contract for example, 'had been for some years in the hands of one man'. Here there was, according to the Select Committee, a disparity between the replies of the managers and the evidence given by Andrew; the former had said that the 'meat contracts were open to competition', whereas Andrew had clearly stated that this was not the case![17]

Once again, the management of the RHI came in for serious criticism, which was reflected in *The Times*; in the section of their report on *Special Hospitals* the RHI received much adverse criticism; the hospital, it was recorded, was 'in receipt of very large support', but 'the authorities of this hospital appear to be incapable of effecting reforms, and are extremely resentful of external observation.' The House of Lords Committee had suggested, the report continued, the following reforms: (i) 'a resident medical officer should be appointed with general control in the absence of the committee, as is the case in the Poor Law Infirmaries'; (ii) a ladies' committee should be appointed (the select committee's report indicated that the Secretary was not convinced of this, and the Matron 'would probably not submit to the supervision of a committee of ladies'); (iii) all nurses should be hospital trained; (iv) 'that the contracts for food, and stores of all kinds, should be by open tender'; and (v) 'that the general supervision by the committee of governors should be greatly increased'. The House of Lords Committee had concluded: 'The objects of this charity are excellent, but until the management

Table 14.1: Suggested grouping of hospitals for purposes of representation on the proposed Central Board

Group of Hospitals, &c.	Number of beds	Number of representatives	Total representatives of Groups
3 Endowed hospitals	1,912	6	–
8 General, with schools	2,613	10	–
9 General, without schools	837	4	–
			20
16 Women and women and children	926	4	–
4 Consumption	511	1	–
2 Dental	–	1	–
3 Incurables	**–**	**1**	**–**
2 Cancer	141	1	–
4 Paralysis and epilepsy	240	1	–
3 Orthopaedic	113	1	–
2 Seamen and accidents	308	1	–
5 Ophthalmic	197	1	–
5 Throat and ear	52	1	–
7; 4 Skin and 3 Fistula, &c	112	1	–
1 Lock [venereal disease]	208	1	–
1 London Fever	180	1	–
4 Lying-in	132	1	–
7 Foreign and pay	249	1	–
Free and part-pay dispensaries	–	1	–
Provident dispensaries	–	1	
			20
General Medical Council	–	1	–
Royal College of Physicians	–	1	–
Royal College of Surgeons	–	1	–
Society of Apothecaries	–	1	–
General Practitioners	–	1	–
University for London	–	1	–
			6
London County Council	–	1	1
Sunday Fund	–	1	1
Saturday Fund	–	1	1
		Total	49

is thoroughly reformed the committee regret that they feel bound to add that the institution is *not* [my italics] one which can be commended.[18] Table 14.1 outlines the suggested groupings of hospital representation on the Central Board as outlined in the House of Lords report.

An internal inquiry in the light of the Select Committee's report

In July 1891 the Secretary (Andrew) received a letter from the 7th Earl of Aberdeen (President of the RHI);[19] this concerned remarks made 'against the Management of the Hospital' by Captain G.A. Webbe (a member of the Board of Management). In an attempt to solve this on-going problem a *Committee of Inquiry* was set up, and in November 'The Secy. presented to the RHI a copy of the Blue Book, containing evidence given by him before the Special Committee of the House of Lords in June last' (see above). In November also 'the Secy drew attention to an Advertisement, inviting persons to send to 106a Crawford St. for copies of evidence given in relation to this Institution before the select Comm[ee] of the House of Lords. He had found the order for a reprint had been given by Mr John Heatley Lewis of 10, Spring St. Sussex Gardens, once an inmate of the Hospital.'[20]

A *Special* Board Meeting was called (at the request of the treasurer – who chaired the meeting) on 2 April 1892. The Earl of Aberdeen had written to the treasurer on the proposed 'inquiry into the management of the Hospital'; this had been the subject of 'a conversation & correspondence [between them] last July.' The Select Committee of the House of Lords had in fact taken its evidence for the report on the management of the Metropolitan Hospitals which was published in June 1892 (see above) in mid-1891. Freshfield, although invited to the meeting, was unable to be present and 'had kindly communicated his views in writing'. The Treasurer then presented to the Board the correspondence which had taken place between Lord Aberdeen and himself and the Secretary of the RHI, as well as Freshfield's letter: five letters in all.

His Lordship had initiated the correspondence. In a letter to Allcroft (which was copied to the Secretary) to the Treasurer dated 28 March 1892 from 1 South Audley Street, W., he claimed that he was 'more convinced than ever [that an internal investigation into the management of the RHI] is in the interests of the Hospital, absolutely and urgently desirable'. He continued by informing the treasurer that in addition to the two Vice-Presidents of the RHI, he had 'secured from two other gentlemen [the Parliamentary Secretary of the Local Government Board in the previous Government, and the present Solicitor General for Scotland] a promise that they will join the Committee'. In a reply to Aberdeen, Allcroft wrote the following day, from 108 Lancaster Gate, W: 'Permit me to observe that you are departing from the understanding of last Autumn by proposing to bring [in] outsiders who know nothing of our affairs … The selection was to be made from among the Vice Presidents of the Hospital.' Aberdeen replied on 30 March that it was, in his opinion 'an *advantage* [my italics] to have ... gentlemen who are in no way connected with the Institution' on the Committee of inquiry. He also alluded to the fact that it might prove difficult to persuade a sufficient number of Vice-Presidents to spare the time to serve on the Committee. He continued: 'Public opinion is at present very sensitive ... to the whole subject of Hospital management [and it] is obviously much better to anticipate this by a voluntary step in that direction.'

Freshfield (writing from 5 Bank Buildings, London E.C. on 1 April) was in entire agreement with the letter Allcroft had sent to Aberdeen on 29 March. He continued:

> ... Please remember that the investigation whatever it may be will be purely informal. Neither the Chairman nor the Secretary will be entitled to administer an oath. The information will be given according to the views of the witnesses and there cannot be any indictment for perjury against any witnesses who should speak untruly; besides this as no oath can be administered and a witness cannot be compelled to speak, cross examination is valueless. To my mind therefore the examination and cross-examination of witnesses must be an absolute failure if it is expected that they will elicit the truth. Beyond this, however, I wish to point out to you the exceeding danger there would be in allowing such statements to be made and allowing them to go un-contradicted. This latter danger, however, is not so great as that which would arise from contradicting, because an issue would undoubtedly have to be raised as to the credibility or reputation of witnesses finding fault with the management, and then everyone connected with the so called defence would be more or less liable to have an action for slander or libel brought against them (there is no protection and no privilege for volunteers). In these circumstances, believe me, I do not fall in with the idea of the compulsory investigation. If the Earl of Aberdeen as President, and you as Treasurer, and the rest of the Board choose to hold an investigation on your own account and to ask certain Vice Presidents to come in and assist you in your considerations, I for one, shall be most happy to attend and go into the matter with you, and should consider it an honour to be asked to attend, but I should absolutely refuse to sit on any Committee unless I had been invited by the Board to do so, and unless all the members not on the Board had been so invited.
>
> I understand that Captain Webbe, a considerable subscriber, thinks the organization and management of the Hospital are defective, and wishes to formulate his views before an independent committee. I also understand that the Earl of Aberdeen is desirous of bringing the management of the Hospital before a Committee. In such a case Captain Webbe would have to take the place of a complainant, and would have to produce witnesses, members of the staff and inmates of the Hospital, to substantiate his complaints; the Board of Management being thus practically placed on their defence.
>
> This is a position which I could not advise them to assume.
>
> Were I conducting the enquiry, I should ask Captain Webbe to attend the

Committee and formulate his complaints. I should have them all taken down, and then, thanking him for the information which he had given, say that the necessary investigations would be made. He will, no doubt, be prepared to name certain people who would support his allegations. After this, the Board would have to see these persons, but not before, and their complaints would be carefully gone into.

Any report must be to the Governors, and not to Captain Webbe.

I am,

My Dear Mr Allcroft

Yours faithfully,

William D. Freshfield[21]

The meeting resolved that this correspondence 'be entered upon the Minutes', and further that the 'Board unanimously approve the opinions expressed in the letter of Mr Freshfield, a Vice-President of the Institution, confirming the arrangement of last July, by which they are prepared to abide', and also that 'a copy of Mr Freshfield's letter and of this resolution be forwarded to the Earl of Aberdeen by the Secretary'. This was duly carried out by Andrew who accompanied these documents with a short note, in which he thanked His Lordship for 'the great interest you take in the affairs of the Institution [but regret that the Board] cannot accept your ... proposal'.

A Board meeting in May 1892 resolved: 'That, in order, if possible, to avoid any differences which might be prejudicial to the best interests of the Institution, it would be desirable that a Deputation [consisting of the Treasurer, William Freshfield and Sir Massey Lopes; it was later agreed to invite Messrs Seaman, Rains or Wickham, also] should propose to meet the President ... and ascertain from him his views with reference to any improvements that might be made in the administration of the Hospital.'[22] Eventually, Aberdeen responded in writing (on 1 June) signifying his willingness to meet the Board, and suggesting that the Earl of Wemyss should join the Committee of Inquiry. Andrew duly responded on behalf of the Board indicating that he would be 'glad to arrange for a special meeting on a day that may be convenient to you.'[23] A *Special* Board Meeting called to 'consider the Report of the Select Committee of the House of Lords upon this Hospital' was held on 30 June 1892. Evidence had been given to the Secretary of the Select Committee as long ago as 29 June 1891: 'a summary of evidence ... relating to their Lordships' recommendations in respect of this Hospital [no 597 – Page 96 of Third Report]' was duly debated.

The 1891-2 RHI *Annual Report* was highly critical of the way the inquiry of the *Select Committee* had been conducted: it 'appeared to be based upon statements privately supplied to their Lordships [who had *not* visited the RHI], although by whom did not transpire ... the particular line of inquiry was not calculated to elicit a full and just account of the conduct of the

Home.' The report, in a preamble, had stated: 'the authorities of [the RHI] appear to be incapable of effecting reforms, and are extremely resentful of external observation …'. The major proposals were (1) a *resident* medical officer should be appointed; (2) a ladies committee should be formed; (3) all nurses should be hospital-trained; (4) contracts for food and 'stores of all kinds' should be by open tender; (5) the 'supervision by the Committee of government should be greatly increased'; and (6) the management needed to be 'thoroughly reformed'. The meeting discussed each conclusion serratum, and concluded that the report was based on a series of misunderstandings, in part resulting from a confusion between its activities and those of a *general* hospital. At the continuation of the adjourned meeting it was resolved unanimously to call a *Special* Meeting of the Governors on 22 July at the Cannon Street Hotel; Freshfield also told the committee that a friend of his was 'strongly in favour of a resident medical officer'. A 'Memorandum' or 'Answer to the Board' (in type) was sent to all Board members, and the 'Secy was directed to have it printed in pamphlet form' to be submitted to an adjourned meeting on 20 July. In summary this document entitled *ANSWER &c* (which consisted of 6 typed pages, signed by the treasurer, and dated 22 July 1892) was considered by the Board to possess no 'justice or validity', and they ventured to suggest that 'their Subscribers and the public will be of the same opinion as themselves'.

At a continuation of the adjourned *Special* Board Meeting, a draft resolution (to be moved by the Chairman of the Special Meeting on 22 July) was agreed to: 'That this meeting of Governors of the [RHI], having heard the explanation laid before it by the Board of Management … approves the same, and feels confident that the Board will continue to adopt such measures as will conduce to the interest and well being of the Institution and its Inmates.'[24]

Continued concerns in the light of the House of Lords report

Aberdeen sent a letter (written from Haddo House, Aberdeen on 20 July) apologising for his absence (in Scotland) from the Special Meeting of Governors and also indicating that he hoped that 'effective steps will at once be taken with a view to carrying out whatever may be found necessary in the directions indicated by the House of Lords Committee'. He was also regretful that he had failed to get a Special Committee appointed (owing to the Board's stipulation that only Vice-Presidents were acceptable) prior to publication of the House of Lords report.

The letter from Lord Aberdeen was duly read to the Special Meeting of Governors, and the above motion was made, to which an amendment (by Captain Webbe) was added: 'That, in the opinion of this Meeting, it is of the utmost importance that the Reforms recommended by the Select Committee of the House of Lords be carried out, and that the Board of Management be requested to take the necessary steps without delay, and further, that an Independent Committee of Governors be appointed to investigate the condition and management of the Hospital.' But, after it was seconded and following further discussion, this amendment was withdrawn, and substituted by one (which was lost): 'That this Meeting places full confidence in the Honour and zeal of the Board of Management, but is of the opinion that in the Interests of the Institution, the recommendations of the Committee of the House of Lords should be considered by a Committee of Governors in conference of the Board'. The original motion was then carried by 62 for and 20 against.[25]

At the August meeting, the Board resolved: 'That an Inquiry into the Management of the Hospital be held before the *Annual Meeting* in November next, and that the following gentlemen be invited to form the Comm[ee] – As President, the Earl of Aberdeen. On the part of the Board – Mr Allcroft, Sir Massey Lopes [who in the event could not serve], Mr Wickham & Mr Seaman. Vice Presidents. Mr W. Fowler, Mr Wm. D. Freshfield, Mr B.L. Cohen, M.P. As Outside Representatives – Lord Sandhurst, Lord Kinnaird, Andrew Graham Murray, Esq. QC, M.P.' Later additions to the Committee were: Sir John Whittaker Ellis Bt, The Earl of Arran, Henry Kimber, and John Rains, Esq. However, prior to the first meeting Seaman died and was replaced by Dr Small, while G.F. White deputised for Lopes. The 'Scope of the Inquiry' was resolved as '… essential that, in a thorough and searching manner, we make sure that everything is done to secure that the Institution shall fulfil in the most effective and complete manner possible the beneficent purpose for which it exists'. This was taken from the final paragraph of Aberdeen's letter to Allcroft dated 20 July 1892.[26]

The *Committee of inquiry* duly met and a report was written; unfortunately the draft had been (in July 1893) 'two months in the hands of the president, the Earl of Aberdeen'! He ultimately replied, and appended an (unsigned) memorandum to the report, in which he intimated that his views were similar to those adopted by the Earl of Arran. The members of the Committee clearly felt that the *Report* was long overdue, and at the end of September they resolved unanimously: 'That, seeing the absolute necessity of being in receipt of the Report of the Committee of Inquiry at the earliest possible time, especially in view of the yearly Report of the Institution, to be presented at the Annual Meeting on 24th of November [1893], Mr Andrew be requested, as Secretary of the Committee of Inquiry to take such steps as he may think necessary to put the Board in possession of the said report.'[27]

In October, a *Special* Board Meeting was called 'to receive and to deal with' the Report of the Committee of Inquiry. It was duly presented, and signed by the following gentlemen:

F.W. Blunt, Esq.
Henry Ellis, Esq.
William D. Freshfield, Esq.
Henry Kimber, Esq., MP
Rt. Hon. Sir Massey Lopes, Bt
John Rains, Esq.
James M. Rücker, Esq.
D.H. Small, Esq.
G.F. White, Esq.
and, Thomas Wickham, Esq.

Also presented was an addendum (letters and memoranda) from the Chairman (The Earl of Aberdeen), and the Earl of Arran.

The meeting agreed unanimously that: (1) the report and addendum 'be taken as read and placed in the Minutes of the Meeting'; (2) at the forthcoming AGM the attention of the Governors be directed to this report 'with such remarks as the Board may think fit'; (3) 'in these remarks it is desirable to guard against an impression … in the memorandum of the Earl of Arran that some change had occurred in the administration of the Hospital, subsequent to the sitting of the Lords' Committee'; and (4) a limited number of copies of the Report be printed, and that a copy be supplied to any Governor applying for one at or after the AGM.

The Board continues to resist change

The Report began by outlining the history of the House of Lords report, including a summary of the criticisms raised concerning the RHI, and the response of the Board of Management of the RHI to these allegations. Regarding the 'five specific reforms recommended by the House of Lords' Committee' the Board had sought and obtained the opinions and experience of: John Langdon Down, G.H. Makins, Richard Armistead, T.S. Clouston, Miss Pyne, S.L. Clift, Dr Coghill, Sir William S. Savory, William Broadbent, and H.C. Burdett. All five criticisms were set out in detail, and the Committee of Inquiry was in favour of maintaining the *status quo* in each case! In his memorandum, however, Aberdeen felt that: (1) a *resident* medical officer should be appointed 'as soon as such [an opportunity] occurs'; (2) Ladies should be 'asked to join the Board or Committee of Management'; and (3) all nurses should be hospital-trained and 'possessed of the highest attainable qualifications, according to the latest developments in that direction for their work'. Arran, in his memorandum, supported the recommendation for a *resident* medical officer, who he felt 'should be the supreme authority of the Hospital'. He also considered that 'the Staff should be recruited from as large a number of hospitals as possible'. He also felt that the Board should 'initiate any change in their mode of supervision which this Inquiry may have shown them to be advisable'.[28] At their October meeting, the Board '... agreed to take Mr Freshfield's opinion as to whether ... ladies were eligible, as Governors, for election as Members of the Board of Management.'[29]

Another *Special* Board Meeting was held in June 1894 'to consider what improvements can be effected in the Management of the Hospital, and to form a Committee to inquire and report.' The Board, however, rejected a formal motion to this effect, by 4 to 8! Moreover, Lopes (a staunch supporter of the inquiry) seconded a resolution that '... the Board form a Committee to inquire into the management and expenditure of the office, and that the House Committee form a [sub] Committee to inquire into the management and expenditure of the Hospital and the Seaside House.'[30]

At a meeting on 5 July, the precise rôles of the staff were 'spelled out' by the House Committee, and this was communicated to the Board a few days later. Clearly Lopes was in favour of a shake up of management, and later in July he moved: 'That it would be desirable to appoint some experienced independent person, who might, with Mr Andrew [the Secretary] go through the Secretariat and the Books of the Hospital and advise whether any alterations or improvements might be made, which would tend to the greater efficiency of the Institution.' However, this too was lost – for two, against six![31]

The rôle of Henry Charles Burdett (1847-1920)

Henry Burdett had given advice both to the House of Lords Select Committee, and also to the RHI's Committee of Inquiry. But he was by no means entirely in support of the RHI.

In April 1883, for example, he had applied for 'plans of the Hospital, and details of administration'. At that time, Andrew had replied on behalf of the Board that '... publication of the required particulars was [unlikely] to benefit the Institution' and the request was declined (Chapter 1). Later that month, Burdett made a further application, but this too was rejected by the Board. In August 1891 (in relation to the Select Committee's report) Burdett is recorded as saying that 'he was refused a plan of the Hospital, and ... impediments were put in his way.' 'Even in Russia [he claimed] they gave him greater facilities for entering a hospital than he could get from the [RHI] at Putney.' In August, a letter was received (by the Secretary) from Mr Kimber, MP 'inquiring into the circumstances under which Mr Burdett, as alleged, was refused access to the Hospital [see above], of which he desired certain details.'

It is not too surprising therefore, that this extremely powerful and well-informed Hospital Administrator was somewhat sceptical of the way in which the RHI was being managed. Amongst other rôles, Burdett was the Editor (and founder) of a weekly journal of hospital administration – *The Hospital*. In February 1893 (presumably in the light of the two inquiries – see above) this journal stated: 'We are glad to learn that in all probability better things will obtain before very long at the [RHI], Putney Heath … The time has passed when large endowments or large revenue from any sources is to exempt institutions from conforming to modern requirements in regard to management and other matters.'[32]

In December 1893, 'the Secy presented [to the Board] a copy of *"The Hospital"* of the 2nd inst containing an editorial article, commenting upon the proceedings of the recent *Annual Meeting*, principally upon the Report of the Commission of Inquiry then presented.' Sir Massey Lopes, although regretting the article, reaffirmed his opinion that a resident medical officer was desirable. The following January, 'A copy of this serial of the 30th ult. was presented, containing an unfriendly notice in relation to the management of the Hospital at Putney, according to an "informant from within the walls", as contrasted with the Management of the Seaside House at St Leonards, described in a letter from a "Visitor" – No name(s) given.' However, the issue of 13 January contained a letter (prefaced by 'a few lines by the Editor') from an 'Inmate', writing 'in favour of the conduct of the place'![33]

In retrospect, it seems extraordinarily tactless of the RHI Board of Management to have antagonised this powerful figure in the first place. But there was yet more 'flak' in other publications; e.g. in December 1893, the Board minutes read: 'The Secy. submitted a paragraph from *'Truth'* (see below) of the 21st inst. referring in unfriendly terms to the proceedings of the late Annual General Meeting.'[34]

The voting system under attack once more

As long ago as 1873, *The Times*, reporting on a meeting held at the Mansion House, had expressed its view(s) on the voting system; Lord Shaftesbury had said (the anonymous writer recorded), 'I heartily hope that the present system of voting for Charities may be got rid of,' while Lord Salisbury's contribution was: 'I should be sorry to join in any expression of opinion with regard to the system of Charity Voting which did not condemn it altogether.' There, we have an assessment of the voting system from two extremes of the political spectrum!

And in 1914, an anonymous writer to the *Lancet* summarised his (or her) views, which seem to have been at that time widely felt, on the *voting system* at the RHI:

> The system of election to the benefits of certain charities by a poll of subscribers has some obvious drawbacks as well as some advantages. One of the latter is the contact which it establishes between the subscribers and the nature of the work which is carried on by their money.
>
> The [RHI], for instance, sends out twice a year a voting paper, revealing an amount of human misery calculated to appal far more callous persons than those

who subscribe to that splendid charity. Medically speaking, the column headed 'Disease or Disability' is full of interest. At first sight it is surprising to find among the 192 candidates for the benefits of the society at the recent election not a single case diagnosed as malignant disease or as pulmonary tuberculosis. The explanation is probably to be found in the delay which necessarily ensues before a patient can be accepted; it always takes months, and generally years, to reach this much coveted haven of refuge, either as an in-patient or as a pensioner. Heart disease, again, is less prominent than might be expected; seven cases alone appear, and in most of them some other condition is superadded. Aneurysm and Bright's disease are absent from the list altogether. Turning to the common causes of disability, 'rheumatoid arthritis' is diagnosed in 58 cases, and chronic rheumatism, osteo-arthritis, and rheumatic gout account for another 14 – an eloquent proof of our therapeutic helplessness for these intractable disorders. The other main group is that of the paralyses, which includes at least 73 cases, and probably more. The diagnoses of these disorders are so confused that in the majority of cases it is impossible to identify the extent and nature of the disease. In a few cases disseminated sclerosis, locomotor ataxia, myelitis, and paralysis agitans are specified; but 'paralysis' is the only label attached to the bulk of the cases. The point is of minor importance, no doubt, because most subscribers do not trouble themselves about the complaint of the candidate they vote for; but it does occasionally happen that a medical man is asked to advise upon the relative disabilities attaching to various diseases.

There are further instances of unsatisfactory diagnosis on the list. 'Internal trouble' appears two or three times; not, by the way, from a false delicacy, for 'fibrous tumours' are specified in another case. 'Debility after surgical operation' may be a euphemism for something more tangible, especially as the candidate is in her sixth year of application; but it is ambiguous and therefore objectionable. Graves' disease as a qualification for an incurables' charity may be a slight shock both to some physicians and to some surgeons. 'Creeping paralysis' is a curious phrase in a list of presumably derived from medical certificates, and 'nervous debility' is equally vague and meaningless. Haemophilia, myxeodema, and anaemia with enlarged spleen are some of the more uncommon and interesting diagnoses put forward. Doubtless the investigations of the society's officers exclude all except really urgent and deserving cases; but there is room for improvement in the system of setting forth the diagnosis and in the information thereby supplied to the electors.[35]

A letter from the *BMA* was at a Board meeting held in March 1906; it had been sent via Lord Northampton (the then President). Its receipt was acknowledged, but the Board regretted that 'they [were] unable to alter the [voting system] which had been in use so many years'.[36]

Continuing criticism of management
In 1927, *Truth* (see above) published a further critical assessment of the management of the RHHI. A patient who had suffered from depression had

walked out of the hospital and had committed suicide in Richmond Park – by drinking Lysol. This, the reporter considered, pointed to poor management at the RHHI, and he/she suspected 'threats of expulsion' had been used by the staff when a patient objected to an occurrence. The 'voting system' was also again criticised.[37] The Board (and others) took violent objection to these 'recent paragraphs published in *Truth*', concerning the management of the RHHI'. The obnoxious article referred to patients being 'afraid to ventilate their grievances'. The acting Chairman (T.C.E. Goff) wrote to the editor of *Truth* on behalf of the Board: '... the statements made in your paper give an entirely wrong impression of the management of [this] Institution ...'. He continued: 'The publication of charges such as these is ... an offence against suffering humanity ...'. However, the matter was considered serious and a *Special* Board Meeting was called for 12 January 1928, when it was decided that the best way forward was for a deputation from the Board to meet the Editor of *Truth*, when the matter seems to have been amicably resolved.[38]

References and Notes

1. [R.R.], 'The Royal hospitals', *Times, Lond.* 19 November 1862: 6; Anonymous, 'A death at a Board meeting', *Hospital* 21 November 1914; Anonymous, 'London charities' [Eleventh Article] (the Royal Hospital for Incurables) *Athenaeum*, 241, 24 August 1867: 239; Board minutes. Book 7: 113-14, and 191-3.

2. F. Andrew, 'Royal Hospital for Incurables', *Athenaeum* 31 August 1867: 274-6; Op.cit. See note 1 above (Board minutes), Book 7: 114; Anonymous, 'Royal Hospital for Incurables', *Athenaeum* 7 September 1867: 304; W.T. Gairdner, 'Miscellanea: Medical aid', *Athenaeum* 14 September 1867: 348.

3. Anonymous, 'The Royal Hospital for Incurables', *Athenaeum* 21 September 1867: 366-7; Op.cit. See note 1 above (Board minutes), Book 7: 134-5, 144-5, 159-60, 165-6, 178-9, 191-3.

4. R. Wilkinson, 'Royal Hospital for Incurables', *Athenaeum* 12 October 1867: 466; R. Wilkinson, W. Banting, 'Royal Hospital for Incurables', *Athenaeum* 2 November 1867: 575-6; Op.cit. See note 1 above (Board minutes), Book 7: 179, 191; M. A. Westbrook, 'Royal Hospital for Incurables', *Athenaeum* 2 November 1867: 576.

5. C.T. Cantuar, 'Royal Hospital for Incurables', *Athenaeum* 30 November 1867: 724; op.cit. See note 1 above (Board minutes), Book 7: 213-5. **Charles Thomas Longley** (1794-1868) was Archbishop of Canterbury from 1862 until his death. Educated at Westminster School and Christ Church, Oxford, he had become headmaster of Harrow (1829-1836) and subsequently Bishop of Ripon (1836-56), Durham (1856-60), and Archbishop of York (1860-62). *See also:* E. Carpenter, *Cantuar: the archbishops in their office* (London; Cassell, 1971) 312-33.

6. Op.cit. See note 1 above (Board minutes), Book 7: 212-3.

7. Anonymous, 'Royal Hospital for Incurables', *Times, Lond.* 1 June 1872: 11; Anonymous, 'Charity electioneering', *Times, Lond.* 22 November 1872: 10.

8. Op.cit. See note 1 above (Board minutes), Book 9: 334, 358; Anonymous, 'Literature: London Charities', *Athenaeum* 18 January 1873: 75-6; 1 February: 141-2.

9. **Alfred Tennyson, first Baron Tennyson** (1809-92), was born at Somersbury, Lincolnshire. He subsequently attended Trinity College, Cambridge and became a prolific poet; he published *The Princess* in 1847. On the death of William Wordsworth (1770-1850) he became poet laureate. Tennyson lived at Farringford, Isle of Wight. He was buried in Westminster Abbey.

10. Op.cit. See note 1 above (Board minutes), Book 10: 107, 109-11, 112-13.

11. Ibid: 113-14.

12. Ibid: Book 12: 238-9, 246-50; Anonymous, '"Asylum" or Workhouse', *Times, Lond.* 11 April 1879: 4; T. Sanders, '"Asylum" or Workhouse', *Times, Lond.* 11 April 1879: 4; F. Andrew, '"Asylum" or Workhouse, *Times, Lond.* 11 April 1879: 4.

13. F. Andrew, 'The Hospital for Incurables', *Times, Lond.* 12 April 1879: 7; Op.cit. See note 1 above (Board minutes), Book 12: 249-50, 251-4.

14. Ibid: 264-6.

15. Ibid: 276-7; F.W. Costar, 'Asylum or Workhouse', *Times, London* 14 April 1879: 4; Anonymous, 'Asylum or Workhouse', *Times, Lond.* 18 April 1879: 11.

16. Op.cit. See note 1 above (Board minutes), Book 13: 186-7, 197-8; Book 17: 164, 397.

17. Anonymous. *Third Report from the Select Committee of the House of Lords on Metropolitan Hospitals, &c. together with the Proceedings of the Committee, minutes of evidence, and appendix.* London: HM Stationery Office 1892; 21 June: 63-65.

18. Anonymous. Metropolitan Hospitals. *Times, Lond.* 1892; 24 June: 13.

19. **John Campbell Gordon**, KT, GCMG, GCVO, seventh Earl of Aberdeen, and from 1915 first Marquess of Aberdeen and Temair (1847-1934) was an eminent statesman. He was born in Edinburgh and educated at St Andrew's University and University College, Oxford. His grandfather (George Hamilton Gordon – 1784-1860), the fourth Earl, had been Prime Minister. From 1893-8 he served in Canada as Governor-General; this ended his presidency of the RHI; he resigned in September 1893 (See Board minutes, Book 19: 250). Much of his work was however carried out in Ireland. In addition, social welfare was a major preoccupation and he was in 'constant association' with the seventh Earl of Shaftesbury and later Henry Drummond. *See also: Dictionary of National Biography* (1931-40): 347-9; *Times, Lond.* 8 March & 19 April 1934; Op.cit. See note 1 above (Board minutes), Book 18: 440-1, 461-4.

20. Op.cit. See note 1 above (Board minutes), Book 17: 417-8, 479, 494.
21. Ibid: Book 18: 80-92, 98-9, 112.
22. Ibid: 132-3, 136-7, 144-5.
23. Ibid: 145-8.
24. Ibid: 160-4 (a minute some years previously had indicated that all provisions were to be purchased at current prices instead of by contract). Book 12: 452); *See also: Answer &c:* Book 18: 165-6, 178-9, 179-180).
25. Ibid: 181-7.
26. Ibid: 196, 197-8, 208, 242-3, 309.
27. Ibid: 422-3, 434-5, 435-6, 449, 464-5.
28. Ibid: 479-81; Royal Hospital for Incurables: *Report of the Committee of Inquiry,* adopted 13 October 1893:11; *Annual Report* 1892-3.
29. Op.cit. See note 1 above (Board minutes), Book 18: 488.
30. Ibid. Book 19: 137-8, 156.
31. Ibid: 162-5, 170.
32. **Sir Henry Charles Burdett,** KCB, KCVO (1847-1920) was an outstanding hospital administrator. Following six years at the Queen's Hospital Birmingham, he became Secretary of the Seamen's Hospital Society, Greenwich; he was later appointed to the Share and Loan Department of the Stock Exchange. Burdett was a pioneer of the cottage hospital movement, and introduced pay beds and wards into London's teaching hospitals. Burdett also played a major part (following Nightingale) in establishing nursing as a 'respectable' profession. He also established the (Royal) National Pension Fund for Nurses. Burdett also founded *The Hospital*, which he edited. *See also*: G.C. Cook, 'Henry Charles Burdett (1847-1920): outstanding hospital administrator, successful Secretary of the Seamen's Hospital Society, and notable philanthropist', *J med Biog* 2001; 9: 195-207; Anonymous, *The Hospital* 1893; 13: 314; Op.cit. See note 1 above (Board minutes), Book 14: 170, 178; Book 17: 435; Book 18: 208-9; Book 19: 16.
33. Op.cit. See note 15 above: 16-17; Anonymous, 'The Royal Hospital for Incurables, '*The Hospital* 1893, 15: 129-130, 143-4; Anonymous, 'The Royal Hospital for Incurables', *The Hospital* 1893, 15: 194; Anonymous, 'The Royal Hospital for Incurables: Voices from the Interior', *The Hospital* 1894, 15: 232. Op.cit. See note 1 above (Board minutes), Book 19: 16.
34. Ibid: 33.
35. Anonymous, Leading article, *Times, Lond.* 31 October 1873: 9; [MD Cantab] 'A catalogue of suffering', *Lancet* 1914, i: 358-9.
36. Op.cit. See note 1 above (Board minutes), Book 23: 250.
37. Anonymous, 'The lot of the incurable', *Truth* 26 October 1927.
38. Op.cit. See note 1 above (Board minutes), Book 25: 406, 408-10, 413-16.

CHAPTER 15

State intervention:
the National Health Service Act
(1946) and its possible consequences

DURING THE FIRST HALF of the twentieth century, the voluntary hospitals were desperately short of funds; many had to close a significant number of beds, because they simply could not afford to pay for their continuing occupancy.[1] The King's Fund was extremely useful to many, but the RHI had never received support from this charity, or in fact from the Metropolitan Sunday Fund. To many, state intervention seemed the only way forward – but this would inevitably lead to a loss of identity and individuality. An opposing view was aired by Sir Thomas Barlow, when speaking in early 1909 to the annual meeting of governors of the London Fever Hospital:

> ... some of their academic friends [he said] were ready to put the whole hospital administration into the melting pot and put doctors and nurses under ... the iron hand of the State. It would in his opinion be the greatest possible calamity to this country if the hospitals were all put into the hands of either the State or the municipality ... the greatest advances in practical medicine had been made [he claimed] under the aegis of voluntary hospitals.[2]

Barlow, as President of the Royal College of Physicians from 1910 to 1914, was to witness, at close quarters, a great deal of controversy over the National Insurance Act. An RHI minute in January 1914 records, for example, that 'the Secretary be instructed to make enquiries from a number of hospitals as to the method of dealing with the question of payment of sick allowance under the National Insurance Act [1911]'. And in February it was resolved that '... during sickness, salaries will be paid in full (up to a month) but that the Board of Management will expect to retain the sick pay due under the Act. At the same time the Board will be willing to consider each case on its merits, if application is made for such consideration.' The *Daily Graphic* outlined in 1914 some of the effects of the Insurance Act; more patients were attending their panel doctor than the local outpatient department. This meant that subscriptions to the voluntary hospitals had declined, with the inevitable consequence that facilities for in-patients and research were increasingly under-funded. The result would be that many smaller hospitals would have to close or amalgamate. And, in 1920, the Government proposed building *new* hospitals. But as was pointed out in correspondence in *The Times*, while the voluntary hospitals had long waiting lists, the Poor Law Infirmaries always had a large number of vacant beds. Therefore, the latter should be utilised in any new building scheme.

The Local Government Act of 1929 meant that numerous institutions (many of them under the auspices of the Metropolitan Asylums Board) were transferred to the (LCC) Act. By the end of 1931, there were 44 general hospitals (with 27,553 beds) in London and 31 special hospitals (with 13,390 beds). The sum total was that there were good as well as bad legacies from the Board of Guardians.[3]

The National Health Service Act

There must have been a great deal of uncertainty at the RHHI (with a serious resultant effect on the Home's financial situation) and anxiety in the months and years immediately after the introduction of the National Health Service (NHS) Act of 1946; this event was several years *before* the centenary of the RHI. The Minister of Health (Aneurin Bevan [1897-1960]) appropriated almost every hospital in the land. Thus, the Midland Counties Home for Incurables at Leamington, and Strathclyde House, the Carlisle home for incurables, for example, were immediately taken over. The *Annual Report* for 1947 began: 'At the time of writing ... it is not known if this Hospital and Home will be included in the new [NHS] ... Should the decision [be affirmative], it will come, on 5th July 1948 [the 'appointed day'], under the remote control of the South-West Metropolitan Regional Board and the immediate control of a Hospital Management Committee, which will probably be composed in the main of the present members of the Board.' The *Annual Report* the following year was equally unclear as to where the future lay, but it added: '... subscribers will be informed directly the result is known.' In 1949, the *Annual Report* indicated to the subscribers that 'the Board of Management had decided to *resist* [my italics] inclusion in the [NHS] and to have the matter settled by arbitration, it being thought that a Home of this nature can best serve its patients by remaining [like most other well-known Homes for Incurables] a voluntary body.'[4]

Board meetings: 1946-50

The Board decided, at a meeting in March 1946, to set up a Sub-committee to 'keep a careful watch on events appertaining to the [NHS] Bill'; it was made up of the following Board members: Sir Edward Maclagan, Lt-General Sir Ernest Bradfield, Mrs Wilson Black, Howard T. Cross and Norman Morris.

At a Board meeting on 25 April 1946 there was considerable discussion on the NHS Bill; it was decided 'that a letter to the Minister ... asking for the exemption of the Hospital from the Bill, under clause 6(3), be signed by the

Chairman [Sir Edward Maclagan], and its dispatch be notified, together with an intimation of the Board's general acceptance of the views of the British Hospitals Association, the Voluntary Hospitals Committee & the Association of Special Hospitals.' It was also decided that information should be 'communicated to Mr [Hugh] Linstead, Member of Parliament for Putney.'[5] The following day, Maclagan duly wrote to Bevan on behalf of the Board of the RHHI, asking for *exclusion* of this institution from the NHS under clause 6(3) – which stated under the heading *Transfer of hospitals to the Minister*:

> If it appears to the Minister that, in the case of any hospital to which the foregoing provisions of this section apply, the transfer of the hospital or of the interests referred to in subsection (I) of this section *will not be required for the purpose of providing hospital and specialist services* [my italics], he may, at any time before the appointed day, serve a notice to that effect on the governing body of the hospital or, as the case may be, on the local authority in which the hospital is vested, and thereupon the foregoing provisions of this section shall cease to apply to that hospital:
>
> Provided that if the governing body or local authority, within such period (not being less than twenty-eight days from the service of the notice) as may be specified in the notice, serve a notice on the Minister stating that they wish the hospital or interests to be transferred to the Minister, the foregoing provisions of this section shall apply to the hospital.

Maclagan wrote:

> … The term 'Hospital', as applied to this Institution, is in some ways a misnomer. No patient is admitted unless his or her disease is certified to be incurable, although all that is possible is done, under the supervision of a visiting doctor, to alleviate the ailments of the patients. The Institution was started in 1854 as an 'Asylum' and it has regularly been refused pecuniary help from bodies like the King Edward Hospital Fund and the [Metropolitan] Hospital Sunday Fund, on the grounds that it is not in line with other hospitals. It is, in fact, a Home and it has always aimed at providing greater amenities to its patients than would be provided in a hospital.
>
> The nomination for admission to the Institution lies in the hands of subscribers and its funds consist mainly of the subscriptions so received and of legacies left for the benefit of the Institution. The Board has always felt itself under an obligation to maintain its patients for life and has gradually put together a reserve, now bringing in about £18,000 a year, with a view to meeting this obligation in future years. It has also an entirely separate branch of its activities, under which it distributes cash pensions of £20 and, latterly, £42 a year to some 450 certified incurables at their homes throughout the British Isles.
>
> The management is based on a fine tradition handed down for close on a century from the Founder, Dr. Andrew Reed, and it has always been ready, when funds were available, to extend its activities. It has at the present moment a number of useful schemes in view which were only delayed by the want of

labour consequent on the war and it would always be ready to listen to official advice as to its future extensions.[6]

The Minister immediately replied that he 'would be prepared to consider the question of the exclusion of the Home from the Service under the relevant section at the appropriate time.' At its June meeting, the Board resolved unanimously 'that the Board attaches great importance to the Hospitals for Incurables in this country acting together in regard to the [NHS] Bill and, with this in mind, invites the Chairman to approach the Chairmen of the other Hospitals for Incurables with a view to arranging a Meeting for the discussion of policy at an early date.' The Chairman decided that before the proposed meeting it would be expedient 'to have a small exploratory meeting with [the British Home and Hospital for Incurables (BHHI)] Streatham in the first place'. At this meeting, it transpired that the BHHI 'intended to take no action [with regard to the NHS Bill] until Regional Board [RB]s had been set up.' Following this, *if* the BHHI and RHHI fell under the same RB 'joint action by the two hospitals was [considered] highly desirable'. The Board approved of this course and felt that for the present 'no further attempt [should] be made to hold a combined meeting of hospitals for incurables.'[7]

Linstead produced a memorandum, which was debated by the Board on 28 May 1947; in this he 'gave his views on the grounds on which he considered the Hospital should apply for exemption'. In June of that year, the Board also received a draft memorandum from Linstead; in this he emphasised the enormous experience at the RHHI in caring for the chronic sick – a theme which those shaping the NHS, he claimed, probably failed to appreciate; the social and nursing aspects, especially, were under-recognised by them! It was, he felt, important that 'this Hospital [the RHHI] should contact the Ministry & lay their views fairly and squarely before the appropriate officials.' The Board considered that an amended letter, in the light of remarks made concurrently by Dr S. Henning Belfrage, MD, MRCS, LRCP (to the effect that not all 'chronic' cases are *incurable*), 'should be sent to the Ministry by the Chairman as soon as possible, & a copy … to the RB, when that Board should be set up.'[8]

At the November meeting of that year, an informal visit to the RHHI by Dr Stark Murray and Mrs Feiling (members of the South-West Metropolitan RB) was reported. It was emphasised, however, 'that before any decision to take over the Hospital was made, the Board still desired to have an opportunity of meeting the RB on a *formal* occasion.' At the January (1948) meeting, with Mr Norman Morris and *not* Sir Edward Maclagan (who had resigned from that office, but continued on the Board) in the chair, it was reported that Morris, Maclagan and Linstead (with the Secretary in attendance) had that morning interviewed the Finance & General Purposes Committee of the South West

Metropolitan RB and 'put this [i.e. the RHHI's] case for [a] disclaimer under the [NHS] Act'. The 'impression left with the delegation was [however] that exemption would be unlikely.' At the March meeting a letter from the Minister was read to the Board, indicating that 'he did *not* [my italics] propose to disclaim the Hospital under the [NHS] Act.' A letter addressed to the Board from a Mr Seymour urged that 'all possible steps should be taken to obtain a reversal of this [totally unacceptable] decision.' Meanwhile, the House Committee had suggested that Linstead be 'invited to see the Minister & that the opinion of Sir Valentine Holmes K.C., should be obtained as to whether this Institution [the RHHI] was, in fact, covered by the Act, whether the Minister had acted ultra vires in refusing exemption &, if so, what further measures were open to the Board to take'; this action was approved.[9]

Uncertainty continues

Holmes, and Mr H.E. Francis evidently felt that 'the Home had good grounds for going to arbitration', and this was conveyed to the Board at their April meeting, when 'Mr Burrell, of Farrer & Co ... gave his advice on certain aspects of the matter'. The Board resolved that '... the Solicitors should be instructed to take such steps as may be necessary to implement the recommendations [made by Holmes and Francis, who should be retained 'to advise & represent the Royal Hospital & Home (RHHI) throughout this matter'] & to further the claim that the [RHHI] is not a hospital within the meaning of the [NHS] Act, 1946.' The Board also approved of a letter being sent to the Minister and the Secretary of the RB, informing both that they intended going to arbitration and 'that any information or returns required ... would be given without prejudice'. A Sub-Committee, consisting of Morris, Linstead and Mrs Henry Arnold (also a member of the Board) was set up to act for the Board 'in co-operation with ... Holmes & Messrs. Farrer & Co'. The Board also agreed that the names of Morris, Mrs Arnold, Lady Webb-Johnson, Linstead, H.T. Cross (members of the Board) and Dr J.M. Badenoch (the Medical Officer) be put forward for service on the Management Committee of the RB. A subsequent letter from the Secretary of the RB informed the Board that 'the Arbitration Tribunal would [it was hoped] hear the Home's case before July 5th' [the appointed day]. And, at the June meeting it was agreed that 'notices to staff & patients should be put up, telling them of the Board's action in going to arbitration.'[10]

At the Board's July meeting 'it was reported that the Solicitors of this Home [the RHHI], of the Streatham Home & of the Jewish Home at Tottenham [whose case would probably be heard first], all of whom are going to arbitration, had had a meeting'. 'Should the Jewish Home be successful [the minute continued], it was proposed to ask the Minister to discontinue the proceedings.' There seems to have been some doubt as to whether 'the

Minister had power to disclaim *after* [my italics] the appointed day & to drop the arbitration proceedings'.[11]

The Home and Hospital for Jewish Incurables [HHJI], Tottenham

This institution had been formed in 1889, in order to deal with 'the care, maintenance and nursing of the many foreign Jewish immigrants who might otherwise have to spend their remaining years (if suffering from incurable diseases) in local authority infirmaries, which lacked a Jewish atmosphere and the facilities for religious observances.' Incidentally, it will be recalled from Chapter 1 that the RHI had rejected a request to house members of the Jewish faith in 1888! By 1972, the Home housed 114 patients.[12]

In November 1947, J.A. Wolfe KC (the Honorary Counsel) of Lincoln's Inn had formed the opinion that this was *not* a hospital as defined in Section 79 of the NHS Act, and therefore 'the provisions of that Act do not apply to it'. Consequently, the Honorary Solicitor (Malcolm Slowe) wrote, on behalf of the HHJI, to the Minister requesting a disclaimer under Section 6(3) of the Act. The Minister ruled (and the North East Metropolitan RB apparently agreed with him) that '... having given careful consideration to the request [he had] decided not to disclaim it.'[13] A joint opinion of Wolfe and Sir Cyril Radcliffe KC (also of Lincoln's Inn) subsequently agreed that the institution was *not* a hospital 'as defined by Section 79 of the Act', and arbitration proceedings were therefore commenced.[14] In a letter marked 'private and confidential' addressed to Sydney Gilbert (Secretary of the HHJI), Slowe mentioned that: '... the Opinion of Sir Valentine Holmes, KC for the [RHHI] is favourable to the Home, but the Opinion of Mr Havers KC for the [BHHI], is not so favourable.'[15]

A difference of opinion at the RHHI

Not all members of the RHHI Board supported the decision to go to arbitration. In August 1949, for example, 'Letters were received from Mr T.G. Marriot & Sir Richard Winstedt, advocating the abandonment of the arbitration proceedings ...'. These members of the Board favoured an endeavour to 'come to terms with the Ministry of Health, on a basis of at least a partial retention of the Home's endowments while joining in the [NHS].' On the contrary, a letter from Colonel G.F. Phillips advocated 'a continuation of the Home's endeavour to remain independent'; Colonel A.T. Maxwell too was in favour of a continuation of the 'policy regarding the arbitration,' although he was seriously concerned about the deteriorating financial situation. Following a general discussion, the Board decided to proceed with their present policy and to ask Sir Walter Monckton KC 'to represent the Home at the arbitration, in succession to ... Holmes [who had retired]'. A further letter presented to this meeting, from Linstead, advocated a deputation of 'those Homes going to arbitration' meeting 'the Lord Chancellor personally, with the request that the arbitration proceedings should be expedited in view of the financial embarrassment being caused [as a result of] the prolonged delay.' The meeting agreed, subject to Monckton's approval, of this course of action; however, the RHHI Solicitors subsequently advised (and this was accepted) that a deputation to the Lord Chancellor at that time would serve 'no good purpose'.[16]

What action to take?

So delayed were the arbitration proceedings and so perilous was the financial position becoming, that a 'Special Board Meeting' of the RHHI was convened on 9 January 1950; this took place in the offices of Messrs. Farrar & Co. Mr Burrell, a partner in that firm, outlined a possible course of action. He confirmed that the case of the 'Home and Hospital for Jewish Incurables' would be heard first (but probably not until May or June of that year) and 'it was to the advantage of this Home [the RHHI] that it should be so.' Under Section 6, Clause 1, of the Act, 'the Minister was entitled to take over those endowments of a hospital held by the Governing Body solely for the purposes of that hospital.' The relevant section of the Act is as follows:

> Subject to the provisions of this Act, there shall, on the appointed day, be transferred to and vest in the Minister by virtue of this Act all interests in or attaching to premises forming part of a voluntary hospital or used for the purposes of a voluntary hospital, and in equipment, furniture or other movable property used in or in connection with such premises, being interests held immediately before the appointed day by the governing body of the hospital or by trustees solely for the purposes of that hospital, and all rights and liabilities to which any such governing body or trustees were entitled or subject immediately before the appointed day, being rights and liabilities acquired or incurred solely for the purposes of managing any such premises or property as aforesaid or otherwise carrying on the business of the hospital or any part thereof, but not including any endowment within the meaning of the next following section or any rights or liabilities transferred under that section.

It was (Burrell continued) the contention of Counsel (i.e. Monckton) that 'this Home's pensions were a charge on the general funds, that it followed that these funds were not solely for the purpose of the Home & that therefore the Minister was not entitled to them.' It was therefore necessary to ask a Judge in the High Court 'for a declaration [and it would be necessary to plead as a *hospital* and not a *home*, but this would 'in no way affect the Home's case before the Arbitrator'] that the endowments of the Home did not vest in the Minister on the appointed day. Should the Judge's decision be favourable, 'the need for arbitration would [he maintained] disappear.' The Board resolved unanimously that 'Mr Burrell should be instructed to open proceedings in the

High Court', and he was 'asked to inform the Jewish, Midland & Streatham Homes of the decision come to at this meeting'.[17]

Arbitration at last

The date of the arbitration proceedings of the Jewish Home for Incurables was eventually set for 27 February 1950. The RHHI solicitors suggested that the main witnesses (i.e. the Chairman, Secretary and Medical Officer) would be well advised to attend these proceedings 'in order to acquaint themselves with the procedure'.

At long last proceedings got under way – before Mr Harold Christie KC. This was not before the Chief Rabbi (Sir Israel Brodie [1895-1979]) had both visited the Home and written (on 6 January 1950) a letter to Aneurin Bevan imploring him to 'disclaim' the HHJI from the NHS Act. Monckton was retained on behalf of the HHJI. The proceedings, which duly began on 27 February, took five days to complete; the result was entirely in favour of the HHJI. The arbitrator also awarded 'party costs'.[18]

At a Board meeting on 6 March: 'The [RHHI] Secretary reported that he had attended at the Jewish Home & Hospital for Incurables' arbitration case and gave a short report on the proceedings. Meanwhile, Linstead asked the Minister (Bevan) in a House of Commons debate about his 'future intentions regarding outstanding arbitration proceedings'. However, the reply he received was considered unsatisfactory, and Farrer & Co 'suggested [and this was approved by the Board] that a more definite question should be put, mentioning this Home by name.'[19]

As far as the RHHI was concerned, the matter was finally clinched on 5 June 1950, when the Chairman read to the Board the following letter from the Ministry addressed to Farrar & Co:

Dear Sirs,

Royal Hospital & Home for Incurables, Putney.

Referring to previous correspondence, I am instructed by the Minister of Health to inform you that he has now been able to give careful consideration to the reports he has received relating to this Institution in the light of the recent decision by the Chairman of the Panel of Arbitrators on the case relating to the Home & Hospital for Jewish Incurables & the evidence upon which such decision was given. As the result of such consideration he has decided not to pursue his contention that the above Institution was transferred to him as a Hospital on 5th July, 1948, & his claim to the premises & the endowments is hereby withdrawn.

Yours faithfully
H.C. Talbot
Assistant Solicitor.[20]

The British Home for Incurables was also exempted from the NHS.[21]

As a finale to this prolonged saga, the Board recommended at its November meeting 'that £250 should be paid to the Jewish Home towards their arbitration expenses ...'.[22]

At long last, the subscribers were informed of the successful outcome in the *Annual Report* for 1950: 'In May this year ... the Minister of Health withdrew all his claims on this Home. This news was received with considerable relief by the patients and friends of the Home, who, with the Board, believe that the comfort and happiness of the patients will be best secured by the "personal" administration of a voluntary committee, which alone can avoid a tendency towards regimentation and can give day-to-day consideration to the innumerable problems ... which arise in so big a community as this.' Nevertheless, the report stressed the 'very heavy financial obligations' of the Board![23]

Aftermath

In March 1954, the Court of Appeal allowed an appeal by the then Minister of Health (Iain Macleod) against the Royal Midland Counties Home for Incurables (RMCH) at Leamington. This case was heard by the Master of the Rolls – Lord Justice Denning. The outcome again depended largely on the description of a *hospital* in section 79 (entitled: 'Interpretation') of the Act, and what constituted 'treatment' as opposed to 'care'. In effect this appeal confirmed that the then Minister was within his rights in taking over the RMCH on the 'appointed day'. Obviously this decision created renewed anxiety at the RHHI, but the 'Hospital Solicitor ... advised that it did not appear likely that, as a result of this appeal, the Minister would try to take over disclaimed Homes for Incurables, and that this would need a special Act of Parliament.' It was thus minuted that: 'the Board decided to take no action in the matter at present.[24]

The Chairman of the Board of Management (Norman Morris) is minuted a decade later, in 1959, as claiming that the decision to steer clear of the NHS was 'greatly to the benefit of the patients'.[25]

Therefore, the RHHI remained a voluntary institution outside the NHS, and that continues to this day.

References and Notes

1. [Economy]. 'The London Hospitals', *Times, Lond.* 10 February 1909: 11; 12 February: 10; G. Rivett, *The Development of the London Hospital system 1823-1982* (London: King Edward's Hospital Fund for London: 1986): 133-227; D. Fraser, *The Welfare State* (Stroud, Gloucestershire: Sutton Publishing Ltd. 2000): 35-59.
2. **Sir Thomas Barlow**, Bt, KCVO, FRCP, FRS (1845-1945) was educated at Owens College, Manchester, and University College London. After a

series of appointments at the Hospital for Sick Children, he became (briefly) Assistant Physician to Charing Cross, then the London Hospital, and eventually University College Hospital (UCH). From 1884-8, he had also been on the staff of the London Fever Hospital. In 1895, he was appointed to the Haldane Chair of Clinical Medicine at UCH, which he held until 1907. His research interests ranged from meningitis, scurvy, rickets and rheumatism in children to Raynaud's disease. At the RCP, Barlow was a Censor, and President from 1910-14; in 1916, he was Harveian Orator. He was also Physician to the Royal Household (1896-1900), Physician-Extraordinary to Queen Victoria, King Edward VII, and King George V. *See also: Lancet* 1945; **i:** 132-2, 164; *BMJ* 1945: **i:** 99-100, 134; *Munk's Roll* **4**: 270-1; Anonymous, 'Voluntary Hospitals', *Globe* 13 February 1909.

3. Board minutes. Book 24: 113 and 116; Anonymous, 'Hospitals and The Insurance Act', *Daily Graphic* 30 January 1914; C.M. Wilson, 'New hospitals', *Times, Lond.* 5 May 1920; J. Murray, 'New hospitals: the Ministry of Health's intentions', *Times, Lond.* 3 May 1920: 10; Scriba, 'Voluntary hospitals: debt due from the State', *Times, Lond.* 1 June 1920: 12; E.A. Attwood, 'Voluntary Hospitals', *Times, Lond.* 2 June 1920: 12; Anonymous, 'Future of hospitals: removal from town to country urged', *Times, Lond.* 19 June 1920: 16; J.C. Buchanan, 'The voluntary hospitals', *Times, Lond.* 21 June 1920: 10; Anonymous, 'LCC Hospitals: defects of "general" institutions: good and bad legacies from guardians', *Times, Lond.* 16 January 1933.

4. Parliamentary papers: Chapter 81: *National Health Service Act,* 1946. 9 & 10 Geo. 6. 1119-1214; Anonymous, 'The ministry to take over Home for Incurables', *Evening Telegraph* 1948; Anonymous, 'Strathclyde will pass to the state: personal touch will be maintained', *Carlisle Journal* 21 May 1948; RHHI *Annual Reports:* 1947: 5; 1948: 5; 1949: 5; Op.cit. See note 1 above (Rivett) 264-78; Fraser 60-4. *See also* Anonymous, *Times, Lond.* 5 July 1948; F. Honigsbaum, 'Evolution of the National Health Service', *Trans Med Soc Lond.* 2000-1; 117: 73-7.

5. Op.cit. See note 3 above (Board minutes), Book 27: 214, 216. **The Rt. Hon. Aneurin Bevan** PC, MP (1897-1960) was the Labour MP for Ebbw Vale, and Minister of Health (August 1943 – January 1951). He also served as Minister of Labour and National Service in 1954. [*See also:* M. Foot, *Aneurin Bevan 1897-1960* (London: Victor Gollancz. 1997) 634]. **Lt General Sir Ernest Bradfield,** FRCS, KCIE, OBE (1880-1963) was educated at King Edward's School, Birmingham and St Mary's Hospital (which he represented at rugby and cricket), London, qualifying in medicine in 1903. The same year he joined the Indian Medical Service (IMS), and in 1908 served on the North-west Frontier. In 1924, Bradfield

was appointed to the Chair of Surgery at Madras Medical College, and from 1937-9 was Medical Director General of the IMS. In 1939, he returned to England as President of the Medical Branch of the India Office, and medical adviser to the Secretary of State; he held these offices until 1946. He was largely instrumental in the formation of the Indian Army Medical Corps. Although he had passed the FRCS Ed. in 1911, he was not elected FRCS until 1962. **Sir Edward Douglas Maclagan,** KCSI (1864-1952), spent most of his professional life in India: Under-Secretary, Government of India, Revenue and Agricultural Department (1892); Chief Secretary to the Government of Punjab (1906); Secretary to the Government of India, Revenue and Agricultural Department (1910-14); Secretary to the government of India, Education Department (1915-18); Lt. Governor of the Punjab (1919-21), Governor (1921-4). He was also (twice) President of the Royal Asiatic Society. **Sir Hugh Nicholas Linstead,** OBE, MP (1901-87) was both a pharmaceutical chemist and a barrister of the Middle Temple. From 1942-64 he was Conservative MP for the Putney Division of Wandsworth.

6. E.D. Maclagan to the Rt. Hon. Aneurin Bevan, Minister of Health 26 April 1946: 2.

7. Op.cit. See note 3 above (Board minutes), Book 27: 217, 219-20, 226-7.

8. Ibid: 248-9, 253-4.; Linstead, *The R.H.H.I.'s place in the National Health Service,* May 1947: 1; H. Linstead, *Outline of a Memorandum on the Care of the Chronic Sick,* (1947): 6; S.H. Belfrage, *Notes* 1 June 1947.

9. Op.cit. See note 3 above (Board minutes), Book 27: 265, 270, 277-8. **Valentine Holmes Kt (1888-1956)** was educated at Charterhouse and Trinity College, Dublin and was Called to the Bar in 1913. From 1935-45 he had been Junior Treasury Counsel.

10. Op.cit. See note 3 above (Board minutes), Book 27: 280-2, 284, 287.

11. Ibid: 289-290, 291, 314.

12. Anonymous. *The Jewish Home & Hospital at Tottenham.* 19 October 1972: 1. [University of Southampton Library Archives and Manuscripts].

13. J.A. Wolfe, *Opinion* 18 November 1947: 2; M. Slowe to The Secretary, Ministry of Health 19 October 1947: 2 [University of Southampton Library Archives and Manuscripts].

14. C. Radcliffe, J.A. Wolfe, *Joint Opinion* 25 April 1948: 2 [University of Southampton Library Archives and Manuscripts].

15. M. Slowe to S. Gilbert, *National Health Service Act* 16 July 1948: 1 [University of Southampton Library Archives and Manuscripts].

16. Op.cit. See note 3 above (Board minutes), Book 27: 321-2, 324, 326. **Walter Turner Monckton, Viscount Monckton of Brenchley,** MC, KC, MP, PC, GCVO, KCMS (1891-1965) was educated at Harrow and Balliol College, Oxford. He had a distinguished legal career, and was

appointed Solicitor-General (1945), Minister of Labour and National Service (1951-5), Minister of Defence (1955-6), and Paymaster General (1956-7). He was created first Viscount Monckton in 1957.

17. Op.cit. See note 3 above (Board minutes), Book 27: 333-6.
18. M. Slowe to S. Gilbert re: *National Service Act* 7 March 1950: 1 [University of Southampton Library Archives and Manuscripts].
19. Op.cit. See note 3 above (Board minutes), Book 27: 341, 345, 347, 350.
20. Ibid: 354.
21. Anonymous, 'Incurables' Home is exempted', *South Lond. Press* 26 May 1950; P.H. Steel, 'The Incurables Home', *Streatham News* 9 June 1950.
22. Op.cit. See note 3 above (Board minutes), Book 27: 374; *See also:* M. Slowe to S. Gilbert. *Arbitration* 5 October 1950: 1. [University of Southampton Library Archives and Manuscripts]; Anonymous, 'Minister gives up his claim to Home', *South Western Star* 2 June 1950; T.G. Pilcher, 'The Royal Hospital and Home for Incurables', *Wandsworth Borough News* 2 June 1950; Anonymous, 'Anxious year', *Richmond Herald* 23 February 1952; *See also:* G.C. Cook, 'Transfer of hospitals and "additional premises" to the State: questionable morality in the implementation of the National Health Service Act (1946)', *Postgrad. med J* 2004 (in press).
23. RHHI Annual Reports 1950: 5.
24. **The Rt. Hon. Iain Norman Macleod,** PC, MP (1913-70) was Conservative MP for Enfield West and was appointed Chancellor of the Exchequer in the year of his death. He was Minister of Health from May 1952 until December 1955. He had been educated at Fettes College, Gonville and Caius College and the Inner Temple; Court of Appeal, 'Home for Incurables "hospital" within health act: Minister of Health v. General Committee of the Royal Midland Counties Home for Incurables', *Times, Lond.* 26 March 1954: 4; Op.cit. See note 3 above (Board minutes), Book 27: 498-9; Anonymous, 'State claims Royal Midland Counties Home: application of committee fails', *Birmingham Post* 8 June 1950.
25. Op.cit. See note 3 above (Board minutes), Book 28: 170-1.

CHAPTER 16

Funding of the Charity, and abandonment of the Voting System at last

THE MAJOR SOURCE of income was of course from the subscribers (Chapter 14) and from legacies. The voting system was, from the outset of the Charity, highly controversial. In January 1871 it was resolved that 'In the payment of legacies one Life Vote shall be given for each sum of Fifty Pounds, the votes to assigned as the Executors may direct.' In August 1873, a Board minute states: 'The Secy. presented copies of the *Christian World* of the 22nd & 29th date, containing a letter condemning the voting system, and referring specially to [a specific case].' There can be little doubt that the voting system was subject to much abuse. For example, a case of *locomotor ataxia,* caused by a syphilitic infection acquired some years before (and caused by 'his own misconduct'), and supported by a doctor and a priest could (if he acquired sufficient votes) lead to the exclusion of a more deserving candidate! There is no doubt however, that this system encouraged subscriptions.

Direct payment was also a debated issue. At a Board meeting in June 1860, i.e. six years after foundation of the RHI, Osborne proposed: 'That in consequence of the number of Patients now in the Hospital, the admission of Inmates on payment be, for the present, discontinued.' An amendment 'That cases continue to be admitted on payment of not less than £30 per annum' was rejected (by 3 to 8). However, a further amendment: 'That in consequence of the number of patients now in the hospital, the admission of Inmates on payment, except such as pay at the rate of £50 a year, be, for the present discontinued' was carried 'nem. con.', 'put as a substantive motion, and carried.'[1]

Fund-raising Sermons

Fund-raising sermons were also the source of substantial income. For example, there are numerous references to charitable preaching, e.g. 'Mr Goulburn promised [to preach] a sermon at his church at Paddington some time in the next year [1859].' This was duly delivered in March 1860 at St John's Church, Paddington when the collection yielded £127.1*s*.2*d*. And in February 1862, the Revd. Daniel Hatterns (sic) preached at Marc St. Chapel Hackney. There are many other examples in the early minute books.[2]

Metropolitan Hospital Sunday Fund
This fund had been set up by several philanthropists and hospital administrators, including Canon John Miller (1814-80) and Henry Burdett (1847-1920). The fund had, as its underlying principle, that Sunday collections on certain days of the year would be devoted to assisting *ailing* hospitals.

In March 1873 the Board decided: 'That an application [should] be made to the Committee of the Hospital Sunday Fund [HSF], claiming to participate in the benefits of the proposed Collection.' In a reply from W.H. Ramsay, the Board was asked for details of their financial position, especially the number of legacies exceeding £100 received over the previous three years. This, they agreed to do! However, 'the officials of the [HSF replied] that the Committee of distribution ... had decided that Institutions for the Incurable should *not* [my italics] participate.' As a result, a motion was put at a Board meeting: 'That an advertisement to the following effect be inserted in the Morning Papers [*The Times, Daily News & Morning Post*] on the two following Mondays]': "[HSF]: 'A communication has been received by the Board of the Royal Hospital for Incurables that this Charity is not to participate in the benefits of the [HSF]".' This motion was slightly amended, and the Board supported it unanimously. Following publication of the advertisement 'a notice ... appeared in the *Echo*, and subsequently an article in the same paper headed "facts about Hospital Sunday".'

In November, a 'circular letter from [the] Chairman of the Metropolitan Free Hospital, stating that at a recent meeting in which free Charities were represented, it had been resolved to form a Committee of Observation to investigate future distributions of the [HSF] and inviting the cooperation of the Board [of the RHI] if they were dissatisfied with the late distribution of the Fund.' It was resolved to send a deputation! However, this was of no avail, for they were told that the RHI was excluded from the HSF on the ground that 'the Institution was not a Hospital in the true sense of the term, but a permanent Asylum for Incurable Persons'. The Board decided to contest this decision, and in January 1874, it was resolved: 'That a communication be addressed to the Committee of the [HSF] in reference to the exclusion of this Hospital from a participation in the collection of 1873, and asking that a deputation from the Board be allowed an interview to represent the claims of this Hospital to a share in 1874.'

A month later, a reply was received. It stated that 'the admission of Hospitals to benefit rested with the Committee of Distribution, to whom the application of the Board would be referred', but the writer felt that exclusion of the RHI was due to several reasons. '1. That it was an Asylum, 2. that the Beneficiaries were entitled, by election, to the benefit; 3. That pensioners were admitted; 4. That the income was not all expended; [and] 5. The Cost of staff.' A deputation from the RHI duly met the Distribution Committee in July 1874, and although they seemed to have had a fair hearing, 'the members feared [that] the reply, when it came, would be unfavourable'. This pessimism was borne out by a subsequent letter dated 13 July of that year.

In March 1875, 'the Secy. drew the attention of the Board to the report of a Public Meeting of [the HSF], convened by the Lord Mayor, at the Mansion House, at which a Resolution was passed, determining that … Hospitals for the Incurables should in future participate in the Fund, upon the basis of the benefits enjoyed by the Inmates.' A later minute records: '… it has never been clear to the Board why the method of nominating its beneficiaries should be selected as disqualifying this Institution to a share in the Collection.' However, this minute concluded: 'The Board have no intention of re-opening the question [but they] most earnestly commend the Institution to the sympathy of ministers of religion …'.

The 'exclusion of this hospital' from the HSF was also contested by the Vicar of St Paul's, Chiswick. Another deputation from the RHI (which included the Secretary) subsequently attended the Annual General Meeting (AGM) of this fund in December 1879. Although the Chairman, Sir Sydney Waterlow, MP, assured them 'that the Council would consider the case of the [RHI] …', his remarks were not considered encouraging because he went on to say that the institution was 'regarded rather as an asylum than a Hospital' and also that 'it appeared to be a National instead of a Metropolitan Institution.' At another meeting, this time with the Bishop of London presiding, the claims of the RHI were again declined. The Board did not easily give up this struggle, and at yet another Annual Meeting in December 1883 an attempt was made to suspend Rule 7 (which referred to the exclusion of all 'elective institutions') but 'at the suggestion of the chairman, Sir Risdon Bennett', the whole question was referred to an adjourned meeting, which seems not to have taken place until May 1884. At the adjourned meeting, the representatives of the RHI lost their case once again! Persistence had not therefore paid off![3]

The King's Fund (the Prince of Wales' Fund prior to Queen Victoria's death in January 1901)

There was also obvious disgruntlement that the RHI was *not* eligible for funding from King Edward's Fund for London, on account of its designation *incurables*. The Board had applied for funding in February 1897, but they were told that during that year, distribution would 'rely upon the criteria used by the Distribution Committee of the Metropolitan Hospital Sunday Fund'. A letter from Sir Sydney Waterlow, President of the Fund, was read to the Board in April 1897. In it he stated that: 'no definite arrangements had been arrived at indicating the manner in which the Committee of his Fund could best assist the Council of the Prince's Hospital Fund.' Clearly, the Board were unhappy with the uncertainties surrounding the method of distribution and as to whether the RHI would be eligible. Shortly after the death of Queen Victoria, in January 1901, a letter was read to the Board indicating that '[this] fund only existed for relieving the sick and therefore no grant could be made to this Hospital.' On 25 June 1903, however, it was again resolved 'to make application for participation in [the King's Fund] distribution.' In July 1916 the Board was informed that the King's Fund 'have now the matter [of Pensions to old Hospital Servants] under consideration, with a view to drafting a general scheme.' The Board agreed 'to postpone further discussion until the Secretary [reported] that King Edward's Hospital Fund had arrived at some decision that is likely to be acceptable to all Institutions.

So desperate for funds were the financial heads of the London voluntary hospitals that the King's Fund made an emergency distribution in 1920 of £250,000 but once again the RHHI was *not* included. In January 1929, a communication was received: '... the demands of the Fund from hospitals in the ordinary sense of the term have so far grown more rapidly than its resources.' However, the Secretary of the King's Fund clearly stated: '... that it is not the desire to [sic] the Fund to exclude any class of institution.' The working of King Edward's Fund and details of the method(s) of distribution can be found in *Times* reports of 1918 and 1931; in the latter article the anonymous reporter recorded the substance of a speech by the Prince of Wales.

A rather bizarre scheme for boosting the income of the Fund was outlined in the *Daily News* for 1922: special packets of cigarettes were to be offered for sale, priced at one penny (which would go to King Edward's Fund) above the normal rate. The brain behind this idea was a Mr J. Inger of High Holborn.[4]

Improved relationships
At a Board meeting in March 1947, 'The Chairman stated that King Edward's Hospital Fund for London had written to say that their policy towards institutions for the treatment of incurables was being reviewed and had suggested that this Hospital [the RHHI] should apply for financial assistance.' This revelation came about during a discussion on a proposed 'Building Fund to be used for the erection of a Paying Patients' Home'. Managers of the fund allocated £1,000 for improvement of the heating system, and £500 for cubicle curtains; in their letter, they also suggested that the RHHI should appoint a small medical committee, because they were in some doubt as to 'whether the patients were having full benefit of modern advances in treatment'. Almost two years later, Colonel A.T. Maxwell (a Board member) met Sir Edward Peacock (see below), Treasurer of the King's Fund, 'with regard to possible financial assistance from the King's Fund' and had received an encouraging response. In July 1949, however, the Board was informed that the King's Fund had refused financial assistance, but it was 'open to the Home to apply for

grants for specific purposes should the arbitration [with regard to the National Health Service – Chapter 15] be decided in the Home's favour.'

In March 1950, the Board agreed to make a further approach (through Maxwell) to the Fund; however, an informal meeting with Peacock was far from encouraging, owing to the fact 'that the King's Fund had entered into heavy commitments and it was unlikely that any large sum would be made available to this Home.' Certain members of the Fund's Committee were apparently of the opinion that the Home 'had acted unwisely in obtaining exemption from the [NHS].' In June, Sir Henry Tidy and Mr Patterson (of the King's Fund) visited the RHHI and were met by the Chairman (Norman Morris) and Lord Amulree, FRCP. The following month, 'A grant of £10,000 towards the reduction of the current year's deficit [which was largely a result of uncertainty regarding the future of the RHHI in the light of arbitration regarding the NHS Act].'

In an accompanying letter, it was 'urged that the Home should abandon the voting system and enter into contractual relations with Regional Boards and local authorities', the implication being that 'compliance or otherwise with this suggestion would affect the Fund's policy in making future grants.' However, at the same meeting (in July 1950), 'The Secretary reported that he had heard from the South West Metropolitan Regional Hospital Board that, as the Home had remained outside the Act on the grounds that it was not a hospital, the Board would be unable ... to enter into contractual arrangements with the Home'! Later that year the Fund's Committee made an offer, which was accepted by the Board, to 'lend a financial expert to examine and report on the Home's finances, administration and expenditure.'

In June 1951, Mr Clive Morris, a member of the Board, visited the King's Fund, when he 'gathered that [they] were less inclined than formerly to make maintenance grants for general purposes but would probably consider a request for help with some specific project, such as a new building for occupational therapy.' This was later modified to 'a combined occupational and physiotherapy department', which would necessitate a 'new wing'. However, as was pointed out, if such a department was in fact built, 'its maintenance would be a further charge on the general funds'. This seems to have been the 'limiting factor', for the Finance Committee did *not* feel able to ask the King's Fund for a capital *as well as* a maintenance grant. The Secretary (J.G. Pilcher) too 'thought it likely that the King's Fund and other big charitable Trusts would be more willing to give a substantial sum for a specific purpose rather than for general maintenance.'

The fund subsequently 'suffered a severe drop in legacies [in 1957]; they received only £15,000 ... compared to over £100,000 in the previous year.' Nevertheless, four representatives [had] visited the Hospital and Home in 1959, and this seems to have been a great success, for in May 1962, 'The Board was glad to note that the grant of £5,000 promised by the King's Fund earlier in the year has now been received'. And in May 1966, the Secretary applied for a grant of £3,061.10s.0d. (of which they were awarded £1,240) for the purchase of 21 hoists and 405 slings. The Fund Committee also threw out several helpful suggestions, e.g. that the Home's Medical Officer (Dr Badenoch) might attend an International Hospital Congress in Brussels, and that 'various staff and catering officers' courses [were] open to hospital officers'.[5]

Annual Dinners

Annual dinners were, from 1854, a major source of income. This was always a high profile affair with 100-200 guests present, and distinguished persons were requested to preside. These dinners, which were on a sumptuous scale, were usually held at the London Tavern, and ladies were invited to dine! At a meeting in February 1861, for example, Dr Reed announced that 'His Grace the Duke of Wellington had consented to preside at the Annual Dinner to be held at the London Tavern [in] March of that year.' However, he subsequently declined.

It was by no means easy to persuade prominent citizens to take on this duty, as the Board minute books make clear. In 1862 for example, Sir Robert Peel, the Marquis of Huntington and Lord Dufferine were all approached, but declined, although the last did eventually accept – and as a result was, like other Chairmen, made a Vice-President of the Charity. Other invitations were duly sent to the Lord Mayor, the Duke of Cambridge and Viscount Enfield MP; the last accepted. A few years later (1866-8), Lord Taunton, Lord Elcho and the Duke of Argyll (all of whom accepted invitations and as a result were also made Vice-Presidents) presided at successive dinners. A later chairman was the speaker of the House of Commons – in 1871.[6] Thus, although there were several refusals, a number of celebrities did in fact accept; these included: Charles Dickens, the Duke of Argyll, Lord Malsbury, and Lord Justice Darling.

During the Great War (1914-18), a Festival lunch was held instead.

Other fund-raising activities

As the nineteenth century progressed, there seems to have been less reliance on Charity sermons and annual subscription dinners. In 1868, Frederick Temple (1821-1902), headmaster of Rugby and later Archbishop of Canterbury, made an appeal for funds. Garden parties, fêtes, concerts, firework displays and the annual Christmas appeal took on a far higher profile, while Royal visits became increasingly important in raising the profile of the Charity. Many other strategies were also resorted to (fig 16.1) – bazaars, an annual sale of patients' work (organised by the Lady Visitors), readings and broadcast appeals. Appeals of all types were organised, but still much depended on the income from subscriptions and the Annual Dinner. Bazaars were a source of substantial income; for example, a successful one took place in 1862. From

The Lord Mayor of London

(The Rt. Honble. Sir Horace Brooks Marshall, M.A., LL.D.)

has promised to take the Chair at a Festival Luncheon in aid of the funds of the Royal Hospital and Home for Incurables, Putney, and in this Peace Year he hopes to create a record by helping to raise a larger sum than has been raised on any such occasion hitherto in the sixty-five years' history of this noble Institution.

Will you help him?

For years he has been a valuable member of the Board of Management of this Institution, and he desires to do a specially good turn to suffering humanity while he holds the responsible office it is now his privilege to fill.

But he must have help!

The Royal Hospital and Home for Incurables, Putney, is doing a splendid and wonderful work. The Board give you their word of honour upon that point. Charles Dickens poured out his heart on this subject when he presided at one of our festival dinners in the year 1854. And since then the work has increased.

We believe you will help.

If you can visit Putney, go and see the Institution and behold with your own eyes what is being done for men and women who are incurably helpless: men and women who for years have been too ill to feed and dress themselves. See the tender and loving care they receive in this <u>huge monument to civilization</u>. You will come away from Putney better and more grateful citizens of a mighty Empire.

The Festival Luncheon will be held at Grocers' Hall on Thursday, June 5th. Please write for full particulars to the Secretary of the Institution at the City Office: Bond Court House, Walbrook, E.C. 4.

To SIR HENRY LOPES, BART., *Treasurer,*   *Date*_____ 1919
ROYAL HOSPITAL AND HOME FOR INCURABLES, PUTNEY.
BOND COURT HOUSE, WALBROOK, E.C. 4.

From*_____

*Address*_____

Sir,
Enclosed you will find a _____ *for* £_____
which _____ send you __ { an Annual Subscription } in aid of the funds of the
a Donation
a Life Subscription

ROYAL HOSPITAL AND HOME FOR INCURABLES, PUTNEY.

*(Signed)*_____

AN ANNUAL SUBSCRIBER *has one Vote at each Election for each Half Guinea.*
A DONATION *entitles to Votes at the next ensuing Election, Four Votes being given for each Guinea contributed.*
A LIFE SUBSCRIBER *has One Vote for Life for Five Guineas, and an additional Vote for Life for every additional Five Guineas.*
* *Please write name as it should be printed in the List of Governors and Donors.*
† *Please strike out the words not applicable.*
PLEASE CROSS CHEQUES "*Messrs* GLYN, MILLS, CURRIE & CO."

Fig. 16.1: Appeal for funds – 1919.

234

1872 until the Second World War (1939-45) the Christmas appeal was an annual event, usually organised by the Secretary (Andrew or Cutting) and outsiders were often asked to write a suitable text. Amongst others were: the Reverend Paxton Hood, Rosamond Oliphant, Ruby Aures, and Hesta Stretton. Also, a group of Charles Dickens' descendents provided entertainment in 1911. On 9 December 1944, (i.e. while the Second World War was still being fought), a fund-raising Ball was held at the Dorchester Hotel. In addition to the entertainers listed in Chapter 13 should be added Sir John Betjeman (1906-84).

In 1865, the Board resolved: 'That a special appeal be sent, at the close of the year, to 5,000 members of the medical profession, the detail being left to the Appeal Committee.'

And, there was also the problem of competing interests. For example, in an appeal for funding by the British Home for Incurables (BHI), it was apparently stated that this was the 'first established' and the 'only' Hospital for Incurables of the Middle Classes. These statements were demonstrably untrue, and it was decided by the Board to send a reply disagreeing with this![7]

Gifts from Queen Victoria
There may have been some difficulty with Royal patroncy in the early days of the Charity (Chapter 9), but Queen Victoria was fundamentally a supporter. In July 1882, the RHI received a gift of £30 from the Queen; the accompanying letter was from Gen. Sir Henry Ponsonby. And in November 1884, 'the Queen … sent a copy of *More Leaves from the Diary of a Life in the Highlands* for the Inmates.'[8]

The Charitable Trusts Bill
In April 1881, a circular from J.D. Allcroft, Esq., Treasurer of Christ's Hospital, was presented to the Board; this invited a deputation to a meeting to 'consider steps to be taken in reference to [the Charitable Trusts Bill then] before the House of Lords.' The 'sum total' was that the voluntary Charities sought 'exemption from the Bill'. Although it passed through the Lords 'with some material amendments', it was held up by the Commons, and was not proceeded with at that session. The Bill did not ultimately come before the House of Commons until May 1883; on the recommendation of Freshfield, the RHI submitted a petition *against* the Bill, and as a result, the Board was invited to send a representative to a meeting of Charities. It was reported in June 1890 that 'a Deputation to the Prime Minister, in opposition to the passing of this Bill' had taken place, but it was 'gathered from Lord Salisbury [1830-1903, the Prime Minister], that the measure [i.e. the Charitable Trusts Bill] was not encouraged by the Government.' The Board therefore decided that 'it was not … desirable to petition against the Bill, as it did not appear,

upon reading it with the related Acts, that the Voluntary Charities were immediately affected by it'. However, another deputation to the Prime Minister subsequently took place, and an assurance [was given] that 'the Bill would not advance a further stage [during the 1890] session.'[9]

The election (voting) system – a major source of funding

This system has been outlined in Chapters 13 and 14. As early as 1890, several subscribers (who had doubtless been influenced by the Charity Voting Reform Association) indicated that they would discontinue subscriptions 'unless the Board took steps for the adoption of some other mode of admission to benefit'. In 1920, the *Methodist Recorder* had asked for spare votes for a particular individual, and this was echoed by the *Pall Mall Gazette* the following year. And as late as 1947, the *Sunday Pictorial* referred to the voting system (which was still held every May and November) as 'a public scandal'. To collect votes, the reporter continued, either the candidate or a relative must: (1) canvass subscribers; (2) seek recommendations from doctors or other professional men; (3) ask friends to donate to the hospital and thus obtain four votes for each guinea; (4) organise whist drives and concerts (in order to obtain votes or (5) to 'use up their own savings and even sell their belongings to buy votes for themselves …'. About 2000 votes were required to be successful, and if <400 were obtained in 10 consecutive elections an individual's name was removed from the list.

Many years later (in 1949) Lord Amulree, a Board member, raised the matter yet again. The King's Fund Committee had suggested in July 1950 (see above) that the voting system should at last be abandoned!

It is probable that it was the intervention of the King's Fund committee that acted as a catalyst for a serious discussion by the Board on a 'future system of admission of patients'. Discussion might have started a month or so before the King's Fund letter had been received; uncertainty must remain about this. Sir Edward Maclagan had compiled a memorandum on the voting system which the 'Secretary was instructed to circulate' to Board members. This system, it will be recalled, had led to severe criticism of the RHI (not least by the House of Lords Select Committee) in the nineteenth century (Chapter 14). In July 1950, the Finance Committee informed the Board that they were 'on the whole, in favour of abandoning the voting system and did not anticipate any appreciable financial loss if this were done'. They had been in touch with the BHHI (at Streatham) and the St Monica Home of Rest (at Kilburn) to find out how they dealt with their admissions.

After a lengthy discussion, the Board were undecided on the issue, and 'The Secretary was instructed to obtain the advice of the Home's solicitors regarding the possibility under the Charter of abandoning the voting system and taking payments from patients.' In September, further discussion took place, and the

Treasurer (F.M.G. Glynn) was 'asked to see the King's Fund before their next Distribution Committee Meeting and sound them out on their intentions towards the Home if the voting system was continued or if it was abandoned.' Two alterations were deemed necessary: '(1) That admission to the Home should not depend on election by subscribers, [and] (2) That patients may, in suitable cases, be asked to contribute periodic payments to the Home's funds as a condition of admission.' Meanwhile, the Home's solicitors had written to say that in their opinion it would be 'necessary only to alter the Bye-laws and not the Charter' in the event of the voting system being discontinued; however, there was evidently a degree of uncertainty about this and they advised that Counsel's Opinion should be taken.

Counsel agreed with the solicitor, and the Board agreed to this course, but with the provisos that 'a new Bye-law will not take effect unless and until it: (a) has been sanctioned by a majority of the Governors at a duly convened Annual or Special General Meeting, and (b) has been allowed by the Privy Council [which Counsel did *not* consider presented an insuperable problem].'

Yet a further discussion took place at the end of November, when it was decided 'that the voting system should [in fact] be discontinued, subject as the Charter required, to the approval of a Special General Meeting of Governors and of the Privy Council.' Since this would take a while to execute, they decided also to 'suspend the May [1951] Election'. At the February 1951 meeting of the Board, the question of proxy voting at the Special General Meeting, which had been fixed for 7 March, was referred to the Home's solicitors, and the Board also agreed to ask their solicitor, Mr Burrell, to be present at that meeting.

The *Annual Report* for 1951 succinctly summarised the outcome of this meeting:

Admission of Patients
The system of admitting patients by the votes of subscribers, in force since the founding of the Home, was abandoned by an overwhelming vote at a well-attended general meeting of subscribers in March. Successful applicants will in future be admitted in order of application and asked to pay what they can reasonably afford; the patient will be spared the expense and trouble of circularising voters and no one will be handicapped in obtaining admission through lack of friends or money, which was the main objection to the former system. It was, of course, realised that this move might lead to a falling off in donations, but it was felt that it was a risk that had to be taken. In fact, the falling off has not been serious and many people have increased their subscriptions to show their appreciation of the change.

Thus, the voting system which had been in force for almost 100 years, and which had been widely criticised in the early days of the Charity, was at last abandoned.[10]

References and Notes

1. Anonymous, 'A nice point', *Hospital* 27 November 1915; Anonymous, 'The voting system', *Hospital Gazette* January 1911; Board minutes Book 3: 106; Book 8: 422; Book 9: 83.

2. Op.cit. See note 1 above (Board minutes), Book 2: 348, 434; Book 4: 149, 380, 394; Book 5: 9, 464; Book 6: 45-6, 107, 133, 213, 325; Book 7: 179-80; 447; Book 8: 143, 220, 235-6, 366; Book 9: 48, 53-4, 513-4; Book 10: 32, 83, 139, 149, 243-4; Book 11: 197-8, 427-8; Book 12: 82, 134-5, 412-3; Book 13: 370-2; Book 14: 72-4, 213, 281-3, 480-2; Book 16: 107, 306; Book 17: 22, 256-7, 481-2; Book 19: 249; Book 20: 205, 457; *See also*: Annual Reports 1892-3, 1899-1900.

3. Op.cit. See note 1 above (Board minutes), Book 9: 358, 417-8, 428, 437-8, 446, 488, 502; Book 10: 63, 161, 171. *See also:* G.C. Cook, 'Henry Charles Burdett (1847-1920): outstanding hospital administrator, successful Secretary of the Seamen's Hospital Society, and notable philanthropist', *J med Biog* 2001; 9: 195-207.

4. Op.cit. See note 1 above (Board minutes), Book 20: 291, 310, 318-9, 340-1; Book 23: 34; Book 24: 216-7; Book 25: 476-7; Anonymous, 'Urgent needs of the London hospitals: £250,000 emergency grant', *Daily Telegraph* 6 July 1920; Anonymous, '£190,000 for hospitals: Work of King Edward's Fund', *Times, Lond.* 15 May 1918; Anonymous, 'Hospital Saturday Fund', *Daily Telegraph* 14 January 1918; Anonymous, 'Royal Hospital for Incurables: no help from public finds', *City Press* 17 June 1922; Anonymous, 'King Edward's Fund: £294,313 for the Hospitals: The Prince's speech', *Times, Lond.* 12 December 1931; Anonymous, 'To aid hospitals: how smokers might raise nearly £4,000,000 a year', *Daily News* 15 March 1922.

5. Ibid. Book 22: 378, Book 27: 243, 251-2, 311, 314, 343, 346, 357, 361, 363-4, 374, 377, 384, 392, 394, 397-8, 401-2, 405-6; Book 28: 119, 139, 264, 400, 406.

6. Op.cit. See note 1 above (Board minutes), Book 3: 318; Book 4: 148-9, 159, 211, 222, 236, 295, 301, 308, 317, 334, 356, 380, 394; Book 6: 69, 83, 363; Book 7: 251; Book 8: 377-8, 415; *See also*: Anonymous, 'Royal Hospital for incurables', *Morning Post* 5 May 1911.

7. Op.cit. See note 1 above (Board minutes), Book 4: 295, 401; Book 5: 484; Book 16: 108; Book 24: 68-9; *See also*: Anonymous, 'Prima donna at Putney', *Wandsworth Borough News* 26 June 1909; Anonymous, '"Keep cheerful": recipe for long life: Mrs Kendal and happy incurables', *Daily Mail* 3 November 1910; Anonymous, 'Spirit of Charles Dickens: author's descendents give an entertainment: audience of invalids', *Chronicle* 19 January 1911; H. Lawson, 'A monument to civilization', *Times, Lond.* 8 March 1911; 'Miss Ellen Terry's magic: the smiles and tears of the incurables', *The Standard* April 1911; Northampton, H.J. Allcroft, C.

Cutting, 'Too sadly true', *Daily Telegraph* 13 April 1911; R.J. Lesslie, 'Help for the Incurable: urgent appeal', *Daily Telegraph* 5 April 1916; Anonymous, 'Charity appeals: War influences in peace: suggestions for public guidance', *Times, Lond.* 15 December 1922; Anonymous, 'Putney Home for Incurables: plea for the institution', *Morning Post* 24 May 1924; Anonymous, 'Royal Hospital and Home for Incurables: record collection of £10,203', *City Press* 27 June 1924.

8. Op.cit. See note 1 above (Board minutes), Book 14: 34, 468.

9. Ibid. Book 12: 166, 446, 507; Book 13: 254, 268; Book 14: 189, 201, 214, 309, 336, 379-80, 386-7; Book 17: 157, 169, 315, 321, 485; *See also*: Anonymous, 'Hospital Sunday Collections', *Morning Post* 26 December 1913; Anonymous, 'Hospital Sunday Fund', *Daily Telegraph* 22 December 1916.

10. Anonymous, 'Hospital for Incurables – Voters wanted', *Furniture Record* 6 May 1910; Anonymous, *Methodist Recorder* 18 November 1920; Anonymous, 'Appeal for votes', *Pall Mall Gazette* 25 November 1921; J. Garrity, 'Votes for sale – to invalids', *Sunday Pictorial* 16 February 1947; Op.cit. See note 1 above (Board minutes), Book 17: 95; Book 27: 312, 358, 364-5, 368, 370-1, 375-6; Annual Report 1951: 7.

CHAPTER 17

The patients 100 years after
the foundation of the Charity

TABLE 17.1 GIVES DETAILS of 100 consecutive entries for individuals who 'presented' for assistance – as either 'inmates' or 'pensioners' in 1954-55 (i.e. exactly 100 years after foundation of the RHI).[1]

By then, the era of 'paying patients' had begun. In January 1953, '... three paying patients had ... been accepted by the House Committee [but] no application for male patients had been submitted.' Two wards for this purpose had already been made available '[and] the first paying patients [had been] admitted on the 9th February 1953'. In 1956, fees for *new* paying patients were 'increased from 9 guineas ... to 10 guineas a week', although this did *not* apply to patients currently in the hospital, or 'those whose applications [had] been accepted or [were] under consideration by the House Committee.'[2]

Appendix 4 sets out rules for patients as they stood in 1926. There has, over the years, been a change in the lowest age for admission; it was originally 16, then 20, later 30 years and now reduced to 18. In the early days it was not uncommon to transfer patients from the pension to the 'inmates' list, and *vice versa.*

There was now an overwhelming majority of women applicants – outnumbering men by 71 to 27. From 1955, the age limit(s) for new patients was lowered from 30 to 21 years, and the House Committee had been asked 'to look with especial care at applications from anyone over the age of 70'.[3] Interesting also is the proportion of individuals seeking *inpatient* as opposed to *outpatient* care; only four sought an outpatient pension.

Neurological disease was the major cause for application to the RHHI; in 29 of the 98, the diagnosis given was *disseminated (multiple) sclerosis,* an entity which possibly consists of several diseases under one 'umbrella'. In 1970, the *Annual Report* stressed that no fewer than 40 per cent of the patients were suffering from disseminated sclerosis. However, Parkinson's disease and rarer entities (some of them genetically determined) also account for a significant number of cases. Eighteen suffered from rheumatoid arthritis. Seventy of the fully documented cases were accepted; this represents a massive increase compared with the two other samples previously analysed (Chapters 4 and 13).

In 1920, the *British Medical Journal* published an article emphasising the enormous difficulty involved in giving a precise prognosis; the anonymous report quoted the Westminster Coroner's recollection of a patient at the RHHI who had lived until 90 years – after being admitted as *incurable* 50 years before![4]

240

Table 17.1: Details of 100 individuals who 'presented' to the Board exactly 100 years after the RHI's foundation

No.	Sex	Date of Birth (nineteenth century unless in bold)	Diagnosis	Duration of illness (yrs)	Date presented	Category[+]
1	F	30 6 64	Fractured right femur; Blood pressure; Angina	(approx 20 yrs)	10 3 54	I
2	F	26 10 **1904**	Disseminated sclerosis	17	24 3 54	I
3	F	19 10 **1918**	Huntingdon's chorea	7	"	I
4	F	4 5 95	Syringo myelia & thyrotoxicosis	5	2 6 54	I
5	F	13 7 82	Chronic cholicystitis [sic] & arthritis	>10	14 4 54	P
6	F	21 10 **1910**	Disseminated sclerosis	3	12 5 54	I
7	F	21 12 **1901**	Friedreich's ataxia	35	19 5 54	I
8	F	7 5 **1906**	Friedreich's ataxia	(since 10 yrs old)	"	I
9	F	26 5 91	Disseminated sclerosis; gold poisoning	30/15	23 6 54	I
10	M	27 10 **1919**	Congenital hydrocephalus	(from birth)	7 7 54	I
11	F	24 5 81	?Stroke	10	?	I
12	F	26 1 95	Disseminated sclerosis	28	18 8 54	I
13	F	'1884'	Spinal deformity & hiatus hernia; kyphoscoliosis	3/several years	25 8 54	I
14	F	26 8 67	Arthritis	(approx 25)	18 8 54	P
15	F	26 8 83	Rheumatoid arthritis	8	1 9 54	I
16	F	17 5 72	Chronic rheumatoid arthritis	(approx 45)	–	I
17	F	6 7 **1910**	Disseminated sclerosis	8	–	I
18	F	6 6 94	Rheumatoid arthritis	5	15 9 54	P
19	F	24 9 65	Rheumatoid arthritis	10	"	P

No.	Sex	Date of Birth (nineteenth century unless in bold)	Diagnosis	Duration of illness (yrs)	Date presented	Category[+]
20	F	2 11 **1911**	Disseminated sclerosis	7	3 11 54	I
21	F	23 11 **1921**	Rheumatoid arthritis	28	"	I
22	F	2 11 **1902**	Amyotrophic lateral sclerosis	3	17 11 54	I
23	F	15 7 75	Gastrectomy; heart failure; paralysis of legs	>15	24 11 54	I
24	F	17 1 **1906**	Disseminated sclerosis; diabetes mellitus	8/14	19 1 55	I
25	F	12 6 96	Syringomyelia	10	1 12 54	I
26	[see no 23]					
27	F	5 8 92	Un-united fracture neck of left femur; left hemiplegia	4	5 1 55	I
28	M	26 4 **1918**	Spastic diplegia	(from early childhood)	17 11 54	I
29	F	27 1 **1918**	Disseminated sclerosis	14	8 12 54	I
30	F	5 11 86	Hypertension; paraplegia approx	5	"	I
31	F	29 10 85	Arterio sclerosis	6	19 1 55	I
32	F	25 12 97	Rheumatoid arthritis	36	"	I
33	M	18 6 **1917**	Disseminated sclerosis	5	"	I
34	F	12 9 70	Osteo-arthritis	>2	30 3 55	I
35	M	7 12 **1915**	Disseminated sclerosis	9	19 1 55	I
36	M	27 6 84	Rheumatoid arthritis; heart disease	50/1	16 2 55	I
37	M	3 1 **1907**	Paraplegia	30	"	I
38	F	7 3 93	Cerebral thrombosis	2	2 2 55	I
39	F	6 12 **1907**	Disseminated sclerosis	11	16 2 55	I

No.	Sex	Date of Birth (nineteenth century unless in bold)	Diagnosis	Duration of illness (yrs)	Date presented	Category[+]
40	F	26 5 **1914**	Disseminated sclerosis	13	16 2 55	I
41	F	5 6 72	Cerebral thrombosis	?	"	I
42	M	2 2 **1912**	Diplegia	(since birth)	2 3 55	I
43	F	13 3 97	Locomotor ataxia	31	16 2 55	I
44	M	5 5 **1916**	Rheumatoid arthritis	20	23 2 55	I
45	M	22 10 **1924**	Muscular dystrophy	20	9 3 55	I
46	F	17 4 86	Osteo arthritis; muscular dystrophy; diabetes approx	9	6 4 55	I
47	F	5 12 95	Parkinsonism	10	16 3 55	I
48	F	10 6 97	Disseminated sclerosis	10	30 3 55	I
49	F	12 10 68	Osteo-arthritis	>20	6 4 55	I
50	F	'1877'	Parkinson's disease	10	9 3 55	I
51	M	7 7 **1903**	Disseminated sclerosis	12	30 3 55	I
52	M	16 3 85	Right hemiplegia & aphasia	5-6	4 5 55	I
53	M	11 9 **1911**	Multiple sclerosis	13	25 5 55	I
54	M	24 8 **1924**	Spastic hemiplegia	(since birth)	–	I
55	M	16 7 **1910**	Disseminated sclerosis	Approx 2	27 4 55	I
56	M	8 2 **1916**	Post-encephalitic Parkinsonism	31	11 5 55	I
57	F	20 9 **1904**	Disseminated sclerosis	9-10	18 5 55	I
58	M	22 1 **1912**	Osteomyelitis; blind	40	29 6 55	I
59	M	23 3 **1908**	Rheumatoid arthritis & amputation of legs	15	13 7 55	I
60	M	6 11 91	Rheumatoid arthritis	27	6 7 55	I
61	[see no 59]					
62	F	16 1 **1904**	Progressive muscular atrophy	5	8 6 55	I
63	F	18 11 85	Dislocated hip & arthritis	(since birth)	1 6 55	P

No.	Sex	Date of Birth (nineteenth century unless in bold)	Diagnosis	Duration of illness (yrs)	Date presented	Category[+]
64	F	16 1 **1911**	Disseminated sclerosis	13	27 7 55	I
65	M	16 5 **1906**	Rheumatoid arthritis	33	17 8 55	I
66	M	10 12 **1905**	Disseminated sclerosis	23	13 7 55	I
67	F	31 3 **1918**	Post encephatic Parkinsonism	(from birth)	19 10 55	I
68	M	10 1 **1904**	Disseminated sclerosis	19	17 8 55	I
69	F	14 1 92	Rheumatoid arthritis	32	12 3 58 [sic]	I
70	M	? 11 81	Parkinson's disease	–	24 8 55	I
71	F	14 10 **1908**	Disseminated sclerosis	2-3	17 8 55	I
72	F	20 12 78	Left hemiplegia	6	7 9 55	I
73	F	6 2 76	Rheumatoid arthritis; fractured femur	40	"	I
74	F	1 11 95	Peroneal atrophy	10-12	"	I
75	F	24 2 **1902**	Functional paraplegia of lower limbs	30	"	I
76	F	29 10 **1905**	Congenital deformity of legs & arms	(since birth)	"	I
77	F	18 10 81	Crippled following poliomyelitis in infancy	(since 2 years old)	21 9 55	I
78	F	9 6 97	Rheumatoid arthritis	Approx 20	24 8 55	I
79	F	14 2 **1914**	Disseminated sclerosis	10	7 9 55	I
80	F	? 2 67	Arthritis	Approx 15	21 9 55	I
81	F	1 5 **1912**	Paralysis – post poliomyelitis	27	7 9 55	I
82	F	12 5 86	Parkinson's disease	Approx 7	20 9 55	I
83	M	22 9 **1902**	Rheumatoid arthritis	12	7 9 55	I
84	F	3 4 99	Hemiplegia	2	–	I
85	F	7 9 **1909**	Disseminated sclerosis	9	28 9 55	I
86	F	18 10 81	Poliomyelitis	(since 2 years old)	21 9 55	I
87	F	4 1 **1909**	Disseminated sclerosis	17	20 9 55	I

No.	Sex	Date of Birth (nineteenth century unless in bold)	Diagnosis	Duration of illness (yrs)	Date presented	Category[+]
88	F	30 3 **1922**	Spina bifida	(since birth)	5 10 55	I
89	F	6 6 **1905**	Disseminated sclerosis	17	19 10 55	I
90	F	27 9 **1905**	Disseminated sclerosis	16	21 9 55	I
91	F	28 2 **1915**	Disseminated sclerosis & apoplexy	10	"	I
92	F	2 6 **1906**	Rheumatoid arthritis	20	19 10 55	I
93	M	7 7 94	Parkinsonism	4	28 9 55	I
94	F	13 2 72	Coronary thrombosis; gangrene leg	1	"	I
95	M	23 4 **1901**	Rheumatoid arthritis	(since 12 years old)	26 10 55	I
96	M	10 3 99	Disseminated sclerosis	4	12 11 55	I
97	M	2 6 **1906**	Muscular atrophy	42	9 11 55	I
98	F	20 2 99	Disseminated sclerosis	15	5 10 55	I
99	F	9 7 93	Parkinson's disease; fractured femur	12/1.5	"	I
100	F	30 12 00	Rheumatoid arthritis	16	14 12 55	I

*Those accepted are in bold. [+]I = inmate; P = pensioner.

References and Notes

1. Royal Hospital & Home for Incurables. Case book No 17 (14501-15500). [RHN archive].
2. Board minutes. Book 27: 458; Book 28: 59.
3. Ibid. Book 28: 40.
4. Anonymous, 'What the soldier said', *Brit Med J.* 1920, **i**: 716.

CHAPTER 18

The Hospital in recent times:
changes, expansion, and Royal visits

THE RHHI UNDERWENT serious problems in the early part of the twentieth century. During the Great War (1914-18) the building was significantly damaged by anti-aircraft shells. During that war, Board discussions centred on whether the benefits of the Charity could be extended to 'victims of the War'. However, at a subsequent meeting, 'It was agreed that it is not desirable at the present time to go further in the matter.' Some two years later (in 1917), the Hon. Sec. of the Ladies Association asked: 'What steps, if any [are being taken], with regard to the admission to the Hospital of men rendered incurable by the War?' A minute states: 'A reply pointing out the difficulties' was sent!

In 1928, the House Committee considered that the accommodation for male patients was not ample enough. Richard M. Pigott FRSBA, who had designed the Nurses' Home, was called in, and decided that an extension involving the 'full width of the Restall Wing' (Chapter 8) would cost £6,000 to £7,000. This would include 'increased verandah accommodation for the women patients'. Since this scheme provided for only eight extra male beds, and the cost was high, the matter was referred back to the House Committee. During a lengthy discussion, Gregg (a member of the Board) proposed that raising the pension from £20 to £25 or £26 a year might be better than paying for this extension! A later letter referred to a 'serious lack of dining room and sitting room accommodation for the women patients'. It was agreed by the Board (on 27 June 1935) that 'after the new Nurses' Home is occupied' (Chapter 11), 'improvements in the Main Hospital building' should be authorised.

The Second World War (1939-45) also brought problems for the RHHI. Aerial attacks were a great threat. On 23 August 1944, the Board was informed, 'that ... seventy-two evacuated patients and the staff who went with them were located in Lennox Castle Emergency Hospital, Lennoxtown, Stirlingshire, near Glasgow, where they arrived some time on Sunday 20 August'. The patients remaining at the RHHI should (the minute continued), 'remain on the ground floor, using the dining rooms and dormitories, the North sitting-room, and two maids' rooms in the basement, leaving the first floor absolutely vacant.' Immediately after the war, like so many voluntary hospitals, the RHHI was hit by severe financial problems; the voluntary (hospital) system (Chapter 15) was in fact in disarray!

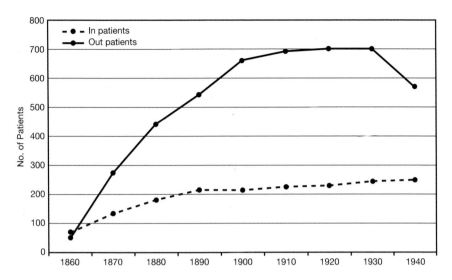

Fig 18.1: Numbers of in-patients and out-patients from 1860 until 1940.

Royal associations (see below) were maintained: in July 1932, for example, King George V and Queen Mary visited the RHHI, and were conducted on an extensive tour of the rooms.[1]

Despite difficult times in the early days of the century, numbers of inpatients were maintained (fig 18.1); the greatest change was in the number of outpatients supported by the Charity. During the 1930s this began to decline owing largely to a significant rise in pensions. In 1937, the pension was raised from £20 to £42 per annum, and in 1967 to £52. In 1952, support for outpatients came to an end.

There is little doubt that the introduction of the National Health Service (NHS), followed by the fight to remain a voluntary organisation, was the most momentous happening in the history of the RHHI in the twentieth century (Chapter 15). But there were other important events as well, not least that involving land development. Also, there was a problem of 'overlap' with activities of the Regional Board which had come into being with the introduction of the NHS in 1948.

Fund-raising dinners had of course taken place since the Royal Hospital's foundation; the 1936 festival dinner – which was held in the Mansion House with the Lord Mayor presiding – was documented in detail in the press of the day. Founder's Day in 1953 was also recorded in detail; it was pointed out on that day by the Chairman – then Norman Morris – that when the RHH had been founded, the cost of keeping one patient was £1 weekly, but a century later this figure had risen to £9.[2]

The Centenary
In 1954, centenary celebrations took place. There was a reception, and the ambitious programme of events planned for that year included: a variety concert at the Royal Albert Hall; a garden party (it was envisaged that this should be attended by either HM the Queen or the Queen Mother – see below); and a Thanksgiving service. The Garden Fête duly took place in July with more than 2000 guests present, and a service with a sermon by the Bishop of Kingston on 27 July.[3]

A local housing initiative and compulsory purchase of RHHI land
The possibility of compulsory purchase of RHHI land had been on the cards for several years. As long ago as 1958 (i.e. a decade after the NHS controversy), it had been suggested by the Board of Management that 'consideration should be given to the development of some of the land belonging to the Hospital which might be suitable for building ...' The Secretary (Villiers) had undertaken a preliminary meeting with a surveyor to discuss this possibility. A Director of Site Improvements Ltd subsequently visited the Hospital and duly reported. The next move was to appoint a sub-committee, which consisted of Sir Cyril Black, C.H. Villiers and W.B. Clowes – all members of the Board) 'to examine the report of the surveyor [dated 3 December 1958] and to consider any other proposals connected with the development of Hospital property or with the re-building of the Hospital and Home ...' However, a London County Council (LCC) decision 'dated 15th November 1959 [had at that time refused] to permit development for *residential* [my italics] purposes of part of the site forming the grounds of the Hospital and Home.' It was proposed though, in 1960, 'to re-zone the area concerned, primarily for residential use.' [4]

In early 1960, Black considered that one of the duties of his sub-committee was 'to advise how much the Board might expect to receive if it decided to sell approximately 13 acres of land at Putney now devoted to Orchards and Kitchen Garden.' Black's sub-committee recommended that 'the *freehold* [my italics] of the land should *not* be sold, and that the best financial return would probably be achieved by offering a 99-year lease to a firm of building development.' Black continued by informing the Board that the LCC 'could make a compulsory purchase of the land in question' but they would only be interested in the freehold (and not a lease), and, in his opinion this course 'was most unlikely to be followed'. At the same meeting the Secretary reported that the Marie Curie Memorial Foundation [MCMF] had an interest in the land for use as 'a headquarters coupled with a Home for 50 cancer patients'. Black, felt however that this would involve obtaining alternative town planning approval (since this would not be a *residential* development); that would be a problem for the MCMF and *not* the RHHI if they were to purchase the land.[5]

No fewer than twenty-eight objections were raised concerning the LCC's proposal that '13 acres of Hospital property should be re-zoned for residential purposes'. Therefore, an inquiry took place at County Hall on 6 October 1960, at which the RHHI was represented by their Counsel, Mr David Widdicombe. A later Board minute refers to 'The Minister of Housing's decision to a proposed modification to the original plan.'[6]

However, shortly afterwards (on 28 June 1962) the Wandsworth Borough Council did in fact serve a *compulsory purchase order* for the land. The courses open as a result of this development were outlined by Black: (i) to make no objection; (ii) to ask the Wandsworth Borough Council to withdraw the compulsory purchase order (Black felt that if they did this the LCC [who were also interested in the land] would probably 'serve a similar order on the Board'); or (iii) to 'continue with the objection which had already been made on behalf of the Board by the Hospital's Solicitors, provided some good grounds could be found for sustaining the objection'. After discussion, the Board decided 'to maintain … its objection to the compulsory purchase order, until it [was] satisfied as to the type of development [multi-storey flats, which would ruin the outlook from the Hospital, were a distinct possibility] being proposed.'

In September 1962, the Board considered a letter from Messrs Weatherall, Green and Smith, Surveyors (who were negotiating on behalf of the Board) agreeing that the 'objection … to the compulsory purchase order should not be withdrawn at present.' And in July 1963, negotiations for compensation in connection with the compulsory purchase order were still proceeding. As a finale to this saga, in March 1964 'the Board [had] approved the recommendation of the Finance Committee that … £325,000 should be accepted from the Wandsworth Borough Council as compensation for the land which [was] subject to a compulsory purchase order, together with legal costs and surveyor's fees.'[7]

The *Wandsworth Borough News* for 24 December 1964 carried an article about what it called an entirely new initiative – the Beaumont Road Housing Scheme. The *new* London Borough of Wandsworth was to be responsible for this development. It consisted of the erection of a 14-storey structure (Andrew Reed House) containing 270 'dwellings' costing £1.6 million – on RHHI ground. It was estimated (the figures were approximate) that rents would, over the following 60 years: 'be absorbed in maintenance [12 per cent], rates [15 per cent], building costs [17 per cent], land [3 per cent] [and] interest [53 per cent].'[8]

Early the following year, the same newspaper published an article on its front page: 'Royal Hospital to be "streamlined".' This article reported that the RHHI had received the sum of £325,000 from the Wandsworth Borough Council for 'the compulsory purchase of 10½ acres of orchard land …', and with that the hospital was to be modernised taking into account much 'expert advice'. The anonymous writer of the article maintained that this compulsory purchase was a 'blessing in disguise' as the 'orchards were more of a liability than an asset', because the labour involved was costly and the sale of fruit had been 'very difficult to market'.[9] This development led to the establishment of a Physical Medicine Department (Chapter 16).

Research and Development

In 1979 there was news of a new *research unit* (this aimed at work on 'brain damage' resulting from multiple sclerosis, strokes and head injury), which, it was anticipated, would open in the 'autumn of 1980'. The 'new wing' (costing £1.25 million), the report continued, would also include 'modernised departments, for studying speech therapy, occupational therapy and physiotherapy', as well as 'a special gymnasium and a pool in the hydrotherapy department'. There would be close links with 'the National Hospital for Nervous Diseases, Queen Square; the Biochemical Unit, Roehampton; [and] the Disabled Living Foundation and Southampton University'. Of course, this was only part of the new development; the *Chatsworth Wing* – to the west of the main building, and designed by Hammett, Norton and Drew (for 30 young disabled patients) had been opened by HM The Queen in May 1976 (see below) and *John Howard House* (a converted convalescent home containing 34 beds in Brighton) was undergoing conversion. The latter was named after the great eighteenth century philanthropist who accomplished so much for the poor of that era and was arguably the inspiration for Reed's pioneering initiatives.[10]

Rôle and title of the RHI in the latter part of the twentieth century

In early 1985, the Editor of the *Wandsworth Borough News* considered that it was appropriate both to give a short history of the RHHI, and to define its current rôle. Although admission was restricted to individuals of 17-65 years, there were many over that age who had been admitted at less than 65 years, the article claimed. The hospital, the anonymous writer recorded, 'collaborated with other hospitals, not only in this country, but also [throughout] Western Europe, to widen the range of caring facilities and [to] provide the best possible treatment for disabled men and women.' Therefore, its *raison d'être* had not changed fundamentally since its foundation in 1854 as a hospital for long-stay (incurable) as opposed to 'acute' (curable) cases! There was now 'a younger disabled unit (see above), a self-care unit, a rehabilitation unit and a day hospital'. In addition, the hospital possessed the holiday home (John Howard House) in Brighton, to which about 100 patients went every year 'for a 10-day holiday by the sea'; about £60,000 was spent on this project. The overall aim was to 'provide a human, secure and relaxed home', and at the same time to 'use the specialised resources of remedial therapy to prevent deterioration in their physical condition and to provide a mentally stimulating environment'.[11]

The *South London Press* for 23 February 1990 contained an article relating to 'new accommodation of the Royal Hospital'. 'More than 330 nurses [the anonymous writer recorded] look after [and rehabilitate] the 270 residents ... and the 30 residents in the RHH [Putney] Brighton Home'. The hospital, it was claimed, 'now aims to provide an environment where optimum levels of independence can be achieved within a secure, relaxed atmosphere', and it contains, the writer continued, 'Britain's largest single residential group of people suffering from advanced forms of Multiple Sclerosis.' This new building, which contained two 16-bed specialist units – one for the treatment of 'severe disability combined with behavioural disorders' and the other for Huntington's Disease (a genetically determined disease of the central nervous system), was duly completed in mid-1997; it had cost £1.95 million.[12]

In 1995, the *Wandsworth Borough News* conveyed to its readership the information that (not before time) the *name* of the hospital was again to change. On 6 March of that year the hospital had been re-named the *Royal Hospital for Neuro-disability,* a move 'designed to link with their joint hosting of the first international conference on the management of patients with 'Waking Coma' or 'Persistent Vegetative State', at the Royal College of Physicians. 'Neuro-disability', it was stressed, includes: 'Cerebral Palsy, Huntington's Disease, Multiple Sclerosis, stroke and brain damage'. It should be noted that only a short time before (in October 1988) the name had been changed to The Royal Hospital and Home, Putney (RHHP).[13] Incidentally, there was a great deal of controversy regarding the change of name in 1995; not all of the members of the Committee of Management considered the change to *neuro-disability* an appropriate substitute for *incurables* (which had already been dropped a few years before), and many local residents still do not understand what this new term means!

There have, since the Chatsworth Wing was completed (in 1976) been several other extensions (see Chapter 8): the Alexandra Wing (1980) – architect: Hammett, Norton and Drew; Drapers Wing (1985) – designed by Hammett *et al* 1985; and Goodman House – architect: David Cowan Associates (1997). All have been to the east or south-east of the main building. Other recent additions have been several new wards: Devonshire, Clifden, Andrew Reed, Wellesley and Wolfson.

The Hospital has, in recent years, retained a high profile in the local (South London) press. 'Although patients have comfortable rooms with televisions ... they are also encouraged to get around the hospital which houses a bank, chemist, dentist and hairdressers.' The writer of this article continued: 'A range of therapies are available, including physical, occupationals, art and music.' And very recently a writer in the *Wandsworth Borough News* summed up the hospital's philosophy: 'all disabled people should have the opportunity to enjoy the best possible quality of life.' He concluded: 'Plans are now under way for [yet another] new wing and therapy rooms and fund-raisers are hoping to collect £6.3 million for the project.'[14]

Negotiations with the local Regional Board
As a result of the exemption from the NHS (Chapter 15), it was felt by the Board that the Hospital was, to some extent or other, caring for patients who were fundamentally not their responsibility. Black reported to the Board in 1959 on a meeting he had had with the Chairman of the South West Metropolitan Regional Board (RB) on the possibility of obtaining payment 'for medical and nursing care ... provided by the Hospital and Home to certain patients who would otherwise be the responsibility of the [RB].' The chairman apparently agreed that 'there was a moral obligation on the part of the Ministry to pay something ...', and there was apparently a precedent involving the Star & Garter Home at Richmond. The outcome of negotiations proved successful, and the RB agreed to 'meet the cost of 20 patients in the Hospital and Home as from 1st April 1961.'[15]

A herb garden
In 1997, the newly named hospital opened its own herb garden, designed to 'stimulate patients who have suffered serious damage to the nervous system'. It was, the writer continued, 'based on a medieval herbary which provided healing infusions for the sick', and had its origins at the 'Hampton Court Flower Show where [the previous year] it won a coveted Silver Gilt award.'[16]

Closure of the City Offices
The lease of the City office (in Queen Victoria Street) was due to expire early in the twentieth century (on 24 June 1905). Rooms 1 to 5 on the '1st floor in No 4 St Paul's Churchyard were considered 'the most suitable' venue for the future. It was proposed at a Board meeting that these offices 'be taken at a rental of 21 years at £315 per annum determinable at 7 or 14 years by giving six months notice.' And in 1912, 'The Secretary was authorised to have the sign outside the City Office windows re-gilded at a cost of £5.10s.0d.'[17]

In March 1918, i.e. towards the end of the Great War, an important letter was read to the Board; they were informed that 'the War Cabinet Committee on Accommodation, whose chairman was the Rt. Hon. Sir Alfred Mond, Bt, MP [had] decided that it [was] absolutely necessary in the vital interest of the nation to requisition ... your premises in No 4 St Paul's Churchyard [there were nearly nine years still to run' on the tenancy] under the Defence of the Realm Act and regulations.' The Board therefore had to find 'other quarters', and the Chairman (Wickham) considered that 'in his opinion it was advisable that the offices of this Charity should remain in the City.' The Board therefore made an offer of £450 a year for the ground floor rooms of Bond Court

House, Walbrook EC – 'for the duration of the War and one year afterwards'. But the agents for this property were only prepared to let them have their facilities for '£500 a year with an agreement for five years'. The Board agreed *reluctantly* to offer this amount but not before they had written to Sir Arthur J. Durrant, MVO outlining their difficulties. A minute in November 1923 indicates that the Board preferred a 5- or 7-years' lease rather than to continue 'as yearly tenants'. The compensation suggested by the Office of Works (for displacing them from St Paul's Churchyard) was later deemed 'not fair or reasonable' and it was agreed to approach the 'Losses Commission'. The Hospital ultimately received £456.4.3 in compensation, and in December 1919, £864.4s.3d. which included five quarters' rent.[18] In 1936, a sub-committee was set up to look into the necessity for continuing City Offices (in fact, these were retained until 1946). It was decided then that: (i) the present offices (still in Bond Court House) be retained until the end of the lease – March 1938; (ii) the existing arrangements be retained *pro tem*; (iii) the *new* Secretary (Cutting was being compelled to resign as Secretary on account of his age) should spend most of his time in the Hospital itself, and (iv) that the advertisement for applications for a *new* Secretary be made in early January 1937.

In August 1945, the Board decided 'that the office staff should return to the City Offices in January next'. However, the return was a short one, for in July 1946, it was resolved unanimously that the offices should be returned to the Hospital 'as soon as reasonably possible'. Furthermore, all Board meetings should take place in the library every month, on a Wednesday at 5.00 p.m. It was later minuted that on Board meeting days, 'the House Committee should meet at 3.00 p.m., the Finance Committee at 4.15 p.m. and the Board at 4.30 p.m.' However, meetings seem to have briefly reverted to the City, for in February 1948, 'The Board expressed their thanks to the Chairman [Norman Morris] for arranging to have the Board Meetings at [Oceanic House, 1a] Cockspur Street'. They were still held there in November 1959.[19]

Distinguished visitors

The late Queen Mother (1900-2002) was an enthusiastic supporter of the Charity; her first visit (as the Duchess of York) was on 3 June 1924; she had been Patron since the year before. Her Majesty returned to open the newly built Nurses' Home (Chapter 11) on 24 July 1935, which had been erected at a cost of £25,000 (although at that time £10,000 still had to be raised). The President of the RHI (who welcomed her on that occasion) was Viscount Lee of Fareham (1868-1947) and the Chairman of the Board, Sir Edward Maclagan (1864-1952). She was to return on 15 June 1957 to take part in a Garden Party, the President and Chairman on this occasion being the 11th Duke of Devonshire (1920-present) and Mr Norman Morris, respectively; the Matron was Miss C.A. Howard, MBE. On 18 July 1973, the Queen Mother paid yet another visit; this was to celebrate 50 years of her Patroncy of the Institution. Although the President was still the Duke of Devonshire, this time the Chairman was General Sir Leslie Tyler, and the Matron Mrs M.C. Bodington.[20]

On 21 June 1966, the RHHI received a visit from Princess Marina, Duchess of Kent (1906-68); the Chairman at that time was General Sir Horatius Murray GCB (1903-89).[21]

On 19 May 1976, HM the Queen (also a Patron) opened the new *Chatsworth Wing*; this is situated to the west of the main building, and had cost £500,000 to erect. And on 27 October 1989, she was back again – this time to open the new Brain Injury Unit; this comprised two wards at the eastern end of the great extension of 1879-81 – the Devonshire and Clifden – and had cost £2.5 million.[22] On 13 March 1991, Diana, Princess of Wales (1962-97) visited the Hospital to open the Andrew Reed Ward and on 16 March 1994, the Prince of Wales (1948-present) paid a brief visit, the main purpose being to 're-dedicate the recently restored [Andrew] Assembly Room', which had cost £100,000.[23] In 2001 HRH The Princess Royal visited the hospital.

A distinguished non-Royal guest in 1966 was Field Marshal Montgomery of Alamein (1887-1976)[24]; his visit marked the 100th anniversary of Founder's Day. And in March the following year, the Roman Catholic Archbishop of Southwark (the Most Reverend Cyril Cowderoy) both visited and celebrated mass at the hospital.[25]

References and Notes

1. Board minutes. Book 24: 164-5, 168, 231, 240; Book 25: 382-4, 392-6; Book 26: 49, 288; Book 27: 170-1. J. Murray, 'The voluntary hospitals', *Saturday Review* 1918; Anonymous, 'Air raid secrets: many hospitals hit', *Morning Post* 7 April 1919; Anonymous, 'Hopeless outlook for hospitals: heavy deficiencies in funds leads to inefficiency in working: serious cases have to be turned away', *Daily Chronicle* 5 September 1919; Anonymous, 'The hospital crisis: urgently needed buildings being closed', *Times, Lond.* 2 March 1920; J. Reid. The plight of the hospitals', *Times, Lond.* 11 March 1920; M. Mackenzie, 'Hospital Funds: charity in extremis', *Times, Lond.* 8 March 1920; Anonymous, 'Hospital crisis', *Daily Express* 12 May 1921; Anonymous, 'Faltering steps: Royal Hospital for Incurables: a plea', *City Press* 16 June 1923: 5.
2. Anonymous, 'Royal Hospital and Home for Incurables: festival dinner at the Mansion House: Lord Mayor presides: list totals £5,500', *Wandsworth Borough News* 3 July 1936: 12-13; Anonymous, 'Founders Day at Putney Incurables: century contrast of patients' upkeep', Ibid 4 December 1953: 3.
3. Anonymous, 'A Royal Hospital centenary', *Brit Med J* 1954; 1: 529; Anonymous, 'Royal Hospital for Incurables: centenary reception', *Wandsworth Borough News* 12 February 1954: 13; Anonymous, 'Incurables'

centenary garden fete: Centenary thanksgiving service', Ibid 30 July 1954: 3.

4. Op.cit. See note 1 above (Board minutes), Book 28: 119-20, 124, 137, 165-6.

5. Ibid: 180-4; **Sir Cyril Wilson Black** MP, FRICS (1902-91) was a chartered surveyor and had been Mayor of Wimbledon, and was MP for Wimbledon (1950-70). From 1959-62 he was a member of the South-West Hospital Regional Hospital Board. Black was a prominent Baptist and also Chairman of the Temperance Permanent Building Society (1939-73).

6. Op.cit. See note 1 above (Board minutes), 205, 260.

7. Ibid: 270-1, 276-7, 327-8.

8. Anonymous, 'The Beaumont Road Housing Scheme', *Wandsworth Borough News*, 24 December 1964: 6.

9. Anonymous, 'Royal Hospital to be "streamlined": benefit from £325,000 land sale', Ibid. 15 January 1965: 1 and 2.

10. Anonymous, 'New research unit at Royal Hospital', Ibid. 10 August 1979: 5. *See also*: Cowan architects, 'A Conservation study for the Royal Hospital for Neuro-disability (London: RIFN, 2001).

11. Anonymous, 'Historic home of treatment for physically disabled', *Wandsworth Borough News*, 15 February 1985: 14. *See also*: M. Tudor, Caring for the disabled – adversity and caring (Putney and Brighton: RHHI, 1981): 11.

12. Anonymous, 'Royal Hospital to build new accommodation: specialist facilities to help severely disabled people', *South London Press* 23 February 1990: 16: 14; Anonymous, 'Hospital tops out unit site', *Wandsworth Borough Guardian* 24 April 1997: 1.

13. Anonymous, 'New name for Putney Hospital', *Wandsworth Borough News* 10 March 1995: 12.

14. Anonymous, 'Hospital helps make lives happy', *Wandsworth Borough Guardian* 9 September 1999: 16; P. Askew, 'One foot in the past', *Wandsworth Borough News* 4 October 2002: 16.

15. Op.cit. See note 1 above (Board minutes), Book 28: 166-8, 220, 227-8.

16. Anonymous, 'Herb garden helps the disabled', *South London Press* 1997; 20 June: 18.

17. Op.cit. See note 1 above (Board minutes), Book 23: 139,177; Book 24: 39.

18. Ibid: 300-4, 305-9, 365, 401-2, 407; Book 25: 162, 166.

19. Ibid: Book 26: 145-6; Book 27: 197, 222-3, 226, 237, 303, 500; Book 28: 148, 160.

20. Anonymous, 'Duchess of York. visit to Putney Home for Incurables', *Morning* Post 4 June 1924; Anonymous, 'Success of the season: Duchess of York's social triumph: 'Queen Elizabeth' *Daily Express* 4 June 1924; Anonymous, 'Duchess of York at Putney: Her Royal Highness and the

incurables', *Wandsworth Borough News* 6 June 1924; Anonymous, 'The Royal Hospital for Incurables: an eventful week for Putney', *Nursing Times & Midwives' Journal,* 14 June 1924: 217; Anonymous, 'Royal Hospital and Home for Incurables: opening of nurses' home by Duchess of York', *Wandsworth Borough News* 26 July 1935: 8 & 12; Anonymous, 'Putney incurables' Royal Garden Party: sunshine visit by the Queen Mother', Ibid. 21 June 1957: 1 & 8; Anonymous, 'Rain did not deter Queen Mother at Royal Hospital', Ibid. 20 July 1973: 1 & 2; Anonymous, 'Queen Mother visits hospital for incurables. *Clapham and Lambeth News* 27 July 1973: 6.

21. Anonymous, 'Princess Marina at Royal Hospital: delightful surprise for patients, *Wandsworth Borough News* 24 June 1966: 1.

22. Anonymous, 'The Queen opens Royal Hospital's new wing', Ibid. 1976; 21 May: 1; E. Columb. 'Queen opens new Brain Injury Unit', Ibid. 3 November 1989: 4.

23. Anonymous, 'Lost for words when Princess visits', Ibid. 1991; 15 March: 2; Anonymous, 'Prince pays a flying visit', Ibid. 18 March 1994: 13.

24. Anonymous, 'Field Marshal Montgomery at Royal Hospital', Ibid. 9 December 1966: 1 & 2, and 16 December: 5.

25. Anonymous, 'Historic visit to Royal Hospital', Ibid. 17 March 1967: 1.

CHAPTER 19

The ghost of Melrose Hall

THERE IS A LEGEND that the hospital building is haunted. Sir Edward Maclagan has provided details of a possible ghostly presence at Melrose Hall. It is that of a notorious nineteenth century murderess – Mrs Manning. According to Maclagan there is, or was, a figure of Mrs Manning at Madame Tussaud's! In conjunction with her husband, she murdered a former suitor of hers, by the name of O'Connor, in 1849. Mrs Manning was of Swiss ancestry and lived in Bermondsey. Having invited O'Connor to dinner, she and her husband took him to the kitchen, shot him in the head and subsequently buried him under the floor-boards. The trial proved an enormous national sensation, and her execution *in public*, outside Horsemonger Lane Prison was attended by a crowd apparently numbering some 30,000 individuals.[1]

Charles Dickens (Chapter 1) was present at the execution, and protested vigorously against the horrible nature of the spectacle and called for the abolition of public executions. In a letter to *The Times* from his home in Devonshire Terrace he felt that 'the infliction of capital punishment [should be] a private solemnity within the prison walls'. In his descriptive letter about the unpleasant episode, Dickens continued:

> I believe that a sight so inconceivably awful as the wickedness and levity of the immense crowd collected at that execution this morning could be imagined by no man, and could be presented in no heathen land under the sun. The horrors of the gibbet and of the crime which brought the wretched murderers to it, faded in my mind before the atrocious bearing, looks and language, of the assembled spectators. When I came upon the scene at midnight, the *shrillness* of the cries and howls that were raised from time to time, denoting that they came from a concourse of boys and girls already assembled in the best places, made my blood run cold. As the night went on, screeching, and laughing, and yelling in strong chorus or parodies on Negro melodies, with substitutions of 'Mrs. Manning' for 'Susannah', and the like, were added to these. When the day dawned, thieves, low prostitutes, ruffians and vagabonds of every kind, flocked on to the ground, with every variety of offensive and foul behaviour. Fightings, faintings, whistlings, imitations of Punch, brutal jokes, tumultuous demonstrations of indecent delight when swooning women were dragged out of the crowd by the police with their dresses disordered, gave a new zest to the general entertainment. When the sun rose brightly – as it did – it gilded thousands upon thousands of upturned faces, so inexpressibly odious in their brutal mirth or callousness, that a man had cause to feel ashamed of the shape he wore, and to shrink from himself, as fashioned in the image of the Devil. When the two miserable creatures who attracted all this ghastly sight about them were turned quivering into the air, there was no more emotion, no more pity, no more

257

thought that two immortal souls had gone to judgement, no more restraint in any of the previous obscenities, than if the name of Christ had never been heard in this world, and there were no belief among men but that they perished like the beasts.

Dickens ended this letter:

> ... when, in our prayers and thanksgivings ..., we are humbly expressing before God our desire to remove the moral evils of the land, I would ask your readers to consider whether it is not a time to think of this one, and to root it out.'[2]

Dickens obviously felt that further (more detailed) criticism of *public* execution was called for, and he again wrote to *The Times* a few days later. He was not however opposed to capital punishment *per se*. He drew upon history as well as some of the great poets of the past to attempt to justify his remarks. In this letter, he made an impassioned appeal to Sir George Grey, Bt, the Home Secretary, to ban public executions.[3] This received an equally vehement reply a day later, both attempting to justify public executions, and begging Grey to 'do no such thing' as Dickens had suggested![4]

Despite Dickens' pleading however, it took some years before public executions were abolished legally in Britain.

Maclagan however, proceeded in his account to cast doubt as to whether Mrs Manning ever set foot in Melrose Hall! The sole connection, he maintained, was that 'a few years before the famous murder she had been a maid to the daughter of the Duchess of Sutherland' (who it will be recalled [Chapter 8] had occupied Melrose Hall in previous years). At the time of the murder, however, the Duchess had left this building and was living in Stafford House, near St James Palace. Legend has it that she requested the Governor of the Horsemonger Lane Prison to accede to Mrs Manning's wish that she should be hanged in a black satin dress and black silk stockings. It is far more likely, according to Maclagan that 'if her ghost has ever walked it would [more likely] be in Bermondsey ... and *not* [my italics] in [Melrose Hall]'. Thus, although there might be a ghostly presence at the RHN, there is no convincing evidence that Mrs Manning was or is involved!

References and Notes

1. E.D. Maclagan. *The Royal Hospital and Home for Incurables: three lectures delivered to the patients of the Hospital, on the 6th, 13th and 27th November, 1946.* London: RHHI 1946, (5 + 9 + 10).
2. C. Dickens, Letter to the Editor, *Times, Lond.* 14 November 1849: 4.
3. C. Dickens, Letter to the Editor, *Times, Lond.* 19 November 1849: 5; **Sir George Grey Bt**, MP (1799-1882) was a barrister who served as Home Secretary under both Earl Russell (1846-52) and Viscount Palmerston (1855-8 and 1861-6). He also 'carried [the] convict discipline bill, which abolished transportation'.
4. F.B. Head. Public execution – Mr. Dickens letter, *Times, Lond.* 20 November 1849: 5.

Epilogue

THE *Royal Hospital for Incurables* (RHI) was the first hospital specifically designed for this category of patient (in 1854), but by the 1890s (the latter days of Queen Victoria's reign) many similar institutions had arisen throughout Britain. The *Medical Directory* for 1900, for example, lists 10 in London alone. By 1876, it was thus clear that the RHI was leading the incurables movement throughout the land; it was in fact a *National* institution, 'and not merely [a] Metropolitan' one.[1]

Presiding at an annual festival dinner in 1932, the Chairman, Major Sir William Prescott Bt. (1874-1945) first described the RHHI as 'a monument of civilization'.[2]

This and other establishments for *incurables* are described in Burdett's *Hospitals and asylums of the World*. By 1936, the Chairman of the RHHI (Sir Edward Maclagan) was able to report that Homes for Incurables had been formed not only in Britain, but also throughout the world; India was, for example, opening them 'in commemoration of the reign of King George V'.[3]

Recently, *rehabilitation* has been added to long-term care, and in this field also, the *Royal Hospital* has assumed a pioneering position.

Until now, no detailed history of this great foundation (the RHN) has been written. I was invited to fill the gap, which I have attempted to do in this the 150th year of the Charity.

References and Notes

1. Board minutes. Book 11: 202; Anonymous, 'Historic Home of treatment for physically disabled', *Wandsworth Borough News* 15 February 1985: 14; H. Richardson (ed.) *English Hospitals 1660-1948; a survey of their architecture and design* (Swindon: Royal Commission on the Historical Monuments of England 1998) 128-31.
2. Anonymous, 'A place apart: The Royal Home for Incurables', *City Press*, 17 June 1932.
3. Anonymous, 'Royal Hospital and Home for incurables: a great monument to civilisation', *City Press*, 4 December 1936.

Principal office-holders etc. (1854-2004)

Patron(s)
1880-1901   HRH The Prince of Wales
1901-1902   HM King Edward VII; [Vice-Patron HRH Princess Christian]
1903-1905   HM King Edward VII; HRH Princess Christian
1908-1909   HM King Edward VII; HRH The Princess of Wales; HRH Princess Christian
1910.1935   HM King George V and HM Queen Mary. HRH Princess Christian (until 1925); HRH Duchess of York (from 1923)
1936   HM King Edward VIII; HM Queen Mary; HRH Duchess of York
1937-1951   HM King George VI; HM The Queen; HM Queen Mary
1952   HM Queen Elizabeth II; HM Queen Elizabeth The Queen Mother; HM Queen Mary (until 1953)
1953-present HM Queen Elizabeth II; HM Queen Elizabeth The Queen Mother (until 2002)

President(s)
1856-1860   The Rt. Hon. The 2nd Earl of Harrowby
1865-1868   His Grace The Archbishop of Canterbury (Charles Thomas Longley)
1868-82   His Grace the Archbishop of Canterbury (Archibald Campbell Tait)
1882-1892   The Rt. Hon. The 7th Earl of Aberdeen
1894-1897   The Rt. Hon. The Earl Crompton, MP
1897-1912   The Most Hon The 5th Marquess of Northampton, KG
1914-1925   The Rt. Hon. The 4th Baron Wolverton
1925-1927   The Rt. Hon. The 1st Viscount Cave
1928-1939   The Rt. Hon. The 1st Viscount Lee of Fareham
1940-1952   The Rt. Hon. The 7th Viscount Clifden
1954-1992   His Grace The 11th Duke of Devonshire
1992-2001   The Marchioness of Douro
2002-present The Countess of Lichfield

Chairman
1856-1857   Samuel Gurney, Esq. Jr.
1858-1859   The Rt. Hon. The Viscount Raynham, MP

1861-1878	Henry Huth, Esq
1879-1892	John Derby Allcroft, Esq
1893-1910	Herbert John Allcroft, Esq
1911-1923	Thomas W. Wickham Esq
1924-1929	Sir William Clerke Bt
1930-1931	Major T. Clarence E. Goff
1932-1935	J. Turton Wright Esq
1936-1947	Sir Edward Maclagan
1948-1959	Norman Morris Esq
1960-1963	General Sir Douglas Gracey
1964-1971	General Sir Horatius Murray
1971-1975	Major-General Sir Leslie Tyler
1976-1978	John Wedgwood, FRCP
1979-1984	C.G. Vaughan-Lee, Esq
1984-1988	The Rt. Hon. The Baron Bancroft
1988-1998	A.K.S. Franks, Esq
1998-present	Sir Michael Bett

Treasurer

1856-1857	Samuel Gurney Esq, Jnr
1857-1859	The Rt. Hon. The Viscount Raynham
1861-1878	Henry Huth Esq
1879-1893	John Derby Allcroft Esq
1893-1910	Herbert John Allcroft Esq
1911-1937	Sir Henry Lopes, Bt
1938-1949	The Rt. Hon. 2nd Baron Roborough
1950-1961	Sir Francis M.G. Glyn
1962-1986	C.G. Vaughan-Lee Esq
1986-1990	H.O. Howe
1990-1992	M.P. Stanley
1992-2000	J.P.R. Malpras
2000-present	A. Bruce

Secretary/Chief Executive

1856-1857	Provisional Secretary, Dr Andrew Reed [Sub-Secretary, Mr Frederic Andrew]
1858-1859	Gratuitous Secretary Dr Andrew Reed
1860	[Sub-Secretary, Mr Frederic Andrew]
1861-1900	Mr Frederic Andrew
1901-1906	Mr W. David Newton
1906-1937	Mr Charles Cutting
1937-1944	Col B.D. Armstrong
1940-1945	Mr P.W. Bennett [Assistant Acting Secretary]

1946-1951   J.G. Pilcher Esq
1951-1968   Brigadier R.M. Villiers
1968-1970   Mr Niall Campbell, A.H.A.
1970-1981   Col N.F. Gordon-Wilson
1981-1992   Col B.E. Blunt
1992-1993   Capt M.E. Ortmaus and Brig V.J. Beauchamp
1993-2000   Brig V.J. Beauchamp
2000-present Rear Admiral P.M.Franklyn

Principal Medical Officer(s)
1860   Dr J.D. Paul
1861-1866   Dr R.C. Cream
1866-1901   Dr T.J. Woodhouse
1901-1932   Dr J. Gay
1933-1937   Dr G. Duckworth
1938-1946   Dr W.B. Winton
1947-1952   Dr J.M. Badenoch
1952-1961   Dr V. Kendall
1962-1972   Dr V. Kendall; Dr M.A. Tudor
1972-1991   Dr M.A. Tudor
1992-1993   Dr R. Singh
1993-present Dr A. Sayer

Director of Medical & Research Services
1978-1979   C. Evans
1979-1987   J. Wedgwood
1987-2002   K. Andrews (since 2003 Director of the Institute)

Matron/Director of Nursing Services/Chief Nurse
1855-1856   Mrs Crossthwaite
1856-1866   Mrs E. Bellringer
1866-1868   Mrs Haughton
1869-1877   Mrs Darbyshire
1877-1881   Miss E. Mason
1881-1903   Mrs Linicke
1903-1909   Miss J. Stirling Hamilton
1909-1930   Miss L.S. Begg
1930-1935   Miss R.E.A. Potter
1936-1942   Miss D.W. Rosier
1943-1954   Miss K.M. Corbett
1955-1966   Miss C.A. Howard
1966-1982   Mrs M.C. Bodington
1983-1991   Miss M. Blincoe

1991-2000	A. Lyne
2000-2002	D. Monkman (since 2002, Chief Nurse)

*Chaplain**

1858-1900	The Hon and Rev Robert Henley
1903-1907	Rev C.T. Bellairs
1908-1939	Rev Digby Gritten
1940-1941	Rev C.R. Stafford Finch
1942-1949	Rev Hugh N. Keeling
1950-1951	Rev K.T. Makin
1952-1956	Rev B. Loney
1957-1962	Rev K.W. Howell
1962-1963	Rev Canon K.W. Howell
1964-1983	Rev I.K. Savile
1983-1990	Rev T.J. Thomas
1991-2004	Rev G.E.D. Bonham-Carter
2004-present	Rev J. Farnham

Collector

1856-1858	Mr Frederic Andrew
1859-1895	Mr James Best
1895-1900	Mr Frederick Starling
1900-1905	Mr Godfrey B. Hall

Appeal Secretary

1951-1953	Mrs J. East
1954-1955	Mrs C.A. Gurney
1956-1958	Rear Admiral F.R.J. Mack; Mr C.L. Pearson
1959	Air Vice Marshall E.C. Bates
1960	Capt J.T. Kimpton; Capt G. Talbot Smith
1961-1970	Brigadier R.M. Long
1970-1978	Air Commodore D.F. Rixson

City Office

1861-1880	10 Poultry, EC
1880-1903	106 Queen Victoria Street, EC
1904-1918	4 St Paul's Churchyard, EC
1918-1937	Bond Court House, Walbrook, EC
1938-1946	42 Gracechurch Street, EC3

---

*Presently pastoral care involves a permanent Church of England chaplain as well as a visiting Roman Catholic priest, a Rabbi, and a Free Church Minister.

Board Minute Books and their dates

		Date on spine, and front of book
Book 1	13 July 1854 – 14 January 1858	
Book 2	28 January 1858 – 12 April 1860	1858
Book 3	16 April 1860 – 22 August 1861	1860
Book 4	12 September 1861 – 14 May 1863	1861
Book 5	28 May 1863 – 13 July 1865	1863
Book 6	27 July 1865 – 14 March 1867	1865
Book 7	26 March 1867 – 11 February 1869	1867
Book 8	25 February 1869 – 4 July 1871	1869
Book 9	13 July 1871 – 28 November 1873	1871
Book 10	11 December 1873 – 23 December 1875	1874
Book 11	13 January 1876 – 14 March 1878	1876
Book 12	28 March 1878 – 11 March 1880	1878
Book 13	23 March 1880 – 16 June 1882	1880
Book 14	22 June 1882 – 11 December 1884	1882
Book 15	23 December 1884 – 27 May 1887	1885
Book 16	24 May 1887 – 10 October 1889	1887
Book 17	24 October 1889 – 27 November 1891	1889
Book 18	10 December 1891 – 10 November 1893	1891
Book 19	21 November 1893 – 5 December 1895	1893
Book 20	12 December 1895 – 4 March 1898	1896
Book 21	10 March 1898 – 25 January 1900	1898
Book 22	8 February 1900 – 18 December 1902	1900
Book 23	22 January 1903 – 15 June 1911	1903
Book 24	27 July 1911 – 28 April 1921	1911
Book 25	23 June 1921 – 11 July 1929	1921
Book 26	25 July 1929 – 22 December 1938	1929
Book 27	19 January 1939 – 31 May 1954	1939
Book 28	28 June 1954 – 28 November 1966	1954

APPENDIX 3

ROYAL HOSPITAL FOR INCURABLES
Putney Heath.

———

Rules for the appointment of Medical Officer [1902]

———

1. The Medical Officer is responsible to the Board of Management for the proper Medical and Surgical treatment of all the inmates and resident staff of the Hospital and must be qualified in both these branches, – as well as being duly registered.
2. He shall attend daily from 10.30 a.m., to noon and at such other times as the condition of any inmate or member of the resident staff may require.
3. Every inmate must be seen by him at least once in each week, whether actually on the sick list or not.
4. A record of every inmate treated by the Medical Officer must be kept in the book provided for that purpose, which book must be presented personally and a report made on the inmates to the House Committee every Wednesday at 12 noon.
5. A list of all inmates receiving special diets must also be kept and the total number reported to the Committee on Wednesday. Whilst the Board do not prohibit special diets, they rely upon the Medical Officer to keep to the ordinary diets so far as possible, thus avoiding additional work in the Kitchen Department.
6. He shall report to the Committee any inmate who shall have so far recovered as to be able to earn his or her own living either partially or otherwise.
7. The Medical Officer shall have sole charge of the drugs, etc. and shall present a requisition to the House Committee when a fresh supply is required.

The appointment is made for ...... years, subject to re-election at the option of the Board.

Rules for Patients – 1926

Royal Hospital and Home for Incurables,
PUTNEY.

RULES FOR PATIENTS.

1.

Patients may be visited between the hours of 2.30 and 5.30 p.m. on week-days (Saturdays 2.30 to 6 p.m.) and from 2 to 4 p.m. on Sundays.

Parcels containing cake, fruit, jam, eggs, &c., are permitted, but meat, fish, and tinned foods are prohibited.

2.

Patients who are able to go out unattended may do so with the permission of the Matron on week-days from 9 a.m. to 12.45 noon, and from 2 p.m. to 7 p.m., from April 1st to September 30th.

Attended patients must not go out after 6 p.m.

On Sundays unattended Patients must return not later than 5 p.m. Attended Patients must return not later than 4 p.m.

From October 1st to March 31st all Patients must return not later than 4.45 p.m., unless special permission be given. Patients, whether in their chairs or walking, are not allowed to linger in the vicinity of the Entrance Lodge, either inside or outside the grounds.

3.

No Patient may be absent for more than one night without permission from the House Committee and permission for absence for one night must be obtained from the Matron. The names and postal addresses of the friends whom it is proposed to visit must be given in all cases.

4.

Any Patient wishing to make either a complaint or a request may do so either to the Matron, the Medical Officer, the Secretary, the House Committee or the Ladies' Visiting Committee. If an inquiry is desired in the case of any complaint, no time should be lost in giving information, otherwise the inquiry is made less easy. Letters respecting complaints, or requests, which are intended for the House Committee, should be addressed to the Secretary. By this means inquiry can be made into the circumstances raised by the letter before the meeting of the House Committee takes place.

5.

No Patient is permitted to bring, or cause to be introduced, into the Hospital, any intoxicating liquors or drugs, nor is allowed to take any medicines other than those prescribed by the Medical Officer.

6.

Patients must provide themselves with all necessary clothing, keep it in good repair, and always be suitably attired throughout the day.

7.

Patients must keep their presses locked. On admission each Patient will receive a key for the press. If the key is lost one shilling will be charged for a new one. The Committee do not hold themselves responsible for any losses.

8.

No articles of furniture or clothes boxes may be introduced without the permission of the Matron.

Any box or trunk brought into the Home must not exceed 36 in. in length, 24 in. in height, or 21 in. in width, and the owner's name must be painted on each end.

The Head Attendant only is allowed to go to the Male Patients' box room. When clothing is required the box must be opened in the presence of the Patient and locked again in the presence of the Patient.

9.

No Patient may be absent from meals without permission of the Matron.

10.

Patients must retire to bed not later than 8 p.m. Male Patients must be in bed by 8.30 p.m. when the Attendants go off duty.

All lights must be extinguished at 9 p.m.

Helpless Patients must retire to bed any time after 6 p.m. whenever the Nurse or the Attendant is ready for them.

11.

Patients may go out only in the chairs assigned to them.

12.

No Patient is allowed in any circumstances to interfere with the fires, or to remove the fireguards, the Nurse alone being responsible.

13.

No Patient may give a present, either in money or in kind, to any Member of the Staff.

14.

Male Patients must not enter the apartments used by the Female Patients. Female Patients must not enter the apartments of the Male Patients.

15.

Betting is strictly prohibited, and Patients are forbidden to enter any public-house.

16.

Smoking is only allowed in the grounds, verandahs, and room set apart for that purpose.

17.

Male Patients must not visit their bed-rooms during the day without permission.

By order of the Board,
     CHARLES CUTTING, Secretary.
January, 1926.

· Patients and Staff are warned against the possible danger of touching any electric switch while wearing head-'phones.

Index